W9-CCY-704

Collateral Circulation of the Heart

Christian Seiler

Collateral Circulation of the Heart

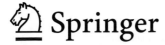 Springer

Christian Seiler
Universitätsspital
Klinik und Poliklinik für Kardiologie
Freiburgstrasse 4
3010 Bern
Switzerland
christian.seiler@insel.ch

ISBN 978-1-84882-341-9   e-ISBN 978-1-84882-342-6
DOI 10.1007/978-1-84882-342-6
Springer Dordrecht Heidelberg London New York

British Library Cataloguing in Publication Data
A catalogue record for this book is available from the British Library

Library of Congress Control Number: 2009921187

Printed on acid-free paper

Springer is part of Springer Science+Business Media (www.springer.com)

Dedicated to Ladina, Luzi, Fia Rageth, Men Maria, my children and to Christina

Preface

The sober explanation for this book is a call by the Springer-Verlag, London, to edit a publication on 'The functional relevance of the collateral circulation' of the heart. Alternatively, it could be 'sold' as the result of my intention to reduce entropy of 18 years of scientific work on the topic of the coronary circulation, which was itself meant to diminish the amount of 'useless' energy. Such a process of reducing disarray in a system with the aim of grasping it better is related to simplification, which carries the risk of introducing error. This can be exemplified by the historic view of angina pectoris, which used to be simplified as being always fatal, thus obscuring for nearly two centuries the view of a 'self-healing' mechanism such as the collateral circulation of the heart. It would be naïve, to assume the present work to be free of erroneous oversimplification, because the very nature of scientific work is related to generating (simple) hypotheses with their subsequent falsification.

In that context and bluntly, my primary interest in the field of the collateral circulation was not initiated with a vision of eradicating the consequences of coronary artery disease (CAD) by promoting the growth of natural bypasses. The time for such sizeable ideas had passed in the 1970s with the start of the work by Wolfgang Schaper. My interest in the area related to maps, geometry charting landscape as a former cartographer and the linked process of minimizing error in doing so. At first sight, landscape is not organized and charting it realistically requires techniques of projecting it on a flat plane, while preserving distances, angles, object size relations. Apparently, biology in the sense of mathematical science is poorly organized. However, patterns of organization can be recognized, and this is even the case in ostensibly chaotic systems. In hindsight, my genuine interest in the field evolved from describing biological patterns with exact means, always including the calculation of the error made during mathematical modelling. Accordingly, one of my favourite occupation used to consist of modelling the coronary artery circulation, the model being a minimal cost function of energy expenditure for the transport of blood, whereby large 'tubes' dissipate little frictional energy but their construction and maintenance is costly because large, and vice versa. The 'maps' of coronary angiograms were crucial for delineating the local territory of 'irrigation', i.e. the so called ischaemic area at risk for infarction. The oversimplification and, thus, error of the system consisted of demarcating different coronary regions, disregarding the possibility of links between them and the assumption that there are no intercoronary anastomoses.

The step between acknowledging inter-coronary anastomoses, links, natural bypasses, collaterals in the human coronary circulation and the structure of this book is small. The following questions, i.e. principle book chapters, arise instantaneously: are they relevant in the sense of life-saving for patients with CAD (Chapter 1); how can they be gauged (Chapter 2); how often are they present and how are they promoted *naturally* (Chapter 3); if present, how do they function physically (Chapter 4), and can they be promoted *artificially* (Chapter 5)? The epigrammatic answers to some of the above questions according to the actual state of (mis)calculation are: yes, they are relevant in every third patient with CAD and in every fourth without CAD; they can be measured invasively; they are able to dilate and constrict and do not function as rigid tubes; and yes, they can be promoted artificially. The demarcation between the main chapters is not absolute, i.e. there are 'anastomoses' among them for the purpose of allowing to read single chapters, and of reflecting the reality of multiple associations between the sub-topics. The potential 'error' of using the design of 'permeable' book chapters is the risk of redundancy, which on one hand, is an essential element of didactics. Conversely, it is anaesthetizing when applied in an overdose. Single- as compared to multi-authorship should reduce rather than amplify the risk of redundancy.

That human coronary collateral vessels are relevant *quo ad vitam* and that they are inducible artificially renders the subject of *collaterology*, which is aimed to be covered by this book, important from a medical standpoint of view. This is even more so considering the epidemiologic and economic burden of CAD and the fact that every sixth to fifth patient suffering from CAD cannot be treated sufficiently by conventional means. *Arteriogenesis*, the promotion of collateral artery growth employed in collaterology is on its way to be a treatment pillar of CAD, but the path is not as straightforward as thought before the first controlled clinical angiogenesis trials. With its winding pattern, it resembles the corkscrew shape of collateral vessels. This hallmark of vascular enlargement is caused by the fact that growth of the vessel is not restricted to one direction (cross-sectional calibre), but is ubiquitous, i.e. also lengthwise. In the absence of cardiac enlargement, an increase in vessel length translates into a meandering route. The latter evokes, again, the way of how scientific work advances with a generated hypothesis pointing into one direction, its (often occurring) falsification, which leads to a temporary retreat, meaning a change of the motion vector.

Acknowledgments

I would like to acknowledge the following: my past and present collaborators Michael Billinger, MD; Stefano de Marchi, MD; Martin Fleisch, MD; Marc Gertsch, MD; Steffen Glökler, MD; Andreas Indermühle, MD/PhD; Pascal Meier, MD; Tilmann Pohl, MD; Markus Schwerzmann, MD; Susanna Senti, MD; Therese Sifeddine, Tobias Traupe, MD; Andreas Wahl, MD; Rolf Vogel, MD/PhD; Tobias Rutz, MD; Hélène Steck, RN; Kerstin Wustmann, MD; Stephan Zbinden, MD; Rainer Zbinden, MD; local, national and international collaborators Janine Antonov, PhD, University of Bern, Switzerland; André Häberli, PhD, University of Bern, Switzerland; Manfred Heller, PhD, University of Bern, Switzerland; Mauro Delorenzi, PhD, University of Lausanne, Switzerland; Rolf Jaggi, PhD, University of Bern, Switzerland; Alexandre Kuhn, PhD, University of Bern, Switzerland; Jan Piek, MD/PhD, University of Amsterdam, The Netherlands; Andreas Rück, MD/PhD, University of Stockholm, Sweden; Christer Sylven, MD/PhD, University of Stockholm, Sweden; Wolfgang Schaper, MD/PhD, Max Planck Institute, Bad Nauheim, Germany; Niels Van Royen, MD/PhD, University of Amsterdam, The Netherlands.

Bernhard Meier, MD, the director of the Cardiology Department at the University Hospital Bern, Switzerland; my mentor in coronary physiology K. Lance Gould, MD, University of Texas, Houston, TX, USA; the Swiss National Science Foundation for Research and the Swiss Heart Foundation for continuous financial support of our work.

Contents

Chapter 1
Relevance of the Human Coronary Collateral Circulation

1.1 Historical Aspects

The symptom of angina pectoris surfaced only in the late 18th century and became more prevalent even 150 years later. For a long time, the view prevailed that angina pectoris was almost always fatal. Conversely, developing tolerance to exercise-induced angina pectoris which could even 'cure' it was described by William Heberden. Structural channels connecting the right and left coronary arteries were first described by Richard Lower of Amsterdam in 1669. In 1757, the Swiss anatomist Albrecht von Haller also demonstrated anastomoses between coronary arteries. The first anatomic observations of anastomoses were possibly made in non-obstructed coronary arteries, because coronary artery disease (CAD) was much less prevalent than today. Using post-mortem imaging of the coronary circulation by a multitude of different techniques, a controversy on the existence of structural intercoronary anastomoses ensued, which was not settled in their favour before the first half of the 20th century in case of the presence of CAD and not before the early 1960s in case of the normal human coronary circulation by William Fulton. Since James Herrik's clinico-pathologic observation in 1912 of the possibility of surviving sudden thrombo-tic coronary obstruction in the presence of intercoronary anastomoses, it has been recognized that the collateral circulation is a very important determinant of the rate and extent of myocardial cell death within an ischaemic zone. However, actual in vivo functional coronary collateral measurements during cardiac surgery and percutaneous coronary intervention (PCI) were first per-formed only in the 1970s and early 1980s respectively. The existence of in vivo functional collaterals in the absence of CAD was not been proven before 2003.

1.1.1 Introduction

In 1983, Proudfit pointed out that ischaemic heart disease could be justly called 'British disease' because of the origin of its pathophysiologic concept being based on William Heberden's description of angina pectoris in 1772, but more

C. Seiler, *Collateral Circulation of the Heart*, DOI 10.1007/978-1-84882-342-6_1,
© Springer-Verlag London Limited 2009

importantly on pathoanatomic observations and their accurate clinical interpretation by Edward Jenner (1749–1823; developer of the smallpox vaccine),
Caleb Hillier Parry (1755–1822), Samuel Black (1764–1832) and Allan Burns
(1781–1844).[1] This 'British team', working over 23 years, established the myocardial ischaemic theory of angina pectoris and clarified the origin of a very
important disease in industrialized countries, but it was only 120 years later that
leaders of the medical profession generally accepted the concept.[1] In parenth-
eses, the question may be raised, why the symptom of angina pectoris was not
described in detail before 1772. This could be due to previous absence or low
prevalence of angina or to the lack of clinical insight to recognize it. It appears
unlikely that clinical inability to detect angina could account for its late manifestation in the literature, and Michaels interpreted probably correctly that this
symptom and, thus, also CAD 'surfaced' only in the late 18th century and
became substantially more prevalent even 150 years later as a result of changing
lifestyle[2] In the context of the pioneering work of the above 18th-century
'British quartet', it is speculative to state that CAD is not called 'British disease'
because one aspect of CAD, i.e. the development of arterial detours around
atherosclerotic obstructions or the growth of natural bypasses, was not built
into the theory of CAD. Quite on the contrary, Parry's observations on angina
pectoris and those of Jenner on the same condition focusing on John Hunter's
case (see below) launched the view that this condition was almost always
suddenly fatal.[3] Thus, while establishing a pivotal part of the concept of
ischaemic heart disease, Jenner, Parry, Black and Burns unwillingly contributed
at the same time to the expansion of the more than 300-year-controversy on the
relevance of the human coronary collateral circulation since its first anatomic
description by Richard Lower of Amsterdam in 1669.[4] This interpretation of
the history of coronary collateral vessels cannot be applied to Heberden,
because he reportedly did not make the link between angina pectoris and
coronary obstruction, but attributed it in individual cases to an unknown
cause or to mediastinal abscess or to 'contraction of the arch of the aorta or
the arteries that go to the arm'.[1] Conversely, Heberden's contribution to the
discovery of the coronary collateral circulation is rated very high as being the
first describing the phenomenon of developing tolerance to exercise-induced
angina pectoris, i.e. the occurrence of 'walking through' angina.[5] Hence, contemporaries and 'compatriots' in the second half of the 18th century simultaneously hold the view that angina pectoris was almost always deadly and could
be well tolerated.

   In this context, several questions related to the discovery and historical
description of the human coronary collateral circulation emerge, which are
subsequently detailed. What were the instruments for the detection of coronary
anastomoses? How and when were the clinical features of CAD related to its
collateral circulation? How and when was the collateral circulation in human
peripheral artery disease discovered? What role did post-mortem detection of
coronary anastomoses play as compared to in vivo assessment with regard to
the debate on the relevance of collaterals? How was the term 'relevance'

interpreted, i.e. as *structural* presence of coronary anastomoses or as the myo-cardial salvaging *function* of structural collaterals? In which context was the term 'relevance' meant, in the presence of obstructive CAD or in normal hearts? How did early animal experiments on the collateral circulation contribute to respective findings in humans? Considering the multitude of these facets alone, it is not unexpected that controversy on the relevance of the human coronary collateral circulation had to evolve in the past.

1.1.2 First Observations of Collateral Vessels

Channels connecting the right and left coronary arteries were first described by Richard Lower of Amsterdam in 1669 (Table 1.1).[4] He detected the anasto-moses by introducing fluid into one coronary artery post-mortem and obser-ving its arrival in the other.[4,6] However, Prinzmetal et al.[7] suggested Thebesius to be the first who revealed by dissection the occurrence of anastomoses between both coronary arteries,[8] whereby the respective anatomic preparations had probably not been performed in normal hearts.[7] In 1757, the Swiss anato-mist Albrecht von Haller (1708–1777; Fig. 1.1) also demonstrated anastomoses of the coronary arteries, whereby he described different origins and routes of coronary arterial detours, such as those going via the pulmonary artery root to the sulcus longitudinalis posterior of the right ventricle, those being located near the ventricular apex or close to the atria as well as extracardiac collaterals.[9] While the technique employed during these early observations of collateral vessels of the human heart was mostly that of mechanical dissection, it remains obscure whether normal or diseased hearts were examined. Considering the possibility that CAD was much less prevalent before the mid-18th century than thereafter,[2] the first anatomic observations of anastomoses were possibly made in non-obstructed coronary arteries.

Before the debate on the existence of structural collaterals started in the mid-19th century, William Heberden (1710–1801, Fig. 1.2) in 1772 systematically and meticulously described his clinical observations in 'nearly a hundred peo-ple' (three women and one boy, aged 12), who suffered from a disorder, '(T)he seat of it, and sense of strangling, and anxiety with which it is attended, may make it not improperly be called angina pectoris'.[5] Of particular importance in an entirely opposite sense for the further course of the history of the human coronary collateral circulation are two pieces of the text: (a) 'The termination of the angina pectoris is remarkable. For if no accident intervene, but the disease go on to its height, the patients all suddenly fall down, and perish almost immediately'. (b) 'With respect to the treatment of this complaint, I have little or nothing to advance: nor indeed is it to be expected we should have made much progress in the cure of a disease, which has hitherto hardly had a place, or a name in medical books. ...I know one who set himself a task of sawing wood for half an hour every day, and was nearly cured. In one also, the disorder

Table 1.1 Historical accounts on the human coronary collateral circulation

Year	First author	Lessening exercise-induced angina pectoris	Non-fatal coronary occlusion	Structural collaterals in 'No CAD*'	Functional collaterals	CAD	No CAD
1669	Lower	–	–	*First description*	–	?	?
1708	Thebesius	–	–	Present	–	?	?
1757	von Haller	*First description*	–	Present	–	?	?
1772	Heberden		–	–	–	Yes**	No
1855	Hyrtl	–	–	Absent	–		Yes
1866	Henle	–	–	Absent	–		Yes
1881	Cohnheim	–	–	End-arteries	–	No	Yes***
1881	Krause	–		Present	–		
1880	Langer	–		Present	–		
1883	West	Walking through a.p.	*First description*	Present	(Yes)	Yes	No
1897	Osler	–		Present	–	Yes	No
1907	Hirsch	–		Abundantly present	Yes	No	Yes
1912	Herrik	–	Yes		Yes	Yes	No
1928	Wenckebach	'Toter Punkt' a.p.	–				–
1938	Schlesinger	–		Absent	Size forbids function	–	Yes
1940	Blumgart	–		Absent at >40 μm	Size forbids function	Yes	Yes
1947	Prinzmetal	–		Extensive (70–180 μm)	–	No	Yes
1951	Zoll	–		Present in 9%	–	Yes	Yes
1956	Baroldi	–		Present (20–350 μm)	No interpretation	Yes	Yes
1959	Pitt			Present in 6%	No evidence	Yes	Yes
1960	Pepler			Present in 35%	–	Yes	Yes
1963	Fulton			Numerous (–500 μm)	–	Yes	Yes
1966	MacAlpin	Warm-up angina			Yes	Yes	No
1969	Gensini	–		Not detected	Yes, in CAD	Yes	Yes

Table 1.1 (continued)

Year	First author	Lessening exercise-induced angina pectoris	Non-fatal coronary occlusion	Structural collaterals in 'No CAD'*	Functional collaterals	CAD	No CAD
1971	Helfant	–	–	–	Yes	Yes	No
1974	Goldstein	–	–	–	*First functional test*	Yes	No
1975	Goldstein	–	–	–	*First functional test*	No	Yes
1984	Feldman	–	–	–	Yes	Yes	No
2003	Wustmann	–	–	–	Yes, in 23–28%	Yes	Yes

*Documented by direct dissection, injection into one coronary artery of H_2O, air, carmine–gelatine, lead–agar, coloured and radiopaque gelatine solution, kerosene, radioactively labelled erythrocytes, glass spheres, wax spheres, bismuth–oxychloride–gelatine; followed or not by unrolling of the heart and dissection.

**Heberden not aware of the existence of coronary artery disease.

***As obtained in the dog heart (!).

Abbreviations: a.p. = angina pectoris; CAD = coronary artery disease.

Fig. 1.1 Portrait of Albrecht
von Haller

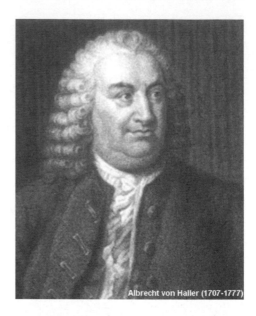

Albrecht von Haller (1707-1777)

Fig. 1.2 Portrait of William
Heberden

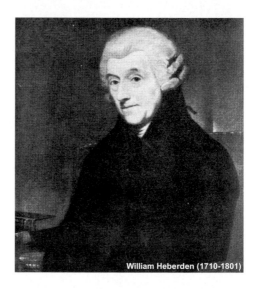

William Heberden (1710-1801)

ceased of itself'. Much more relevant than the internal contradiction between
(a) and (b) was Heberden's firm statement in (a) of a disease with always fatal
outcome, which appeared to be even confirmed by (b). For his contemporaries
and until more than 100 years later, the message of Heberden's description of
angina pectoris was that of an absolutely fatal illness, notwithstanding the
content of (b) that there might be a cure or even spontaneous healing, and
despite a later report in 1785, in which an unknown patient described, 'I have

frequently, when in company, borne the pain, and continued my pace without indulging it; at which times it has lasted from five to perhaps ten minutes, and then gone off'.[10] Thus historically, the development of tolerance against myocardial ischaemia, later attributed to recruitment of the collateral circulation (see also the Chapter 2), was not appreciated. Nowadays, Heberden is cited for his first description of walking through angina (Table 1.1) and not for his judging angina pectoris to be a 100% fatal disease of unknown origin. With regard to post-mortem examination of one of Heberden's patients, he reported,[5] 'On opening the body of one, who died suddenly of this disease, a very skilful anatomist could discover no fault in the heart, the valves, in the arteries, or neighbouring veins, excepting small rudiments of ossification in the aorta'. The 'skilful' anatomist happened to be John Hunter (1728–1793; Fig. 1.3), the famous pathologist and surgeon, who himself was intimately and intricately involved in the history of CAD and the discovery of the collateral circulation, as both scientist and patient.[11] As a patient of William Heberden, John Hunter had suffered from angina pectoris for the last 20 years of his life.[12] So as if to buttress the original notion of Heberden of angina pectoris as a fatal disease, Hunter died suddenly at the age of 65. In the post-mortem examination of John Hunter,[12] the coronary arteries were described as having '...their branches which ramify through the substance of the heart in the state of bony tubes, which were with difficulty divided by the knife, and their transverse sections did not collapse, but remained open'. Nevertheless, the coronary arteries themselves were not suspected as the *direct* cause of Hunter's disease and death[12]: 'From this account of the appearances observed after death, it is reasonable to attribute the principal symptoms of the disease to an organic affection of the heart'. However, Edward Jenner (1749–1823, the discoverer of vaccination), Hunter's former assistant, strongly suspected a relationship

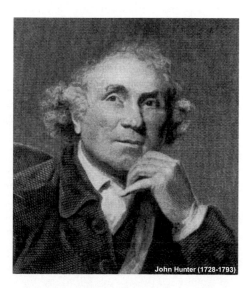

John Hunter (1728-1793)

Fig. 1.3 Portrait of John Hunter

between 'coronary ossification' and angina pectoris, and out of concern for his mentor and friend, he wrote of his opinion long before Hunter's death to his personal physician, Heberden.[1]

Although the role of the late John Hunter as a CAD patient was one delaying the recognition of a clinically relevant coronary collateral circulation, his position as a scientist was essential for the discovery of peripheral natural bypasses.[11] Indeed, the collateral arterial growth was detected in an unusual anatomic area. Aside from his duties as a pathologist, John Hunter became also a surgeon to the British royal family, and one privilege he thereby enjoyed was to hunt in the Royal deer park.[11] He took advantage of that opportunity not to hunt, but to perform an experiment provoked by the extraordinary annual growth of the stag's antlers. To explore the contribution of the arterial supply to that growth, he ligated the major supplying artery on one side. As anticipated, it was cool and the growth of the antler on that side interrupted. However, the influence of the ligation was only transient. After a short time, the antler became warm again and exuberant growth occurred. Hunter identified the fact that a collateral arterial supply had developed to bypass the arterial occlusion created by his ligature, and he went on to demonstrate that the phenomenon occurred elsewhere, e.g. following femoral artery ligation in the dog.[11] In the sense of 'translational' research, he exploited the animal observation to develop a new surgical treatment technique for limb aneurysm by gradually ligating the artery above the aneurysm in the hope that collateral development would render amputation unnecessary, which it did.

It was not before 1883, that the paradigm of the absolutely fatal coronary occlusion was overcome by West's description of several cases in whom at autopsy complete obstruction of a coronary artery was found, yet the patients had long survived this serious lesion.[13] With regard to the existence of a human coronary collateral circulation, this observation has constituted not a sufficient but certainly a necessary condition.

1.1.3   Post-mortem Assessment

In 1855, 186 years following the first description of the existence of human coronary collateral vessels by Lower,[4] Hyrtl denied the occurrence of these anastomoses,[14] and subsequently, Henle[15] and Cohnheim confirmed the findings of Hyrtl, whereby Cohnheim stated that the coronary arteries were true end-arteries.[16] The approximately 100-year era of ever-increasing pathoanatomic studies on the human coronary circulation had begun, whereby a multitude of preparation techniques for imaging the coronary circulation were employed, the fact of which substantially contributed to the partly contradictory findings (Table 1.1). In part, it was not even direct post-mortem evidence in humans which implied the existence of end-arteries as was the case in Cohnheim's study.

1.1.3.1 Imaging Techniques

Post-mortem imaging of the anatomy of coronary arterial anastomoses requires some form of coronary injection technique. As Fulton remarked,[17] a list of injection techniques consisting of over 70 different techniques was far from complete. Following were and still are the frequently employed methods: corrosion technique, clearing technique and arteriography. The corrosion technique leaves only the cast of the arterial lumen after coronary injection of a solidifying mass with subsequent digestion of the surrounding tissue. Using this method, Hyrtl[14] and Henle[15] failed to demonstrate the arterial communications between different supply areas in normal hearts. Clearing in organic solvents after injection with an opaque medium was developed by Spalteholz and is known as clearing technique.[18] This technique achieved the demonstration of even the smallest calibre anastomoses in normal hearts. A disadvantage was the visualization of vessels for only a few millimetre below the surface and the removal of all lipids from the vessel wall. Injection of a radiopaque medium followed by X-ray exposure on film is arteriography. This method has been and is the most widely used post mortem method. Despite the shortcomings of the two-dimensional radiography for the demonstration of small-calibre anastomoses, it was widely used in the past.[17] The distinction of continuity of the arterial lumen (indicative of an anastomosis) from mere overlap in the third dimension of the left ventricular (LV) wall thickness can be very difficult without employing stereoarteriography.

The principle of a considerable part of the arteriographic techniques employed consisted of an increasingly sophisticated injection with or without dissection procedure (Fig. 1.4). Using this technique, the heart is removed and

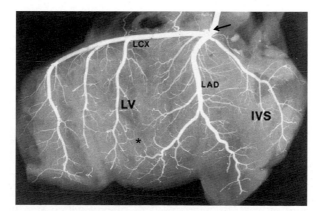

Fig. 1.4 Post-mortem coronary angiography of a canine left ventricle. The left coronary artery circulation was filled with barium sulfate–gelatine mass and dissected according to the method described by Rodriguez and Reiner ('unrolled' heart),[21] whereby the right ventricle was separated from the left ventricle (LV). The barium sulfate-gelatine mass was injected via a flange (→) into the left coronary artery. Some intercoronary anastomoses are visible (*). IVS = interventricular septum; LAD = left anterior descending coronary artery; LCX = left circumflex coronary artery

flushed from intracavitary clots by saline solution. A cannula of suitable size with a flange is then placed into, e.g. the left coronary artery ostium and held in place by a purse string suture (Fig. 1.4). The coronary artery is then flushed with 100–200 ml of physiologic saline solution. A previously prepared injectate, e.g. barium sulfate–gelatine,[19] in a pressurized flask is then injected into the cannulated coronary artery under controlled pressure of, example, 100 mmHg at a temperature of 40°C.[20] The radiographic mixture fills the epicardial arteries and small branches but not the capillary bed because of high viscosity. The extent to which the coronary arterial tree is filled by the injectate depends on its viscosity, the injection pressure, the temperature at the time of injection and the solidifying temperature of the injectate. For example, barium sulfate–gelatine becomes solid at room temperature.[19] Historically, approximately a dozen of various substances were injected into the coronary arteries (Table 1.1), and thus, a wide variety of the degree of coronary filling ranging from capillary crossing to filling of only large coronary arteries was reached. With the exception of pure mechanical dissection studies, one of the prominent reasons for the debate on the existence of structural anastomoses between coronary territories is inherent in the variety of injectates employed in post-mortem studies. In case of obtaining a post-mortem arteriogram, or before the era of radiology as an aid in dissecting the coronary arterial tree, the heart is 'unrolled' so that all of the epicardial coronary arteries can be seen in one plane,[21] thereby also revealing anastomotic connections between the major coronary artery territories (Fig. 1.4). The technique of 'unrolling' the heart consists of making two planes of incision, one to either side of the cardiac septa, so that the branches to the interventricular septum remain in continuity with the parent arteries.[21]

It was not before 1938, that the above-described method of injecting a radiopaque mass into the coronary arteries plus unrolling the heart was described by Schlesinger[22]. Thus, the different method of coronary injection and myocardial corrosion employed by Hyrtl in 1855 was possibly part of the diverging results regarding the existence of structural collaterals, when compared to previous or subsequent studies[14] (Table 1.1). However, the confirmation of Hyrtl's findings by Cohnheim and von Schulthess-Rechberg was based on their experiments in dogs with cessation of the heart beat within 2 minutes of occluding either the left or right coronary artery (RCA).[16] In opposition to the end-artery theory, Krause and Langer[23] again claimed that the coronary arteries communicated through pre-capillary anastomoses (Table 1.1). In addition to West's observation of non-fatal coronary artery occlusion, he provided the following pathoanatomic description indicating the existence of a coronary collateral circulation[13]: 'Cases are not very rare in which the mouth of one coronary artery is completely blocked by atheromatous change in the casts of the aorta, and still the heart's nutrition has for a long time been well provided for. In one such case which I have recently examined, the coronary artery, the mouth of which was completely obliterated, was of normal size and appearance even up to the obstruction, and contained blood which must have been supplied to it from the unobstructed artery of the opposite side'. In 1907, Hirsch and

Spalteholz stated that in dogs there are functionally competent coronary anastomoses and that the coronary circulation in humans is similarly rich in
collateral vessels,[24] whereby the latter investigator based his conclusions on a
method of coronary injection and subsequent treatment of the heart in order to
make the myocardium transparent, thus revealing the coronary anastomoses to
the naked eye (see above, clearing technique).[18]

Similarly as West demonstrated some 30 years earlier, the clinico-pathologic
study by Herrik documented in 1912 that sudden coronary occlusion of even
large coronary branches had not to be fatal[3]: '..., there is, as has been shown by
reference to experimental work, no intrinsic reason why some patients with
obstruction of even large branches of the coronary artery may not recover'.
Herrik is credited to mention coronary thrombosis as the cause of the sudden
vascular obstruction, and he supported this notion by providing the case
histories with post-mortem results of six patients with angina pectoris. With
regard to the potential benefit of coronary collaterals, Herrik remarked: 'The
hope for the damaged myocardium lies in the direction of securing a supply of
blood through friendly neighbouring vessels so as to restore as far as possible its
functional integrity'. However, purely pathoanatomic studies such as that by
Schlesinger did not recognize the size of the structural collaterals to be sufficient
in order to be functional at sudden occlusion[22] (Table 1.1). Schlesinger[22] as well
as Zoll et al.[25] reported an incidence of only 9% of coronary anastomoses larger
than 40 μm in normal human hearts. Based on that result, Schlesinger initially
concluded that no coronary anastomoses existed in the normal human heart.[22]
He later modified that view and stated that interarterial connections in normal
hearts were not larger than 40 μm in the absence of coronary or myocardial
disease.[26] Based on the refinement of pathoanatomic techniques for imaging the
coronary circulation, which was substantially promoted by Schlesinger (lea-
d–agar injection plus unrolling the heart plus arteriography),[22] the existence of
human coronary collaterals in the presence of CAD was undisputable by the
late 1930s (Fig. 1.5[26]). Prinzmetal et al. perfused the coronary arteries of 13
normal hearts with calibrated glass beads sized 70–220 μm and demonstrated
intercoronary anastomoses ranging from 70 to 180 μm[7] (Table 1.1). The technique employed was conventional with injection of the glass spheres into the left
or right coronary artery and collection of the spheres at the opposite coronary
artery, the coronary sinus and the ventricular cavities. Using this method, not
only arterio-arterial (70–180 μm), but also arterio-venous (70–170 μm), arterio-
sinusoidal, arterio-luminal collaterals (70–220 μm) and Thebesian veins could
be found (Fig. 1.6).[7] It was concluded that the normal human heart had an
extensive collateral circulation with anastomotic channels of various types.[7]
To conclude on the basis of four patients with CAD that '...this collateral
circulation is ready to function immediately at which time the anastomotic
communications may become enlarged in the presence of a favourable pressure
gradient' certainly represented an over-interpretation of the purely structural
data obtained.[7] The above-mentioned study by Zoll et al. employed an arteriographic *coloured* lead–agar injection technique followed by unrolling the heart

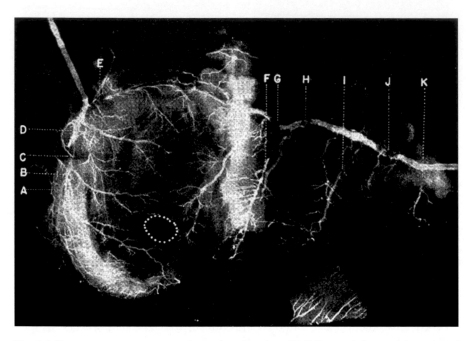

Fig. 1.5 Post-mortem coronary angiography of an 'unrolled' human left ventricle prepared similarly as described for the previous figure. A, B, C, D, E, F, I, K indicate chronic total coronary occlusions. G and H indicate coronary emboli and J indicates a fresh thrombus[26]

and taking a radiograph of the unrolled heart (Fig. 1.7).[25] Of notice, Zoll's investigation was the first large-scale post-mortem study in 1,050 human hearts, thus accounting for individual variations in the coronary anastomotic circulation and allowing subgroup analyses according to various types of potential determinants of collaterals (Table 1.2).[25] The authors in that study concluded that anastomoses were clearly demonstrated and relevantly increased in hearts with coronary artery occlusion or marked CAD, in cor pulmonale, in the presence of LV hypertrophy and valvular lesions, and in normal hearts from patients with anaemia.[25] In 1956, Baroldi et al., using the corrosion method with plastic casts of the coronary vessels, found 'conspicuous' coronary anastomoses in normal human hearts ranging in size from 20 to 350 μm and in length between 1 and 5 cm (Fig. 1.8).[27] Based on the described disagreement about the occurrence of structural interarterial coronary collateral vessels in normal hearts, Pitt re-investigated the problem using an injection technique of wax spheres sized 35–45 μm and 75–90 μm in 75 hearts, whereby anastomoses were present in only 1 of 15 normal hearts examined[28] (Table 1.1). In comparison, anastomoses were found in 41 of the 58 pathologic hearts. In an attempt to elicit possible genetic differences in the occurrence of human interarterial coronary anastomoses in normal hearts, Pepler et al. studied 90 hearts of Europeans and 94 hearts of the South African Bantu population using a

Collateral circulation of the heart

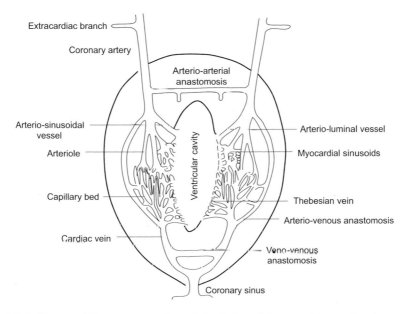

Fig. 1.6 A diagram of the coronary collateral circulation of the normal human heart as seen by Prinzmetal et al. in 1947.[7] All the collateral channels depicted were documented anatomically. Red indicates the arterial bed and blue the venous bed of the coronary circulation

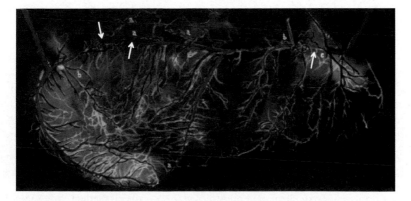

Fig. 1.7 Coloured coronary angiogram of a human 'unrolled' heart with multiple coronary artery occlusions (→) and extensive interarterial coronary anastomoses. Coronary collateral vessels are recognizable by grossly dissectible channels between two arteries (**a**), by injection mass of any colour distal to a complete coronary artery occlusion (**b**) and by admixture of colours of injection mass (**c**)[25]

Table 1.2 Presence of structural intercoronary anastomoses according to disease (Zoll et al.)

Condition	N	Anastomoses present (%)
Normal hearts	101	9
Normal hearts from anaemic patients	89	39
Coronary artery occlusion	275	95
Coronary artery disease with slight arterial narrowing	65	17
Coronary artery disease with moderate arterial narrowing	44	25
Coronary artery disease with marked arterial narrowing	19	63
Cor pulmonale	15	73
Cardiac hypertrophy (normal coronaries and valvular disease)	215	31
Valvular heart disease (without hypertrophy)	13	31
Total of the entire series	1,050	46

Coronary artery disease   **No coronary artery disease**

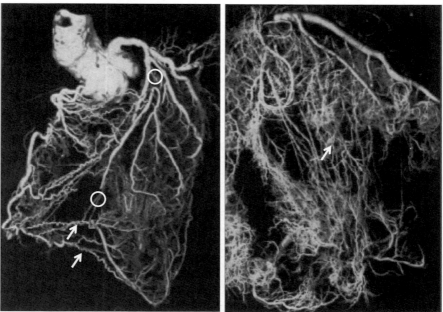

Fig. 1.8 Coronary arterial circulation prepared by the 'corrosion method' (injection of the coronary arteries with a suspension of polyvinyl chloride containing a plastic substance, i.e. Geon Latex 576 and digestion of the surrounding tissue).[27] *Left side panel*: The left anterior descending coronary artery of a 62-year-old male patient is interrupted at its origin and its distal third (circle). The distal part is filled via collateral vessels (→). *Right side panel*: Normal heart of a 19-year-old man showing anastomoses (→) of the interventricular septum

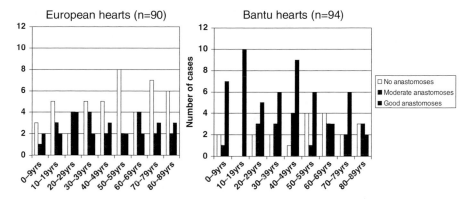

Fig. 1.9 Number of hearts (*vertical axis*) of European (*left side*) and Bantu individuals (*right side*) showing coronary anastomoses of different degrees according to age groups (*horizontal axis*)

method of injecting gelatine–potassium-iodide–barium sulfate plus unrolling the heart with subsequent arteriography.[29] Among the 90 European hearts, 23 revealed so called good anastomoses (23 hearts normal, 8 of them with good anastomoses), and in the 94 Bantu hearts, there were 54 with good collateral channels (49 hearts normal, 26 with good anastomoses; see also Table 1.1 and Fig. 1.9). The higher incidence of good anastomoses in normal Bantu than in European hearts was interpreted as being related to the widespread megaloblastic and iron-deficiency anaemia among Bantu and not to genetic reasons.[29] The better anastomotic blood supply was found unrelated to ventricular hypertrophy, coronary atherosclerosis or gross anatomic differences of the arterial tree, such as the occurrence of an intermediary branch of the left coronary artery.

1.1.3.2 Coronary Collateral Vessels in Neonates

In infant hearts not subjected to the stimuli of anoxia, anaemia or cardiac hypertrophy, Bloor et al. found intercoronary anastomoses ranging up to 80 μm in diameter.[30] The pathoanatomic study by Reiner et al. in a series of 55 neonatal hearts revealed a high frequency from 33 to 78% of communicating arterial channels > 40 μm between the right and the left coronary arteries.[31] The absence of collateral vessels occurred more often in premature than in full-term neonates (Fig. 1.10). Interarterial connections were encountered more often in children of women aged ≤23 at birth than in those of women above that age, and it appeared that collaterals present at birth tended to involute during childhood (Fig. 1.11).[31] While the latter finding can be questioned on the basis of the study's low statistical power in that age group (Fig. 1.11), the result of a high prevalence of coronary anastomoses in neonates appears to be consistent, and they may be interpreted as remnants of the retiform, early stages of arterial development, i.e. of vasculogenesis in foetal life.

Fig. 1.10 Frequency
(*vertical axis*) and degree
(*horizontal axis*) of coronary
collateral vessels in
premature and full-term
neonates

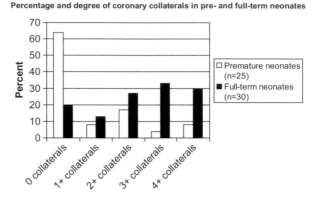

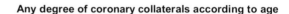

Fig. 1.11 Frequency
(*vertical axis*) of coronary
collateral vessels according
to age of individuals
(*horizontal axis*)

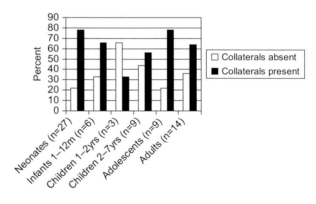

1.1.3.3 Pathoanatomic Studies by Fulton

The issue of whether arterial anastomoses (pre-) exist in the normal heart is
fundamental to the understanding of the collateral circulation in CAD. As
described above, there was a period of ever recurring change in opinion on
the topic of coronary anastomoses for almost 300 years after their first description in the normal human heart. The authoritative statement, in 1881 by
Cohnheim and von Schulthess-Rechberg[16], that the (canine!) coronary arteries
were 'end arteries' substantially blunted the progress in that field for many
years. This could not be overcome by Spalteholz and Hirsch[18,24], by Crainicianu[32] and by Gross[33], who independently found abundant coronary arterial
anastomoses in normal human hearts using a method of coronary injection
followed by myocardial clearing (see above). The knowledge provided by the
latter studies was even obscured by the advent of a simplified technique of two-
dimensional arteriography,[22] whereby the interventricular septum had been
often excised (likely the most important site of anastomoses). Also, the technique of two-dimensional arteriography of the unrolled heart (see Fig. 1.7)
rendered it difficult to distinguish vascular overlay in the third dimension

from vascular continuity between adjacent arterial beds (i.e. anastomoses). Regarding the latter issue, one would spontaneously expect an overestimation rather than an underestimation of coronary anastomoses. However, probably adhering to the principle of conservative assessment, the researchers' finding of *no* or *few* anastomoses likely rejected cases of uncertain anastomoses. It was not until the early 1960s when the debate on the existence of structural coronary anastomoses in the normal human heart could be definitely settled by Fulton using an entirely different pathoanatomic imaging technique for the coronary circulation.[34,35] This method in comparison to previous techniques revolutionized post-mortem arteriography with regard to the quality of the images (Fig. 1.12). The following factors used in Fulton's technique contributed to

No coronary artery disease

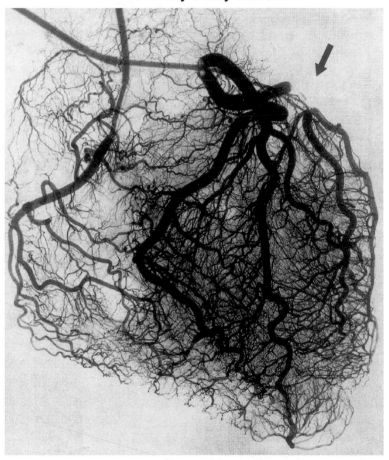

Fig. 1.12 Post-mortem coronary angiogram of a normal heart. Ligation of a branch of the left circumflex coronary artery (LCX; →) was performed before contrast injection. The existence of anastomotic communication was demonstrated by retrograde filling of the LCX distal to the ligation in <20 s[17]

its augmented reliability in detecting coronary anastomoses of any type: the bismuth-oxychloride–gelatine radiographic contrast medium containing uniformly sized particles down to 0.5–2.0 μm (~5 times smaller than Schlesinger's lead–agar medium[19]), which could penetrate vessels down to 10–15 μm in luminal diameter without entering capillaries. For injection into the RCA and detection of the contrast in the left coronary artery, the medium was tinted red with finely divided vermilion suspended in gelatine. One of the two criteria required for the definition of anastomoses was the presence in the left coronary artery of red pigment injected into the RCA.[34] The second criterion was stereoarteriographic, i.e. three-dimensional demonstration of unequivocal communication between arterial branches.[34] Stereoarteriography was the second decisive factor being responsible for the unmatched imaging results. The third factor was immersion radiography,[36] aimed at uniform exposure of the injected vessels, being sustained in varying thickness of tissue. Thus, radiography was carried out with the specimen totally immersed in saline. The fourth factor related to the use of fine-grain X-ray film and stereoscopic viewing at fivefold magnification. Finally, Fulton omitted the excision of the interventricular septum (Fig. 1.13) and examined the entire heart prior to dissection, followed by three 'short-axis' or transverse sections: atrial 'cap', basal block, transventricular section and apex. Employing systematically the described method, 'numerous anastomoses in all normal hearts' (n = 17) as well as in those with CAD (n = 25) were found in a total of 59 human hearts (17 hearts with heart disease other than CAD; Figs. 1.13 and 1.14).[34,35] Coronary collateral vessels were categorized as superficial, i.e. epicardial and deep anastomoses, whereby the latter comprised interventricular septal anastomoses, the sub-endocardial plexus of the left (Fig. 1.15) and that of the right ventricle.

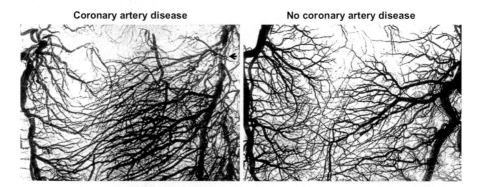

Coronary artery disease   No coronary artery disease

Fig. 1.13 Image of numerous interventricular anastomoses via septal branches of the left anterior descending coronary artery (LAD) in a patient with coronary artery disease (*left side panel*; chronic total occlusion of the LAD →), and in an individual with normal heart (*right side panel*). Small- and medium-sized collateral vessels (50–200 μm in diameter) can be traced between the LAD on the right side of the images and the ramus interventricularis posterior of the right coronary artery on the left side. Image magnification: 2×

Fig. 1.14 Score of coronary arterial anastomoses (*vertical axis*) and their diameter (*horizontal axis*) categorized according to normal hearts and hearts with coronary artery disease (CAD). In the presence of CAD, there is a shift to more prevalent large-sized collateral vessels

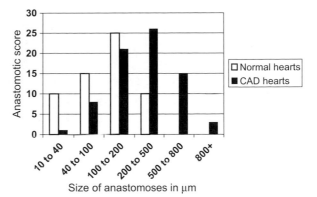

Anastomotic score=Σ of anastomotic indices x 10/# in group

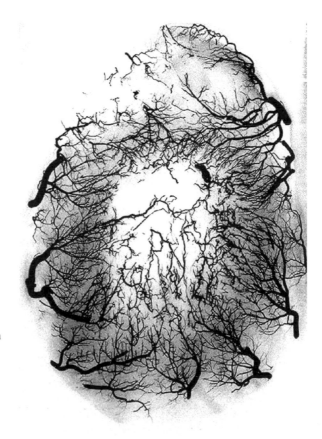

Fig. 1.15 Subendocardial coronary anastomotic plexus of the left ventricle in a heart with a normal coronary circulation. The connections between the epicardial vessels and the subendocardial plexus are displayed. Image magnification: 1.5×

Fig. 1.16 Sum of coronary anastomoses in normal hearts (*vertical axis*) and their diameter (*horizontal axis*) according to the site of occurrence. *a.* anastomoses, *interv.* interventriular, *LV* left ventricle, *RV* right ventricle

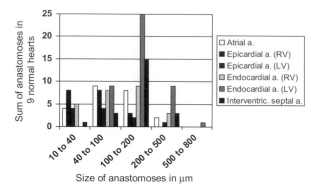

Figure 1.16 illustrates the relative distribution of the different types of coronary anastomoses as determined in nine normal human hearts of Fulton's study.[35] Other coronary collaterals were vasa vasorum (sometimes enlarging to 'bridging' collaterals) and extracoronary connections, i.e. atrial–mediastinal connections.[34] Figure 1.14 also shows the relative distribution of anastomoses as analysed by Fulton in the normal and CAD groups,[35] whereby it was obvious that the difference lay not so much in their numbers but rather in the enlarged calibre of structural collaterals in the presence of CAD.

1.1.4 In Vivo Assessment

1.1.4.1 First Clinico-pathological Associations

Most of the above-described historical work on human coronary arterial anastomoses consists of pathoanatomic investigations. In vivo assessment of the coronary collateral circulation required developing awareness of ante-mortem clinico-pathologic relationships between CAD symptoms and coronary atherosclerosis/coronary anastomoses found at autopsy. Prospective in vivo characterization needed introduction of new techniques for coronary imaging and measurement of coronary haemodynamics, such as selective angiography, functional coronary pressure, flow or flow velocity measurements during cardiac surgery and PCI. While the clinico-pathologic link between angina pectoris and coronary atherosclerotic obstruction was first made by John Wall only 4 years after the first symptom description by Heberden[37], it was not until 1883 that Samuel West retrospectively established the possibility of the patient's survival despite concomitant coronary obstructive disease (thanks to 'anastomosis of the coronary arteries').[13] Since Herrik's account of the possibility of surviving sudden thrombotic coronary obstruction in the presence of intercoronary anastomoses,[3] it has been recognized that the collateral circulation is a very important determinant of the rate and extent of cell death within an ischaemic zone. The time span between the description of initial symptom by Heberden in 1772 and the documentation of an associated 'pathology' was even close to 200 years with regard to 'walking through angina pectoris' and the presence of well-developed coronary collaterals by MacAlpin et al.[38] Following Herberden, the symptoms of adaptation to physical exercise in angina pectoris had also been mentioned by Osler in 1897[39] and by Wenckebach in 1928,[40] and it had been alternatively called 'angina of first effort', and in its forme fruste 'warm-up angina'. However, MacAlpin et al. were the first to even *suggest* the relationship to the angiographically detected, abundant collaterals in five of their eight invasively examined patients (Table 1.1).[38]

1.1.4.2 First In Vivo Coronary Angiographic Studies

Paulin was the second to document 'interarterial coronary anastomoses in relation to arterial obstruction demonstrated in coronary arteriography' during life in humans.[41] The first *systematic* in vivo retrospective angiographic analysis of the coronary collateral circulation was performed in 100 patients by Gensini and Bruto da Costa in 1969.[42] Among the 53 patients with normal coronary angiograms or stenotic lesions of < 50% in diameter, no collateral channels were detected. Since the mentioned study had been performed before the invention of PCI, angiographic collateral assessment was carried out by selective coronary contrast injection without artificial occlusion of the contralateral vessel.[42] In the 47 patients with more severe CAD, 37 cases revealed coronary collaterals, and the authors described several patterns of anastomotic pathways (e.g. Fig. 1.17). A clinico-pathologic association was inferred by the statement that coronary collaterals could account for a normal resting electrocardiogram (ECG) (n = 5) despite the presence of a major coronary artery occlusion.[42] In 1971, Helfant et al. investigated a selected population of 119 patients with

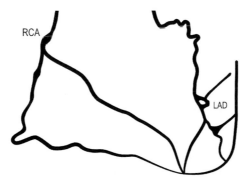

Fig. 1.17 Drawing of an angiogram with right to left coronary artery collaterals in a patient with a 90% stenosis of the left anterior descending coronary artery (LAD; stenosis not visualized; right anterior oblique (RAO) view). Site of injection: right coronary artery (RCA). The contrast agent reaches the distal LAD via a right ventricular branch

severe one-vessel CAD (stenosis in the proximal half of a major coronary artery with > 90% diameter narrowing) with regard to the 'functional importance of the human coronary collateral circulation'.[43] The originality content of the mentioned study consisted of its prospective design with a follow-up of 22 months and the direct comparison between the initial angiographic presence (n = 61 patients) and respectively absence (n = 58 patients) of collateral vessels and several functional clinical parameters and events. No relevant differences were observed between the groups in the level of physical activity before coronary angiography, in the duration of angina pectoris, frequency of prior myocardial infarction or prevalence of ECG, haemodynamic and left ventriculographic abnormalities.[43] However, Helfant et al. observed more frequent abnormal post-exercise ECG in the presence than in the absence of collateral vessels,[43] the fact of which had probably to do with the association of more severe CAD with better developed collaterals. Conversely, death during follow-up occurred less often in patients with (6/44) than in those without (10/45) collaterals, although the rate of myocardial infarction was nearly identical in both groups. The authors concluded that collaterals possibly 'protect not as much against having myocardial infarction as against a lethal outcome of these attacks', and thus, they re-hypothesized rather than verified or falsified the functional relevance of coronary collaterals.[43]

Without obtaining *direct* haemodynamic coronary collateral measurements (see below), several investigations have addressed the functional relevance of angiographically documented collateral vessels in humans. Evaluations of systolic LV function at rest and during exercise have generally indicated that patients with collaterals have better wall motion than those without collateral vessels.[44,45] Measurements of relative myocardial perfusion using thallium-201 have also suggested that collaterals can improve perfusion at rest and even during exercise.[46]

1.1.4.3 Direct Haemodynamic Collateral Measurements During Bypass Surgery

A fundamental question with regard to the relevance of the human coronary collateral circulation relates to its function. The term function has several aspects, i.e. not only the capacity of collaterals to prevent myocardial ischaemia and to salvage myocardium following sudden coronary occlusion but also their haemodynamic behaviour during occlusion as opposed to the structural, angiographic appearance. Furthermore, collateral function can mean the capacity to dilate or reduce vascular resistance in response to increased myocardial oxygen demand or to vasodilating substances. By employing post-mortem or in vivo coronary arteriography, only indirect conclusions can be drawn on collateral function by correlating their structural appearance to certain clinical outcome variables such as that performed by the above-mentioned study.[43] Since the role of human coronary collaterals in the pathophysiology of CAD was not elucidated by that investigation, direct haemodynamic collateral assessment was

first attempted by Goldstein et al. in the early 1970s.[47,48] In 29 patients with
CAD who underwent coronary venous bypass grafting, Goldstein et al.
obtained coronary haemodynamic measurements via the distally but not proximally attached vein graft, while the coronary artery receiving the graft was
totally occluded proximal to the site of graft attachment.[47] An earlier coronary
haemodynamic investigation during bypass surgery did not perform total
occlusion of the grafted vessel, and thus, obtained actual collateral flow parameters only in a minority of patients with chronic occlusion.[49] The measured
parameters in the study by Goldstein et al. were aortic and peripheral coronary
pressure and retrograde, i.e. collateral flow at baseline and after administration
of nitroglycerin.[47] The ratio between mean coronary peripheral (i.e. so called
coronary wedge pressure) and mean aortic pressure rose from 0.39 to 0.43
in response to nitroglycerin, while retrograde flow increased from 2.7 to
2.9 ml/min, which resulted in a significant reduction of collateral resistance.
Also, the authors found a correlation between the angiographic size and
extent of coronary collaterals and physiologic evidence of collateral function.[47] In seven patients without occlusive CAD who underwent aortic
valve replacement, Goldstein et al. obtained the same coronary haemodynamic parameters during a brief proximal occlusion of the right and the left
coronary arteries.[48] The ratio between mean peripheral coronary and aortic
pressures ranged between 0.09 and 0.36 and averaged 0.21 as compared to
an average of 0.50 in the above-mentioned study among patients with CAD
and angiographically well-developed collaterals (Fig. 1.18).[47,48] Considering

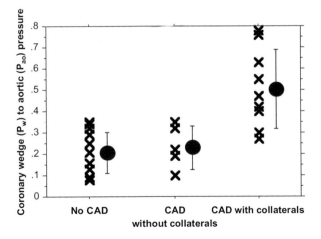

Fig. 1.18 Ratio of distal coronary occlusive pressure (coronary wedge pressure, P_{occl} in
mmHg) to aortic pressure (P_{ao} in mmHg; *vertical axis*) in different groups of patients
(*horizontal axis*) without coronary artery disease (no CAD; patients with aortic stenosis),
with CAD but no angiographic collaterals, and with CAD plus angiographic collaterals. The
ratio provides a continuous estimate of collateral relative to normal antegrade coronary flow
($\neq$ to collateral flow index). Crosses indicate individual values, filled symbols and error bars
indicate mean values ± standard deviation. Plot according to Goldstein et al.[47,48]

the very low number of seven patients recruited for the study, the authors probably concluded prematurely that 'collaterals in patients without diseased coronary arteries have an extremely limited capacity to transmit either flow or pressure'.[48] Notwithstanding, these were the first in vivo functional measurements of the coronary collateral circulation in humans with and without CAD, and were performed even prior to the introduction of coronary angioplasty.

1.1.4.4 Direct Haemodynamic Collateral Measurements During Angioplasty

The advent of PCI using over-the-wire angioplasty balloon catheters principally opened a new option for direct in vivo assessment of collateral haemodynamics in non-anaesthetized conscious humans.[50] However, it was not before 1984 that Feldman et al. reported the results of their study in 19 patients with a proximal left anterior descending coronary artery (LAD) stenosis and present (n = 6) or absent (n = 13) angiographic collateral filling undergoing measurements of aortic and occlusive peripheral coronary pressure as well as great cardiac vein flow[51] (Table 1.1). Coronary collateral vessels were found to be potentially important in a pathophysiologic sense, because clinical, ECG and haemodynamic evidences for transient myocardial ischaemia during balloon occlusion occurred less often, and flow and coronary pressure indices of collateral perfusion were better in men with angiographic evidence of collateral vessels than in those without.[51] The fact that RCA angiography as obtained during LAD *patency* constituted the reference method is the major limitation of this first small investigation using the coronary angioplasty model for functional assessment of the human collateral circulation. Coronary angiography is a much blunter instrument for collateral assessment than haemodynamic measurements, and in the way it was used by Feldman et al. (during patency of the collateral receiving artery), a situation different from that during the comparative occlusive haemodynamic measurements was assessed (spontaneously visible versus recruitable collaterals). The introduction of ultrathin Doppler and pressure sensor angioplasty guide wires has made it possible to obtain coronary flow velocity or pressure in remote vascular areas, and thus, to measure functional variables for studying the pathophysiology of the human coronary circulation, including the relevance of the collateral circulation. While in the case of occlusive coronary pressure measurements, its registration was and is also feasible via an over-the-wire angioplasty balloon catheter, occlusive flow velocity in humans can only be reliably obtained via an intracoronary guide-wire-mounted Doppler sensor. Ofili et al. were the first to detect coronary collateral flow by a Doppler guide wire during angioplasty.[52] The theoretical basis for coronary pressure- or velocity-derived quantitative indices for the

precise invasive assessment of collateral flow in humans was provided
by Pijls et al.[53] and Seiler et al.[54] (see also Chapter 2).

1.1.4.5 Functional Collaterals in the Absence of Coronary Atherosclerosis

The debate on the functional relevance of structural anastomoses in the
presence of normal coronary arteries continued with the above-cited
study by Goldstein et al. in patients with normal coronary arteries.[48] In
2003, Wustmann et al. presented the results of a study in 100 patients
with entirely (n = 51) or partially (n = 49) normal coronary arteries (i.e.
absence of angiographic stenotic lesions), in whom coronary pressure-
derived collateral relative to normal flow was obtained in non-stenotic
vessels during a 1-minute angioplasty balloon occlusion at a low inflation
pressure of 1 atmosphere.[55] Among the 51 patients with entirely normal
coronary arteries, 25% had no angina pectoris and 20% had no ECG signs
of myocardial ischaemia during coronary occlusion, i.e. their collateral
circulation was functional enough to prevent signs of myocardial ischaemia. The issue of briefly occluding a normal coronary artery by an angioplasty balloon was addressed by performing the procedure in the principal
investigator of that study, an individual with normal coronary arteries
(Figs. 1.19 and 1.20). Figure 1.21 illustrates, on the basis of 110 individuals with normal coronary arteries admitted to coronary angiography for
atypical chest pain, that 23% have a recruitable collateral relative to
normal flow of > 1/4, i.e. a value corresponding well to collaterals sufficient to prevent ischaemia during a 1-minute occlusion. In comparison,
28% of patients *with* CAD have a collateral relative to normal flow of >
1/4 (Fig. 1.21).

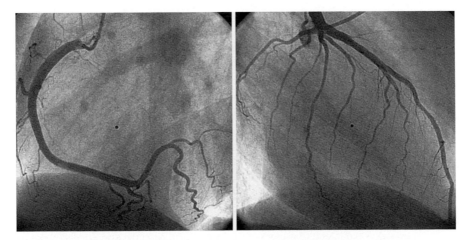

Fig. 1.19 Normal coronary angiogram from an individual without cardiac disease who
underwent occlusive quantitative coronary collateral assessment (see Fig. 1.20)

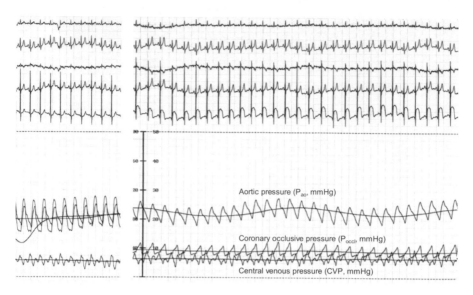

Fig. 1.20 Simultaneous electrocardiogram (ECG) (*upper part*), aortic, coronary and central venous pressure recordings (*lower part* of the tracings) as obtained in the individual from Fig. 1.19 without cardiac disease. *Left side*: recordings during coronary artery patency. *Right side*: recordings during artificial angioplasty balloon occlusion at 1 atmosphere inflation pressure of the mid left anterior descending coronary artery (LAD). On the intracoronary ECG lead (fourth lead from above), ST segment elevations are recognizable during LAD occlusion. These signs of myocardial ischaemia are present despite a value of collateral relative to normal antegrade LAD flow of 0.37 ($= [39-6]/[96-6]$, i.e. collateral flow index, $CFI = [P_{occl}-CVP]/[P_{ao}-CVP]$)

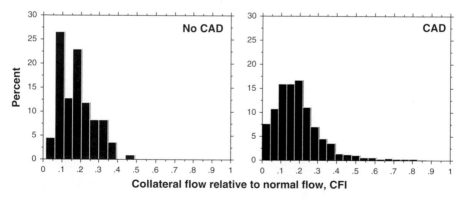

Fig. 1.21 Occurrence in percent of total (*vertical axis*) of collateral relative to normal antegrade coronary flow (collateral flow index, CFI; *horizontal axis*) in the absence and presence of coronary artery disease (CAD). With CAD, a right-ward shift of CFI values towards higher values can be observed

1.2 Interspecies Differences

As a consequence of the long-lasting debate on the relevance of the human coronary collateral circulation, a suitable animal model could not be defined, and arguments persisted until recently as to which species is the most representative of humans. That the pig heart has few collaterals, which are located endomurally and subendocardially, is generally agreed upon. Pathoanatomic studies by Spalteholz suggested already in the 1920s that the dog heart is a more suitable model with regard to preformed epicardial coronary anastomoses than the swine heart. Post-mortem arteriography in pigs that underwent gradual coronary artery occlusion revealed numerous small endomural and subepicardial anastomoses, whereas in dogs a few large interarterial epicardial anastomoses were observed. Accordingly, the infarct size in that interspecies observation by Schaper et al. was larger in pigs than in dogs. Abrupt as opposed to gradual occlusion of a major coronary artery in the pig is known to be related to a much higher mortality of close to 100% than the respective procedure in dogs. The animal model most relevant to the human situation of atherosclerotic plaque rupture is that of abrupt coronary occlusion highlighting the existence of preformed collateral vessels. In 1987, Maxwell et al. quantified the coronary collateral circulation during acute myocardial ischaemia in eight species in vivo using radiolabelled microspheres. The ranking order between species regarding collateral relative to normal myocardial zone blood flow was as follows: guinea pig (collateral = normal zone flow), dog (16%), cat (12%), rat (6%), ferret (2%), baboon (2%), rabbit (2%) and pig (1%). Thus, guinea pigs, dogs and cats are well suited for studies of *vascular* adaptation to ischaemia (i.e. collateral recruitment, collateral remodelling or arteriogenesis); rats, rabbits and pigs which have practically no functionally relevant collateral flow are appropriate for investigations on *myocardial* adaptation to ischaemia (i.e. myoacardial preconditioning). The animal model closest to humans with regard to functional collateral flow is the dog.

1.2.1 Introduction

Before the introduction of angioplasty guide-wire-mounted pressure and Doppler sensors, functional aspects of the coronary collateral circulation in humans were difficult to study, and the problem could be approached only by animal experimentation. With regard to the search for substances, devices or other treatment modalities potentially promoting collateral growth, but also to the investigation of collateral pathogenesis, the animal model is indispensable. As a direct consequence of the long-lasting debate on the relevance of the human coronary collateral circulation (see Section 1.2), i.e. because of the actual absence of the human reference, a suitable animal model could not be defined with certainty, and arguments persisted until quite recently as to which species is the most representative of humans.[56–62] Other general problems in the search for the ideal animal model with regard to coronary collaterals are the age disparity between animal model (often young) and human (patients in their 60 s), the discrepancy of disease state (absent in animals, CAD in patients) and the difference in organ size (often small animals with a higher mitosis rate than in the relatively large-sized human patient). The latter aspect is closely accounted for, if the dog or pig is chosen as animal model. Without particularly focusing on coronary anastomoses, the pig can be and was regarded as an appropriate model for the human being because of the similarities in gross coronary anatomy.[63–65] On the other hand, the dog has been said to be less well suited for this purpose in.[66] Weaver et al. studied the anatomy and distribution of coronary arteries in 65 hearts from domestic and miniature pigs with the goal of establishing adequate and statistically relevant baseline information for using swine in cardiovascular research.[61] Like man, the swine has a left coronary artery which is larger in calibre and longer than the RCA, and the RCA is dominant in 78%, i.e. supplying the posterior septum and atrioventricular node via the posterior descending coronary artery. Intracoronary dye injections showed in that study that 72% of the right ventricular mass was supplied by the RCA and 28% by the LAD, whereas in the LV 49% of its mass was provided by the LAD, 25.5% by the RCA and 25.5% by the left circumflex coronary artery (LCX). The authors of that investigation concluded that not only the coronary anatomy but also the distribution of blood supply to different myocardial regions of the swine heart was very similar to that of humans, and the swine appeared to them an excellent animal model for the study of *normal* coronary physiology.[61] The latter point raises a further important aspect regarding the selection of an animal model: the particular purpose of the study. For example, does the study focus on the development of myocardial tolerance to ischaemia or on vascular adaptation to ischaemia. The former would require an animal without a coronary collateral circulation, the latter a model with extensive coronary anastomoses. In the same context, Weaver et al. found the pig to be an excellent model for the investigation of human myocardial ischaemia, because coronary collateral flow would be practically absent in both species without heart disease.[61]

1.2.2 Pig Versus Dog as a Model for the Human Coronary Collateral Circulation

That the pig heart has few collaterals, which are located endomurally and subendocardially, is generally agreed upon.[59,67,68] The statement by Weaver et al. about the pig being an ideal model for the normal human heart was wrong,[61] and it reflects the lack of knowledge about the preformed human coronary collateral circulation. The observation of small intramural or septal anastomoses was reported similar to those in humans,[56] and so was the lack of vascular communications between epicardial branches, a feature typical for the extensive collateral circulation in dogs.[59] However, the much earlier pathoanatomic studies by Spalteholz strongly suggested that the dog heart is a more suitable model with regard to preformed epicardial coronary anastomoses than the swine heart (Figs. 1.22 and 1.23).[69]

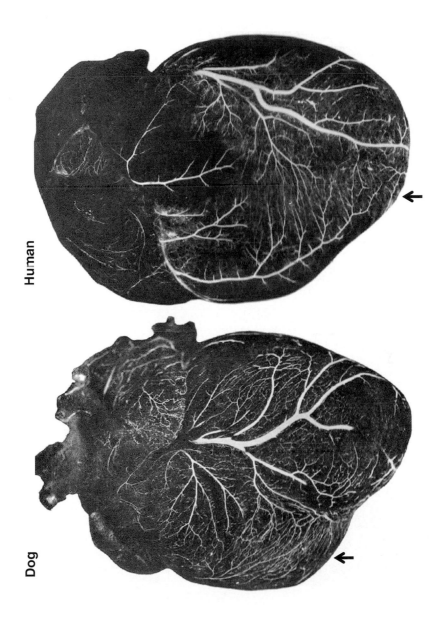

Fig. 1.22 Post-mortem coronary angiograms taken from a normal canine (*left side*) and a normal human heart (*right side*). The left anterior descending and the right coronary artery territories are imaged, whereby numerous anastomoses between them are visible (→)[69]

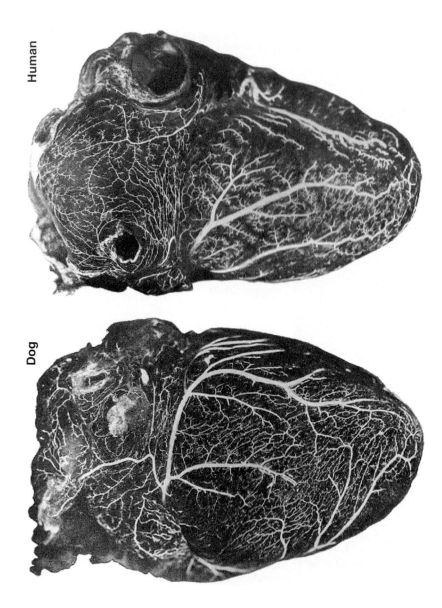

Fig. 1.23 Post-mortem coronary angiograms taken from a normal canine (*left side*) and a normal human heart (*right side*) with the left circumflex coronary artery (LCX) region imaged (posterolateral view). Numerous anastomoses between a marginal branch of the LCX and the main LCX itself are visible[69]

During chronic coronary artery occlusion in pigs by ameroid constriction over the course of an average of 2.5 weeks, Schaper et al. observed a mortality of 30%, which was similar to the 34% in the canine group of the same investigation.[59] In human CAD, the abrupt, thrombotic coronary occlusion as a consequence of an atherosclerotic plaque rupture is a well known and frequent event, and thus, *gradual* constriction of a coronary artery in the animal model represents only the rather safe part of the situation in humans. In this context, abrupt occlusion of a major coronary artery in the pig is related to a much higher mortality of close to 100% than the respective procedure in dogs.[60,70] The rate of myocardial infarction in the study by Schaper et al. was 44% in pigs as compared to 21% in the canine group.[59] The development of arterial back pressure (a measure of collateral perfusion) following vascular constriction occurred after 3–4 weeks and could be measured in only 11 of 25 pigs completing the 12-weeks study protocol, but in all 68 dogs.[59] In this selected group of pigs, it amounted to 60% of diastolic aortic pressure, which was similar as in the canine group. Furthermore, myocardial infarction was large in relation to the ischaemic area at risk in pigs, whereas it was small in dogs. Post-mortem arteriography in the pigs of Schaper et al.'s study revealed numerous small endomural and subepicardial anastomoses, whereas in dogs a few large interarterial epicardial anastomoses were observed.[59] At present, the results of that study can be interpreted to the effect that the minimally conducting small collaterals in pigs caused the larger infarcts as compared to the well-carrying canine collateral arteries (Fig. 1.24). The above-cited study is described in detail because of the paucity of investigations with systematic interspecies comparisons using the identical protocol. Hence, there have been numerous studies focusing on a single species, such as the canine heart and its development of collateral flow following coronary occlusion (Fig. 1.25).[71] However and except for the mentioned study by Schaper et al.[59] and an earlier investigation by Eckstein[64] (pigs with minimal functional collaterals in comparison with dogs), only two other investigations have actually performed an interspecies comparison of the collateral circulation of the heart.[72,73]

Sjöquist et al. compared the residual myocardial blood flow in 8 pigs and 11 dogs by tracer microspheres (85-Strontium) 1 hour after abrupt occlusion of the LAD. Considering the consistent finding of an almost absolutely lethal outcome in pigs following abrupt proximal coronary artery occlusion,[60] it is surprising that only three pigs (but also three dogs) had to be excluded from the study by Sjöquist et al. due to ventricular arrhythmias. In the centre of the ischaemic myocardium in the pig, residual blood flow was 0.01 ml/min/g sub-endocardially and 0.02 ml/min/g subepicardially, whereas in dog it was 0.13 ml/min/g subendocardially and 0.28 ml/min/g subendocardially ($p < 0.01$).[72] Thus, it could be shown by quantitative means that collateral blood flow in the pig is almost nil, and it is extensive and more pronounced by a factor of ≥ 14 in the dog.[72]

Dog   Pig

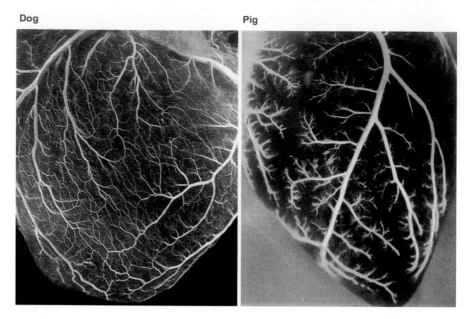

Fig. 1.24 Post-mortem coronary angiograms taken from a normal canine (*left side*; antero-lateral view) and a normal porcine heart (*right side*; anterior view). There is a multitude of coronary anastomoses between the canine left anterior descending and left circumflex coronary artery, but no collateral vessels in the pig heart. Images by J. and W. Schaper

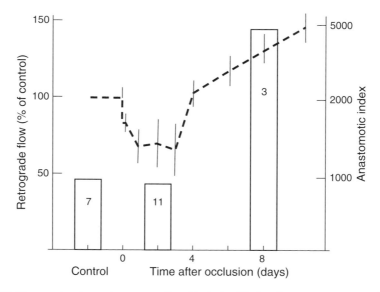

Fig. 1.25 Changes in retrograde coronary flow (*dashed red line*) and coronary anastomotic index (*white bars*; both *vertical axes*) following coronary artery occlusion (*horizontal axis*). Retrograde, i.e. collateral flow values are expressed as a percentage of control values. Mean anastomotic indices are depicted for a control group without occlusion and for dogs with occlusion up to 4 days and with occlusion for 8–12 days. Vertical error lines indicate standard error of the mean

1.2.3 Extensive Interspecies Comparison of the Coronary Collateral Circulation

In 1987, Maxwell et al. quantified the coronary collateral circulation during acute myocardial ischaemia in eight species in vivo using radiolabelled microspheres.[73] In each case, a prominent branch of the left coronary artery was ligated, and within 5 minutes [141]Cerium-labelled microspheres were injected into the left atrium. After killing the animal, myocardial tissue samples were obtained from a non-ischaemic and ischaemic territory, and the radioactivity of the ischaemic samples was measured and related to the activity of the non-ischaemic area (Fig. 1.26).[73] In the guinea pig heart, no zone of relevant underperfusion was detected despite ligation of a major coronary artery (i.e. relative collateral flow = 100%; Fig. 1.26). In the hearts from the other species, coronary collateral flow as a percentage of normal, non-ischaemic flow was 15.9±1.8% (standard error of the mean) in dogs (n − 6), 11.8±1.1% in cats (n = 16), 6.1±0.7% in rats (n = 6), 2.4±0.6% in ferrets (n = 6), 2.1±0.3% in baboons (n = 6), 2.0±0.5% in rabbits (n = 9) and 0.6±0.2% in pigs (n = 6). Similarly as in the canine group studied by Weaver et al.[61], Maxwell et al. found that the border zones of perfusion sharply delineated even in species with good collateral flow (except for the guinea pig).[73] The strength of this work is that collateral blood flow was measured over a wide range of the mammalian realm by the same method, thus rendering the results comparable. The objective was to obtain a reasonable selection of the appropriate animal model for the hypothesis to

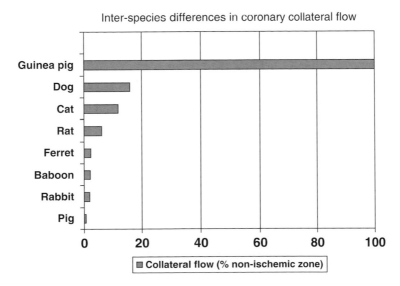

Fig. 1.26 Collateral flow as a percentage of flow to the non-ischaemic myocardium (*horizontal axis*) in eight different species (*vertical axis*) undergoing coronary artery ligation. Myocardial perfusion measurements by radioactive microspheres. Each heart yielded between 2 and 27 tissue samples from the ischaemic zone and a similar number from the non-ischaemic area

be tested: guinea pigs, dogs and cats with their substantial collateral flow are well suited for studies of *vascular* adaptation to ischaemia (i.e. collateral recruitment, collateral remodelling or arteriogenesis); rats, rabbits and pigs which have practically no functionally relevant collateral flow are appropriate for investigations on *myocardial* adaptation to ischaemia (i.e. myoacardial preconditioning). Obviously, such a specification of the animal model according to its purpose is independent of the exact knowledge of the human coronary collateral circulation, and thus, the study by Maxwell et al. mitigated the existing argument as to which species is the most representative of man. As a consequence of that debate, the development and control of myocardial infarction had been studied in widely differing preparations such as dogs,[74,75] cats,[76,77] rats,[78,79] rabbits,[80,81] pigs, guinea pigs[82,83] and baboons.[84,85]

Despite the circumstance that Maxwell et al.'s study elegantly avoided the missing knowledge about the human reference of functional collaterals in the presence and absence of CAD, this information is indispensable for selecting the adequate animal model for the following reason: if an animal model without collateral flow is erroneously chosen to be representative for humans, then the investigation of *myocardial* preconditioning does not take into account the contribution of collateral recruitment (vascular adaptation) in a hypothetical human investigation to the study result; conversely, if an animal model with extensive collateral flow is erroneously chosen to be representative for humans, then the study of *vascular* adaptation to ischaemia (collateral recruitment) does not correct for preconditioning as a contributor to the development of ischaemia tolerance. In this context, Fig. 1.27 illustrates

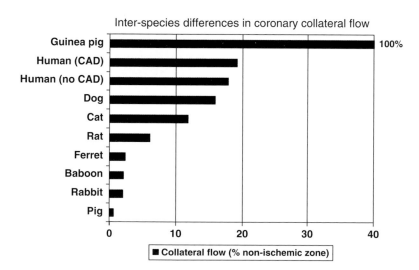

Fig. 1.27 Collateral relative to normal coronary flow (*horizontal axis*) in eight different species plus humans with and without coronary artery disease (CAD; *vertical axis*) who underwent coronary artery ligation, respectively a 1-minute balloon occlusion. Data from animal species are taken from Fig. 1.26 for comparison to collateral flow index values in humans

that on average, the animal model closest to humans with regard to functional collateral flow is the dog (and not the pig as often stated) irrespective of the presence or absence of human CAD: relative collateral to normal antegrade flow in 944 patients with CAD = 0.192±0.132 (mean standard ± deviation) and in 110 individuals without CAD = 0.178±0.092 (data from our collateral flow data base). From the wide spectrum of existing individual collateral flow values in humans (see Fig. 1.21), it follows that a variety of animal models may be representative for humans. However, since the number of animals included in the studies of Schaper et al.[59] and Maxwell et al.[73] is low and does not allow frequency distribution statistics of collateral flow, the question of the animal model most appropriate for the human coronary collateral circulation still awaits an exact answer.

1.3   Individual Relevance

Aside from their myocardial-salvaging effect, well-developed coronary collaterals may also elicit negative aspects, such as the risk of an unwanted extension of myocardial infarction during alcohol ablation of septal hypertrophy in hypertrophic obstructive cardiomyopathy (HOCM), the occurrence of coronary steal during myocardial hyperaemia and the risk of restenosis following coronary angioplasty. A potential problem of septal alcohol ablation in HOCM not recognized is a functional collateral circulation even in the absence of CAD among 25% of individuals, in whom the alcohol injected into a septal branch can reach the right anterior descending coronary artery or LAD.

The physical mechanism leading to restenosis in the presence of well-developed collaterals has been interpreted to be the competition of antegrade with collateral flow leading to reduced flow velocity at the injured site of angioplasty with augmented platelet adherence, thrombus formation, endothelial proliferation and developing restenosis.

The described potential negative aspects of well-developed collaterals weigh much less than their benefit on myocardial salvage.

1.3.1   Introduction

Since the determinants of myocardial infarct size following acute coronary occlusion in dogs were first described (time of occlusion, myocardial area at risk for infarction, absence of collateral supply, absence of ischaemic preconditioning, myocardial oxygen consumption during occlusion),[86,87] it has become recognized that collateral flow is one of the most important factors of the rate and extent of cell death within ischaemic zones. However, individually, well-developed coronary collaterals may also elicit negative as well as beneficial aspects as the subsequent examples illustrate. Coronary collateral steal is clinically less relevant in non-occlusive than in occlusive CAD. In the former, it occurs in about 10%, whereas in the presence of chronic total occlusion almost every second patient shows hyperaemia-induced decrease in the collateral-dependent area.

1.3.2 Collaterals and Transcoronary Ablation of Septal Hypertrophy

The principle of transcoronary ablation of septal hypertrophy (TASH) in HOCM consists of reducing the thickness of the basal part of the interventricular septum, which is responsible for the LV outflow tract obstruction (Fig. 1.28). The hypertrophied septum is thinned by inducing a circumscribed myocardial infarction in the supply area of the first and/or second septal branch of the LAD (Fig. 1.28). Infarction is induced by injecting a small amount (2–5 ml) of pure alcohol into the proximally occluded septal branch, via an over-the-wire angioplasty balloon catheter.[88] Alternatively, basal septal infarction is achieved by implantation of a coil into the septal branch.[89] A potential problem of septal alcohol ablation not recognized so far is the existence of a functional collateral circulation even in the absence of CAD among close to 25% of individuals (see also Fig. 1.21).[55] Collateral arterioles and small collateral arteries are predominantly located at the interventricular septum between the LAD and the RCA.[90] Septal branch balloon occlusion creates a coronary pressure drop distal to the occlusion and an RCA-septal-branch pressure

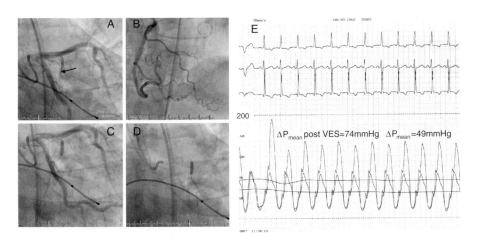

Fig. 1.28 Transcoronary alcohol ablation of a septal branch (→) of the left anterior descending coronary artery (**Panels A, C, D**). The normal right coronary artery is small (**Panel B**). **Panel D**: Inflated over-the-wire angioplasty balloon catheter positioned in the first septal branch with injection of contrast and visualization of the respective myocardial area. **Panel E**: Simultaneous left ventricular and aortic pressure tracing showing a severe gradient across the left ventricular outflow tract

gradient across preformed collaterals if they are present, which induces collateral flow from the RCA to the septal branch. Injection of alcohol into the occluded septal branch represents a counter flow to the collateral flow. This as well as cardiac contraction contributes to the admixture between alcohol and blood, which may eventually reach the RCA territory and cause unwanted inferior, instead of only septal myocardial infarction (Figs. 1.29 and 1.30).[91]

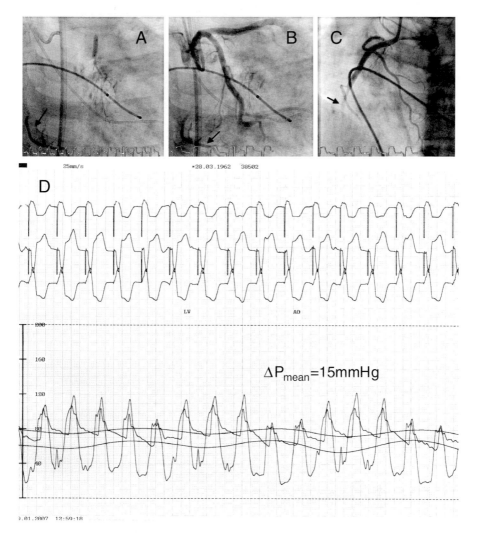

Fig. 1.29 Identical case as in Fig. 1.28. Imaging of the right coronary artery (RCA) following injection of the occluded first septal branch after alcohol ablation via collateral vessels (→; **Panels A and B**). Angiography of the RCA documents occlusion (**Panel C**). Simultaneous left ventricular and aortic pressure tracing (**Panel D**) revealing a markedly diminished mean gradient of 15 mmHg

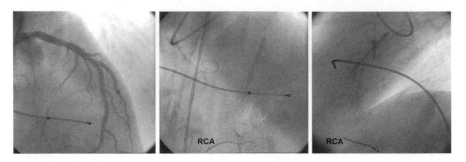

Fig. 1.30 Similar case as in Figs. 28 and 29 of transcoronary alcohol ablation of a septal branch for hypertrophic obstructive cardiomyopathy. An antero-posterior cranial view (*left and middle panel*) shows the first septal branch with a 'milking' sign before (*left panel*) and after alcohol injection (*middle and right panel; right panel*: lateral view) with imaging of the right coronary artery (RCA) during injection of contrast via the over-the-wire balloon catheter

Figures 1.30 and 1.31 exemplify that the described scenario may occur not only in the RCA territory but also in the entire LAD region via existing septal-to-septal anastomoses. In the patient shown in Fig. 1.31, a preformed collateral artery between the balloon-occluded first and the third septal branches of the LAD was responsible for the adverse outcome of complete LAD occlusion following injection of 2.5 ml pure alcohol over 11 minutes. Subsequently, this 60-year-old female patient with initially severe LV outflow tract obstruction developed ventricular septal defect due to anterior wall myocardial infarction requiring emergency surgical intervention (Fig. 1.32).

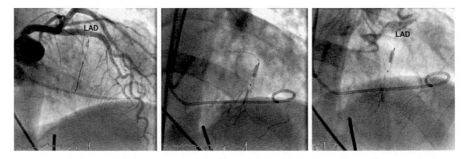

Fig. 1.31 Transcoronary alcohol ablation of a second septal branch (antero-posterior cranial view). During injection of the contrast before alcohol (*middle panel*), not only the septal branch distal of the occluded balloon but also a more distal septal branch of the left anterior descending artery (LAD) is visualized via intercoronary anastomoses. In the context of the subsequent injection of a small amount of alcohol, an acute occlusion of the LAD occurred (*right panel*; LAD)

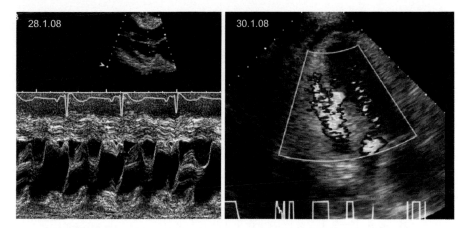

Fig. 1.32 Identical case as in Fig. 1.31. M-mode echocardiographic recording revealing pronounced systolic anterior movement of the mitral valve due to the severe obstruction across the left ventricular outflow tract (*left panel*; before alcohol ablation). Following acute anterior myocardial infarction in the context of alcohol-induced occlusion of the left anterior descending coronary artery, ventricular septal defect occurred (*right panel*), which was successfully operated by patch closure

1.3.3 Coronary Collateral Steal

The myocardial microvasculature downstream of the main coronary arterial supply areas can be schematically imagined as parallel resistances. The microcirculatory resistance regulates coronary blood flow to a certain vascular territory. According to the autoregulatory behaviour of the coronary circulation, microvascular resistance downstream of a stenotic vascular region is lowered already under resting conditions in order to maintain normal myocardial perfusion. Therefore, the capacity to further decrease microvascular resistance in this area under conditions of hyperaemia is reduced. This leads to a diminished or absent coronary flow reserve (CFR: hyperaemic flow divided by flow at rest), if interarterial anastomoses are absent between the post-stenotic and an adjacent normal vascular region (CFR≥1). If it is present, and particularly of well-developed interarterial anastomoses, the uneven distribution of parallel hyperaemic microvascular resistances may lead to coronary flow away from the post-stenotic, collateralized area towards the normal vascular region (steal; CFR< 1; Fig. 1.33; for further details, see Section 4). In animal models and in patients with collateral-dependent blood supply, coronary steal in response to physical exercise or to pharmacological vasodilation has been studied repeatedly.[92–95] Gould et al. defined the following requirements for the occurrence of coronary steal[96]: (a) there is a coronary pressure drop in the epicardial collateral supplying artery due to a stenotic lesion (serial vascular resistance increase), (b) the collateral resistance is not negligible and (c) the microvasculature distal to the collateralized region lacks vasodilatory capacity.

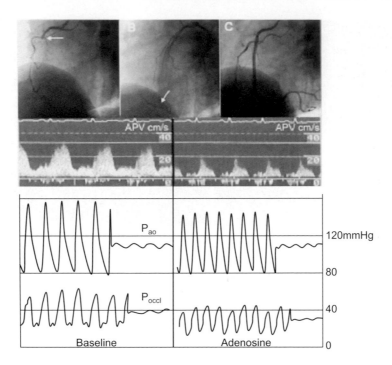

Fig. 1.33 Demonstration of coronary collateral steal in a patient with chronic total occlusion of the right coronary artery (**Panel A and B**; **Panel C** after recanalization of the occlusion). The middle row of the figure shows intracoronary Doppler flow tracings at rest (*left side*) and during adenosine infusion (*right side*) with a decrease in flow velocity during hyperaemia. Accordingly, the aortic (*black curve*) and coronary (*red curve*) pressure recordings (*lower row*) document a constant mean aortic pressure, but a decrease in mean coronary occlusive pressure by approximately 10 mmHg during hyperaemia versus resting condition

Among patients with non-occlusive CAD, coronary collateral steal occurs less frequently (10%) than in those with chronic total occlusion (46%).[94,95]

1.3.4 Risk of Coronary Restenosis and Collateral Flow

The principal driving force of collateral flow through preformed or remodelled coronary collaterals consists of a post-stenotic coronary pressure drop, which itself leads to a pressure gradient between the collateral supplying and the collateral receiving (i.e. stenotic) arteries. Thus theoretically, the removal of the stenotic lesion by PCI instantaneously leads to a diminished or even absent collateral flow, which does not compete with antegrade flow. Nevertheless, it has been repeatedly documented that high collateral supply to a vascular region treated by PCI is associated with increased risk of restenosis[97–99] (Fig. 1.34; see also chapter 4), and the physical mechanism leading to restenosis has been

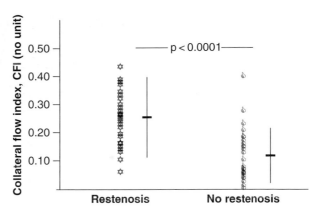

Fig. 1.34 Collateral relative to normal antegrade flow (collateral flow index, *vertical axis*) in patients with and without angiographic restenosis (*horizontal axis*) of an atherosclerotic lesion previously treated by percutaneous coronary intervention

interpreted to be the competition of antegrade with collateral flow leading to reduced flow velocity at the injured site of PCI with augmented platelet adherence, thrombus formation, endothelial proliferation and developing restenosis.[100] However theoretically, it is assumed that in the absence of an epicardial stenotic resistance, collateral flow to the respective vascular area is zero.[101] Practically, this assumption is likely to be incorrect, because it is based on two further suppositions often not found in reality: zero pressure drop along the epicardial path of a normal coronary artery (in reality ~5 mmHg), and horizontal origin and supply or orifice site of the collateral vessel (instead of a frequent proximal collateral origin with mid-vascular or distal contralateral orifice). Also, the sustained existence of functional collaterals despite the absence of stenotic lesions is supported by the finding of sufficient collateral channels in close to one-fourth of the individuals with normal coronary circulation.[55]

1.3.5 Beneficial Effect of Collaterals on Myocardial Salvage

The above-described potential negative aspects of well-developed collaterals weigh much less than their benefit on myocardial salvage (see also Section 1.4). Specifically, unwanted expansion of myocardial infarction during TASH in HOCM has, so far, been described only as anecdotes; in the population with non-occlusive CAD, coronary steal occurs in a minority of patients; the relative risk of coronary restenosis 9 months after stent implantation has been observed to be increased by a factor of only 1.07.[99] In the individual patient, myocardial salvage by collaterals can be safely postulated in the presence of normal LV systolic function, and respectively the absence of regional wall motion abnormalities, despite the total occlusion of ≥1 coronary arteries at the proximal or mid-vascular site. Figure 1.35 illustrates such a case of a 75-year-old patient with normal LV angiography, despite total occlusion of all three major coronary arteries: proximal LAD, proximal LCX (patent large intermediary

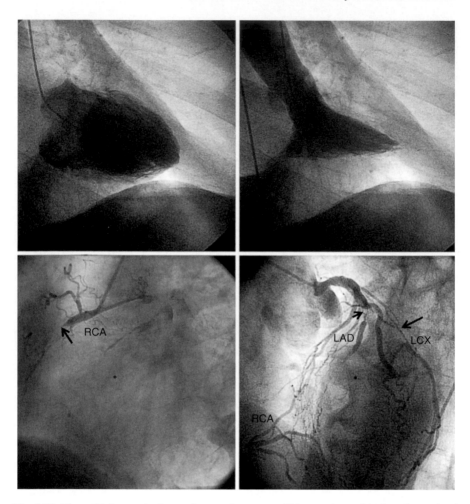

Fig. 1.35 Normal left ventricular angiogram (*upper panels*) in a patient with chronic proximal occlusion (→) of all three major coronary arteries (*lower panels*) providing evidence for the myocardial-salvaging effect of coronary collaterals. The only non-occluded vessel is an intermediary branch. RCA: right coronary artery; LAD: left anterior descending coronary artery, LCX: left circumflex coronary artery

branch) and proximal RCA. In the presence of such a severe degree of CAD, it may be challenging to define the main collateral supply to each one of the occluded arteries. However, the presence of a normal LV global and regional systolic function allows the conclusion that collateral supply at the time of occlusion was sufficient to salvage myocardium. Figure 1.36 shows another case (72-year-old male patient) with sufficiently collateralized LV anterior wall despite proximal LAD occlusion. A single atrial epicardial collateral artery originating from the ostial RCA supplies enough flow to replace the LAD

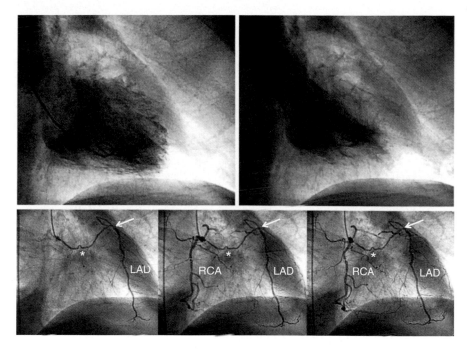

Fig. 1.36 Normal left ventricular angiogram (*upper panels*) in a patient with chronic occlusion (→) of the proximal left anterior descending coronary artery (LAD; *lower panels*, anteroposterior cranial view). Contrast injection into the right coronary artery (RCA) with imaging at first of the conus branch collateral artery to the LAD (*). A second, atrial collateral artery between RCA and LAD (*middle and right lower panel*) fills with contrast from both coronary arteries, thus illustrating competing collateral flow between RCA and LAD

territory, i.e. to reduce the ischaemic area at risk for myocardial infarction of the proximal LAD to zero. Even before the RCA is filled with radiographic contrast, the entire LAD is supplied via the proximal collateral artery, thus illustrating the concept of an inverse relationship between collateral flow and area at risk for infarction.[86] The fact of a normal systolic function of the LV anterior wall in this case allows the conclusion that the determinants of infarct size other than collateral supply, such as time of coronary occlusion, myocardial preconditioning and oxygen consumption played no role because of the replacement of the LAD area at risk by one branch collateral.[86] A second, more proximal collateral artery taking off from the RCA is even in competition with the main collateral vessel, because of the presence of a counterflow originating from a high septal collateral artery (Fig. 1.36). A further example of an individual beneficial effect of collateral supply to an occluded LAD is provided by Fig. 1.37 depicting the left coronary angiogram and LV angiography of a 55-year-old woman, who was admitted for invasive cardiac examination for atypical chest pain. The fact that she did not suffer exercise-induced angina pectoris further indicates the beneficial effect of the very large distal

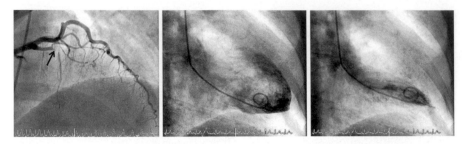

Fig. 1.37 Coronary angiogram (left anterior oblique cranial view; *left panel*) with chronic occlusion of the left anterior descending artery at the first diagonal and first septal branch (→) and a normal left ventricular angiogram (*middle and left panel*) exemplifying another case of saving myocardial function by well-developed collaterals

epicardial branch collateral artery from the RCA to the LAD (Fig. 1.38) apart from the normal systolic LV function. Conversely, absent collateral filling of a chronic mid-LAD occlusion is related to a lack of myocardial salvage with extended LV anterior wall akinesia (Fig. 1.39). Alternatively, extended collateral supply may develop only *after* coronary artery occlusion purely on physical grounds of an existing pressure gradient between the collateral supplying and receiving, i.e. the occluded artery, and thus, it may supply an already infarcted myocardial territory (Fig. 1.40). However, if in the acute phase of myocardial infarction there is already filling with radiographic contrast of the occluded coronary artery via collaterals, the subsequently developing infarct size is smaller than in the situation without preformed collaterals (Fig. 1.41).

Fig. 1.38 Identical case as in Fig. 1.37. Coronary angiogram (slight left anterior oblique cranial view) with contrast injection into the right coronary artery (RCA) and complete filling of the proximally occluded left anterior descending artery (LAD) via a large branch collateral artery (→)

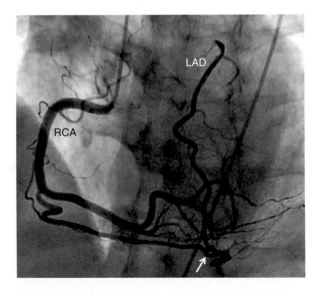

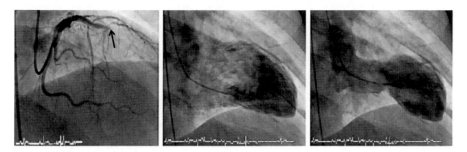

Fig. 1.39 Coronary angiogram (antero-posterior view; *left panel*) with occlusion of the left anterior descending artery (LAD) directly distal to the second diagonal and second septal branch (→). In the absence of collateral supply to the occluded LAD, the left ventricular angiogram (*middle and left panels*) reveals an extensive akinesia of the antero-apical wall

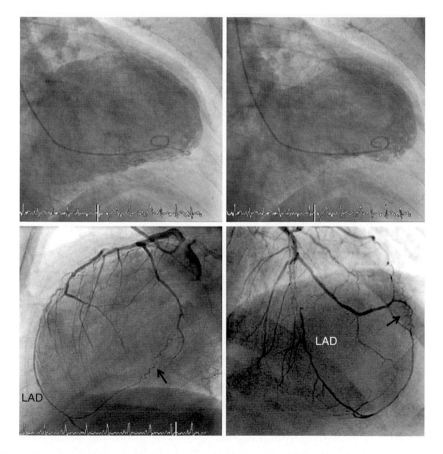

Fig. 1.40 Left ventricular angiogram (*upper panels*) with extensive antero-apical wall akinesia in a case with a well-developed branch collateral artery (→) between the first diagonal branch of the left anterior descending artery (LAD) and the occluded LAD (*lower panels; left panel*: lateral view; *right panel*: antero-posterior cranial view). The collateral artery in this case grew only after the mid-LAD occlusion with anterior wall myocardial infarction, thus providing no myocardial-salvaging effect

Fig. 1.41 Scatter plot of peak creatine kinase (*vertical axis*) in patients with a first acute myocardial infarction and the angiographic collateral degree to the occluded vessel (*horizontal axis*) before primary percutaneous coronary intervention (PCI)

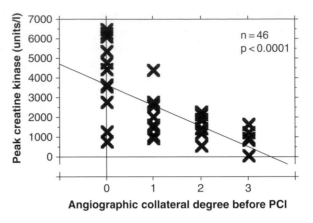

1.4 Collective Prognostic Relevance

Until recently, the collective prognostic relevance of coronary collaterals has been controversial. The debate was related to inconsistent populations examined, to a variably defined term 'prognosis', and to methodological issues such as the low occurrence of study endpoints, the short follow-up and blunt instruments employed to measure collateral supply. Since chronic stable CAD has a low annual mortality of 2%, a meaningful investigation requires a large study population of several hundred patients with a long follow-up. The goal of a statistically relevant study may be better reached in patients with *acute* CAD and its higher mortality rate of up to 9% during the first 6 months following myocardial infarction.

Aside from all-cause mortality, the hierarchy of endpoints consists of cardiac deaths, cardiovascular deaths, myocardial infarction, unstable angina pectoris, repeat revascularization and the combination of those events. Surrogate endpoints employed in studies on the prognostic relevance of collaterals are infarct size, LV aneurysm formation, LV systolic function and myocardial viability.

The beneficial effect of well-developed collaterals on all surrogate endpoints has been recognized. However in order to reduce infarct size, collaterals need to be preformed, whereas they may develop only after myocardial infarction in order to prevent LV remodelling and aneurysm formation.

During the first 3–6 hours of acute coronary syndrome, angiographically well-visible collateral vessels are present in 30–40%, a number increasing to almost 100% in the presence of continuing vascular occlusion. Late angiographic appearance signifies less prognostic benefit, because collaterals supplying necrotic myocardium do not salvage it. Recent studies on the prognostic effect of collaterals in acute myocardial infarction have reported a relevant reduction in cumulative 6-month mortality from 9–23% to 4–7%.

The majority of studies on the prognostic relevance of collaterals in chronic CAD have used angiographic grading for characterizing the degree of collateral perfusion. In a historic study, cumulative survival rates during a follow-up duration between 11 and 19 years in 96 patients with chronic coronary occlusion were 52% at 10 years in patients with angiographically well-developed collaterals and 35% among those with poor collaterals. Using quantitative coronary collateral measurement in 739 patients with chronic stable CAD, cumulative 10-year survival rates in relation to all-cause deaths and cardiac deaths were 71 and 88%, respectively, in patients with low collateral flow index (CFI), and 89 and 97% in patients with high CFI.

1.4.1 Introduction

Despite the fact that the coronary collateral circulation has long been recognized as an alternative source of blood supply to a myocardial area jeopardized by ischaemia, its prognostic relevance for the population of patients with CAD has been controversial until recently. The debate was in part related to diverging focuses with regard to the population examined (acute versus chronic CAD, varying severity of CAD), to the term 'prognosis' and to the methodological issues such as the power of the investigation relative to the occurrence of study endpoints, the duration of follow-up and the instrument employed to measure the determinant of outcome, i.e. collateral supply. For example, two recent studies have documented reduction in non-fatal cardiovascular events among patients with versus those without angiographic coronary collaterals in chronic stable CAD.[102,103] Conversely, data from the same group have indicated an unfavourable prognosis in the presence of well-developed collaterals among patients with more severe chronic CAD.[104] In this context, the collective prognostic significance of the human coronary collateral circulation will be subsequently discussed under the following aspects: various endpoints defining prognosis, relevance in acute and chronic CAD.

1.4.2 Endpoints for Defining Prognosis and Assessment of Collateral Flow

There is a hierarchy of cardiac determinants of prognosis ranging from more 'soft', frequently occurring endpoints to 'firm', rare clinical events. The prevalent endpoints for the definition of prognosis, such as the symptom of angina pectoris or the development of impaired systolic LV function have been employed quite frequently for methodological reasons, whereas prognosis has been rarely assessed on the basis of all-cause mortality, i.e. the ultimate and undisputable event. Since chronic stable CAD has a low annual mortality of around 2%,[105,106] a statistically meaningful prognostic investigation requires a large study population of several hundred patients with a long follow-up duration (e.g. estimated number of deaths during an average of 5 years of follow-up in 500 patients = 50; 2,500 patient-years). The two largest studies on the impact of coronary collaterals on clinical outcome in chronic CAD have overseen, respectively, 5,985 patient-years and 3,907 patient-years,[106,107] and the respective absolute figures of overall mortality have been 295 and 83. The expression of 'patient-years' suggests that the goal of a statistically relevant study may be better reached in patients with *acute* CAD and its much higher mortality rate of up to 9% during the first 6 months following myocardial infarction.[108] Aside from all-cause, total mortality, the hierarchy of cardiac endpoints consists of cardiac deaths, cardiovascular deaths, myocardial infarction, unstable angina pectoris, repeat PCI or coronary bypass grafting, the combination of those major adverse cardiac events, and of surrogate endpoints such as infarct size (see Fig. 1.41), LV systolic function and LV aneurysm formation. It ought to be appreciated that in a long-term follow-up study, cardiac and cardiovascular mortality is a much softer endpoint than total mortality, because its labelling depends not so much on the clarity of a definition but on the acumen of the person directly characterizing the mode of death. On the other hand, a large absolute number of the hardest endpoint possible, total mortality, may be statistically insufficient if the instrument to assess its hypothesized determinant, i.e. the collateral circulation, is blunt. The measurement tool most frequently used for collateral assessment in studies on the prognostic relevance of collaterals is coronary angiography, whereby, mostly, the dichotomous labelling of present or absent collaterals has been employed.[43,102,104,107–116] Only a minority of investigations has employed quantitative means to measure collaterals,[106,117–119] thus methodologically allowing a lower absolute number of events because of better differentiation between well and poorly developed collaterals than by angiographic qualification. Similarly, the number of patients included can be reduced without limiting the statistical power of the study by employing a continuous surrogate endpoint such as LV ejection fraction, because of the detection of more subtle differences between groups of patients with well and poorly grown collaterals.

1.4.2.1 Surrogate Endpoints

The influence on surrogate endpoints of the human coronary collateral circulation is discussed here independently of the population with acute or chronic CAD. The surrogate endpoints employed in most studies are infarct size, LV aneurysm formation, LV systolic function and, rarely, myocardial viability. Principally, these variables are reasonable to select as endpoints, because they all more or less reflect infarct size. The *size* of myocardial infarction most importantly determines the outcome after such an event.[120] Pathophysiologically, infarct size is directly determined by the duration of coronary artery occlusion, the lack of collateral supply to the ischaemic area at risk for infarction, the size of the area at risk, the absence of myocardial ischaemic preconditioning (no angina pectoris prior to the infarct) and myocardial oxygen consumption during coronary occlusion.[86,87] Myocardial infarct size in humans has been traditionally measured by creatine kinase (CK) levels (peak value, area under the curve).[121] Hirai et al. studied the effect of coronary collateral perfusion in 32 patients with acute myocardial infarction who underwent intracoronary thrombolysis, and found a relevant influence of angiographically present collaterals in the absence of reperfusion (n = 6) on the time to peak CK release (= 16 vs. 21 hours in patients without reperfusion and collaterals, n = 7; $p < 0.05$), but not on peak CK level (1,879 vs. 2,707 units/l).[122] Habib et al. performed a similar, but statistically relevant study in 125 patients with failed thrombolysis who either revealed collaterals on coronary angiography (n = 51) or who did not have collaterals (n = 74).[123] Patients with and without collaterals had practically identical peak serum CK levels as in the just previously mentioned study: 1,877 units/l and 2,661 units/l ($p = 0.004$; Fig. 1.42), and the effect of the collateral status was independent of infarct site. Accordingly, pre-discharge LV ejection fraction was 53% in patients with angiographic collaterals and 48% in those without collaterals ($p = 0.02$).[123] Sabia et al. qualified infarct size by an echocardiographic wall motion score (low score: small region of abnormal LV wall motion) 1 month after angioplasty of an occluded coronary artery in comparison to the baseline wall motion score[124] (n = 43 patients). A regression analysis was then performed between the follow-up wall motion score and the percentage of the infarct bed perfused via collaterals as obtained by myocardial contrast echocardiography before PCI of the infarct-related artery. The percentage of the infarct bed supplied by collateral flow at base

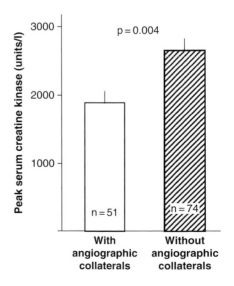

Fig. 1.42 Box plot of peak creatine kinase (*vertical axis*; mean values) in thrombolysis in myocardial infarction (TIMI) patients with and without angiographic evidence of coronary collaterals at initial coronary angiography. Inclusion of patients only in case of failed recanalization 90-minutes after administration of tissue plasminogen activator. Error bars indicate standard error of the mean

line was directly correlated with LV wall function and inversely correlated with the wall-motion score 1 month after successful angioplasty ($p <$ 0.001).[124] In this study population with subacute or chronic myocardial infarction, the degree of improvement in regional systolic LV function was not influenced by the length of time between the acute infarct and the attempted angioplasty (range from 2 days to 5 weeks).[124] The study by Clements et al. employed [99m]technetium for measuring the ischaemic area at risk for infarction, the final infarct size and the salvaged myocardium in 60 patients who underwent primary PCI.[112] Collateral flow to the ischaemic area was scored angiographically. In the absence of antegrade flow through the infarct-related artery, the presence of collaterals was related to a reduced infarct size. Alternatively, Christian et al. assessed collateral supply to the acutely occluded arterial region of 89 patients non-invasively by [99m]techne-tium pixel count (nadir) relative to maximum pixel count in the normally perfused area, and found an inverse relationship between LV infarct size and relative collateral flow (Fig. 1.43).[125] A more recent investigation by Elsman et al. in 1,059 patients with acute myocardial infarction treated with primary PCI found an inverse relation between angiographic collateral score (0/1, 2 and 3) and cumulative lactate dehydrogenase release, 36 hours after chest pain onset.[115] The debate on the relevance of collaterals has been revived very recently by an apparently well-powered study including 501 patients with acute myocardial infarction within 6 hours of symptom onset, who underwent successful primary PCI.[126] Sorajja et al. obtained myocardial infarct size by [99m]technetium and the collateral presence by angiography, and observed an infarct size of 16±16% of the LV among patients with collateral supply as compared to 21±21% in the absence of collaterals ($p = 0.02$).[126] Despite that result, which was supported by an analogue pattern for enzymatic infarct size, the authors concluded that there was no relationship between baseline collat-eral flow and infarct size. The more appropriate interpretation of the study results would have been that the instrument employed for collateral

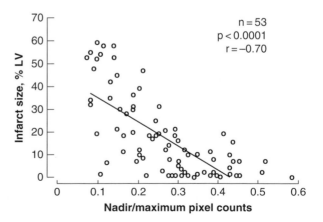

Fig. 1.43 Correlation between infarct size as determined by radionuclide scintigraphy (*vertical axis*) and the ratio of nadir-to-maximum [99m]technetium pixel counts in the infarct area and an adjacent normal myocardial region (i.e. an index of collateral to normal myocardial perfusion; *horizontal axis*)

characterization was too blunt to render the investigation powerful enough for detecting the mentioned differences also in the subgroups of anterior and non-anterior myocardial infarction.

Hirai et al. investigated the effect of pre-existent angiographic collaterals on the prevention of LV aneurysm formation in 47 patients who underwent intacoronary thrombolysis within 6 hours after onset of chest pain during a first anterior myocardial infarction.[122] In 22 patients, thrombolysis was unsuccessful, and among those with collateral supply to the occluded artery (n = 10), LV aneurysm developed in only 1, whereas it occurred in 7 of 12 patients without collaterals ($p < 0.05$). Apparently, even collateral channels developing only after an acute myocardial infarction (n = 11; n = 10 without collaterals 1 month after infarct) may prevent LV dilatation within 2 years of the event,[113] the fact of which is not related to myocardial salvage but probably to a mitigation of LV wall stress by the epicardially located network of 'pressurized' collateral arteries.

The LV ejection fraction as a variable, potentially influenced by collaterals, was co-examined by two of the above-cited studies.[113,123] Habib et al. documented a higher LV ejection fraction of 54% in 51 patients with failed thrombolysis and good collaterals as compared to 50% among the 74 patients without collaterals.[123] It is not unexpected that Kodama et al. did not find a relationship between collateral flow and LV ejection fraction late after myocardial infarction, since they focused on a group of patients in whom collateral channels had developed only after infarct.[113] Similarly, it has been shown recently that recovery of systolic LV dysfunction following revascularization of a chronic total coronary occlusion is not directly related to the collateral supply to that region, because collateral development may occur before or after coronary occlusion.[119] Naturally, the relevance of collateral supply to a region jeopardized by myocardial ischaemia is only given if it exists before ischaemia development, and collaterals do not salvage myocardium if they grow afterwards during the course of 1–2 weeks in response to the existing physical coronary perfusion pressure difference along small preformed anastomoses between a normal and the occluded vessels. Thus, a controversy on the significance of coronary collaterals may also ensue on the basis of failure to distinguish between preformed and subsequently developed collaterals with regard to coronary occlusion. Along the same line of argument, Elhendy et al. were able to predict by low dose dobutamine stress echocardiography, with reasonable accuracy, the recovery of systolic LV function following coronary artery bypass grafting, but recovery was not influenced by angiographic collateral grades in patients with total coronary occlusion.[127]

1.4.2.2 Clinical Endpoints

Studies on the occurrence of clinical adverse events during follow-up in relation to the coronary collateral circulation are presented below and subdivided according to their focus on patients with acute coronary syndrome and with chronic CAD.

1.4.3 Acute Coronary Artery Disease and Clinical Events in Relation to Collaterals

Angiographic collaterals to myocardium distal to an acutely occluded coronary artery have been detected in 334 of 626 patients (69%) during the acute infarct phase (242/626 = 38% with grade 2 or 3 collaterals), whereby the prevalence has been shown to increase between 3 and 6 hours following symptom onset (from 66 to 75%), and the absence of collaterals has been related to the early occurrence of cardiogenic shock in patients with inferior myocardial infarction.[128] Earlier investigations have observed collateral vessels at the onset of acute myocardial infarction less frequently, i.e. in about 40% of patients.[129,130] Schwartz et al. reported an analysis of the coronary collateral circulation in a consecutive series of 116 post-infarction angiograms from patients with persistent 100% occlusion of their infarct artery.[130] Of 42 patients studied within 6 hours of infarction, 52% had no angiographic evidence of any coronary collateral development as compared with only 8% (1 of 16 patients) studied 1 day to 2 weeks after infarction.[130] Virtually all patients studied beyond 2 weeks after myocardial infarction (14–45 days) and later than 45 days had visible collateral flow. As outlined above,[113] collaterals developing late after acute infarct into an area of necrotic myocardial tissue may exert a beneficial effect on LV dilatation or aneurysm expansion, but not on LV systolic function. Conversely, residual blood flow carried by collaterals at the time of acute myocardial infarction implies reduced infarct size and improved residual LV ejection fraction.[123,125] However, whether collateral circulation improves clinical prognosis after acute myocardial infarction remains rarely investigated and seems to be controversial.[108,131] Considering the described, numerous variables influencing the relevance of collateral supply in acute coronary syndrome, such as the time window of study inclusion after symptom onset, the mode of revascularization (none, thrombolysis, PCI), the differentiation of preformed or subsequently grown collaterals, the mode of collateral assessment, the debate is not unexpected.

1.4.3.1 Studies in the Pre-angioplasty Era

In this context, Gohlke et al. investigated the prognostic importance of a residual stenosis of the infarct artery and of collateral flow to the infarct area in a group of 102 young patients who had survived an anterior wall Q-wave acute myocardial infarction.[110] In that study, patients with at least moderate collateral flow had a higher mortality rate of 21% than patients without or with faint collateral flow (8%, $p < 0.05$),[110] whereby this finding did not reflect the absence of a protective effect of collaterals as the authors concluded, but it indicated the diagnostic relevance of collaterals as a marker for the severity of atherosclerotic lesions. Thus, in the study by Gohlke et al., the actual prognostic comparison was between patients with different degrees of residual LAD stenoses and not between different degrees of collateral flow.[110] Similarly, the investigation by Nicolau et al. was not one examining the prognostic relevance of a well-developed coronary collateral circulation at the time of acute myocardial infarction (n = 422 treated with thrombolysis and followed for 8 years) (Fig. 1.44), but one comparing the prognosis in patients with successful (fully restored antegrade flow) and partly or unsuccessful thrombolysis (survival rates of 89 and 80%, $p < 0.04$).[114] By Cox multivariate analysis in that study [114] the following *independent* variables showed significant correlations with long-term survival: global LV ejection fraction ($p = 0.0003$), antegrade flow degree ($p = 0.0006$), collateral flow degree (negative correlation, $p = 0.0179$) and medical treatment (negative correlation, $p = 0.0464$). To perform a multivariate analysis with two variables biologically so intimately linked as residual antegrade flow and the degree of collaterals cannot provide the result of 'independent variables' and is unreasonable. Using a methodologically more favourable study design, Boehrer et al. assessed the influence of collateral filling of the infarct artery on long-term morbidity and mortality in 146 surviving patients of initial acute myocardial infarction in whom the infarct artery was occluded.[111] Of 120 patients with angiographic evidence of collaterals, 16% suffered cardiac death during the average follow-up of 42 months, while 19% died from cardiac causes in the group of 26 patients without collaterals.[111]

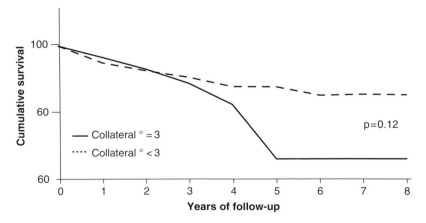

Fig. 1.44 Cumulative survival curves according to the presence (*solid line*) or absence (*dashed line*) of well-developed collaterals to the infarct-related coronary artery as evidenced by angiography

1.4.3.2 Studies in Patients Undergoing Primary PCI

Investigations on the prognostic effect of collaterals in patients with successful primary PCI within the 6-hour window of symptom onset are methodologically advantageous over the above-described pre-PCI studies, because their populations are much more homogeneous and thus better comparable. However, they are scarce and the results appear to be controversial. In a study including 238 patients with acute myocardial infarction due to mid- or proximal LAD occlusion, Pérez-Castellano et al. found a significantly higher in-hospital mortality among patients without as compared to those with collaterals on the angiogram obtained during primary PCI (Fig. 1.45; 58 excluded due to residual antegrade flow).[131] On first sight and compared to, e.g., the above-cited study by Boehrer[111], the one by Pérez-Castellano et al. appears similarly underpowered (n = 146 vs. n = 180; absolute number of deaths: n = 23 vs. n = 31).[131] The principal numerical disparity consists of the varying number of patients with angiographically absent collaterals: 26 of 146 (18%) in the study by Boehrer et al. and 115 of 180 (64%) in that by Pérez-Castellano[111,131]. This difference exemplifies the influence of the time course of collateral development following acute myocardial infarction on their prognostic relevance, i.e. late angiographic appearance is more frequent than early manifestation, but it signifies less prognostic benefit, because collaterals supplying necrotic myocardium do not salvage it. The study by Pérez-Castellano et al. focused on collaterals present during the 6-hour time window after symptom onset, and thus more appropriately, examined the relevance of preformed collaterals.[131] The study by Antoniucci et al.[108] is comparable to that by Pérez-Castellano et al.,[131] since both studied the outcome in patients with acute myocardial infarction who underwent primary PCI within 6 hours from symptom onset, and the rate

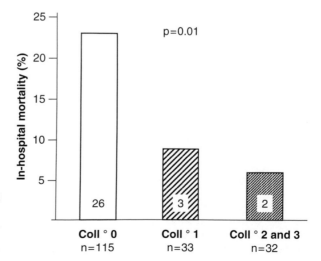

Fig. 1.45 Box plot between in-hospital mortality following acute myocardial infarction (*vertical axis*) and angiographic collateral degree (coll; *horizontal axis*). Numbers in the boxes are absolute numbers of death

of angiographic collaterals in both was similar, i.e. 23% respectively 36%. However, Antoniucci et al.'s work included a much larger study population of 1,164 patients who presented with acute infarct of any territory, and the follow-up of clinical events was registered until 6 months after initial revascularization.[108] At 6 months, 11 of 264 patients in the group with visible collaterals (4%) and 80 of 900 patients without collaterals (9%) had died (Fig. 1.46).[108]. Due to an erroneous inclusion procedure of clinical variables in the multivariate logistic regression analysis, the authors concluded that the coronary collateral circulation did not exert a protective effect in patients who underwent revascularization in the first 6 hours of acute myocardial infarction onset.[108] The variables falsely entered in the regression model were factors not statistically different in univariate analysis between patients with and without collaterals (age, gender, previous myocardial infarction, PCI failure, infarct artery stenting, multiple stents) and factors not independent of each other (collateral circulation dependent on chronic total occlusion, on multivessel CAD). Thus in essence, both studies on the prognostic effect of collaterals in acute myocardial infarction have reported a statistically relevant reduction in cumulative 6-month mortality from 9–23% to 4–7%. However, the above-mentioned study by Elsman et al. in 1,059 patients with acute ST-segment-elevation myocardial infarction treated with primary PCI within < 6 hours of chest pain onset found cumulative 1-year survival rates among patients with angiographic collateral grades 0, 1 and 2 or 3 of 95, 96.2 and 97.2% respectively ($p = 0.66$).[115]

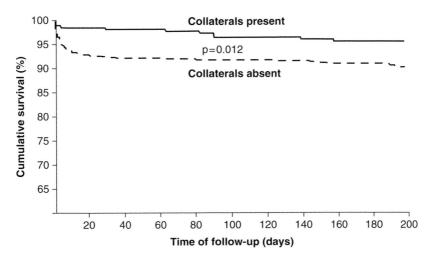

Fig. 1.46 Cumulative survival curves of 264 patients with acute myocardial infarction and angiographic evidence of coronary collaterals supplying the infarct area (collaterals present; *solid line*), as compared to 900 patients without collaterals (collaterals absent; *dashed line*)

1.4.4 Chronic Coronary Artery Disease and Clinical Events in Relation to Collaterals

With regard to the practical dilemma of the collateral circulation being an indicator of the severity of CAD or a predictor of future cardiac events, the setting of acute or chronic CAD does not make a difference. Thus in both situations, an investigation focusing on the prognostic relevance of collaterals should correct for their role as markers for CAD severity, i.e. it ought not be ambiguous whether an unfavourable outcome is due to high coronary athero-sclerotic lesion severity as indicated by extended collaterals or because of well-developed collaterals. For example, the above-discussed study by Nicolau et al. of early infarct artery collateral flow after thrombolysis found conflicting results even *within* itself[114]: antegrade coronary flow grade was observed to be directly, but collateral flow to be inversely related to survival. With regard to myocardial perfusion, this finding does not make sense, because it must be irrelevant whether an ischaemic territory is supplied via native or collateral vessels as long as it is adequately subtended. While in acute CAD, the collateral circulation as an indicator for CAD can be corrected for by primary PCI, thus rendering the study population homogeneous with regard to the variable ste-nosis severity, a similar effect can be reached in chronic CAD by focusing exclusively on chronic total coronary occlusions. However, strictly speaking, chronic total occlusion with downstream *infarcted* myocardium ought to be excluded from such an analysis.

1.4.4.1 Angiographic Collateral Grading

The study by Hansen on the prognostic relevance of collaterals in chronic CAD did account in part for the mentioned pitfall by including only patients with occluded coronary arteries out of a series of 300 patients examined for the presence of chest pain, suspicion of previous acute myocardial infarction and heart failure from 1968 to 1975 (no bypass grafting, no PCI).[109] However, 52 of the 96 patients included in the study had had a history of myocardial infarction (unclear how many in the region of interest). Of the 96 patients, 67 revealed angiographically good and 29 poor collaterals. Cumulative survival rates dur-ing a follow-up duration between 11 and 19 years were 51.5% at 10 years in patients with well-developed collaterals and 34.5% among those with poor collaterals (Fig. 1.47; $p < 0.10$).[109] The majority of studies on the prognostic relevance of collaterals in chronic CAD have used angiographic grading for characterizing the degree of collateral perfusion. Following the work by Han-sen,[109] the subject was re-investigated only after several years using a refined method for collateral assessment, i.e. quantitative, coronary pressure-derived collateral measurement (see below).[117,118] However, it was not before 2004 that the topic regained heightened interest using the tool of angiographic collateral qualification in relation to their prognostic relevance.[102] In 281 patients

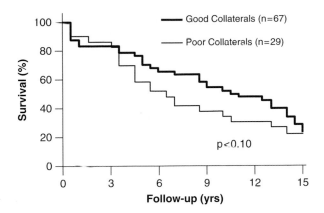

Fig. 1.47 Cumulative survival curves in patients with chronic total coronary occlusion depending on the presence of angiographically qualified 'good collaterals' (*blue line*) or 'poor collaterals' (*black line*). None of the patients had had acute myocardial infarction within 3 months prior to coronary angiography. However, 29 of the patients with well-developed collaterals and 23 of those with poorly developed collaterals had had a history of myocardial infarction

randomized to off-pump or on-pump coronary artery bypass grafting, Nathoe et al. found angiographic collaterals to be present in close to 50%.[102] Cumulative rates of event-free survival at 1 year were 87% in patients with collaterals and 69% in those without collaterals after off-pump bypass surgery ($p = 0.01$), and 66 and 63%, respectively ($p = 0.79$), following on-pump surgery.[102] The protective effect of collaterals in the off-pump group appeared to be conveyed by fewer peri-operative myocardial infarcts than in the on-pump group. In an attempt to untangle the relevance of the collateral circulation as a marker of CAD severity from that as a prognostic determinant, Koerselman et al. performed a case–control study in 244 patients admitted for elective PCI.[104] Angiographic collaterals were absent in 153 and present in 91 patients, and the results indicated that in chronic CAD, the presence of angiographic collaterals may indicate a prognostically adverse outcome, in particular, if present to a limited extent (grade 1 of 3).[104] The authors of that study vaguely proposed that the fate of a patient is determined by the balance between CAD severity and the presence and extent of the coronary collateral circulation. The same research group studied the relationship between angiographic collaterals and cardiac death or myocardial infarction, at 1 year after coronary revascularization, in 561 patients who were enrolled in a randomized study that compared stent implantation with bypass grafting.[103] Collaterals were present in 176 patients (31%). The adjusted odds ratio of cardiac death or infarction was 0.18 (95% confidence interval 0.04–0.78) in the presence of collaterals, and the cumulative survival free of death or infarction with and without collaterals was 1.1 and 5.3%, respectively ($p = 0.01$).[103] Considering the very low absolute numbers of cardiac death and myocardial infarction of 3 and 4, and of 26 and 21, respectively, in both studies by Koerselman et al.[104] and by

Nathoe et al.,[103] the opposing conclusions the authors drew are difficult to appreciate. In comparison to the latter, underpowered investigations, the one by Abbott et al. compared the baseline characteristics and cumulative 1-year event rates of 6,183 consecutive patients who underwent PCI by target vessel collateral status.[107] Collateral status was defined angiographically as absent (n = 5,051), as treated artery *supplied* collaterals (n = 239) and *received* collaterals (n = 893). The major limitation of this study is that the discriminations between the absence of angiographic collaterals to the artery of interest and collaterals taking off that vessel (i.e. supplying another artery) lack any clear definition, and has to be regarded as very difficult especially in the context of a data registry. Compared with the no-collaterals group, those with PCI of a collateral receiving artery had lower adjusted death/myocardial infarction rates (relative risk of 0.72, 95% CI 0.54–0.96, $p = 0.02$) and repeat revascularization rates (relative risk 0.73, 95% CI 0.59–0.91, $p = 0.005$).[107] Cumulative 1-year mortality was 4.7% and 4.1% in the group without and with collaterals, respectively, to the vessel undergoing PCI ($p = 0.70$). Due to the weird angiographic collateral definition, the important all-cause mortality data are not usable.

Very recently, Grobbee et al. (first author: Regieli) retrospectively analysed the data from a lipid-lowering trial involving 879 male participants who underwent coronary angiography and being followed for 24 months.[132] Presence of coronary collaterals spontaneously visible on angiography was assessed. Event-free survival after 2 years was 84% in patients without collaterals and 92% in patients with collaterals ($p = 0.0020$; events: CAD death, myocardial infarction, repeat PCI, coronary artery bypass grafting; Fig. 1.48). Despite the fact that the absolute numbers of death and myocardial infarction were still very low and similar to the above-mentioned figures (eight deaths, 19 infarcts),[132] the authors now firmly concluded that the 'protective effect is independent of disease burden, and remains present in patients with extensive CAD'.

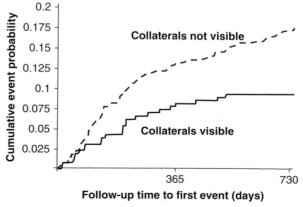

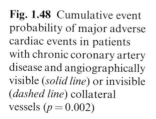

Fig. 1.48 Cumulative event probability of major adverse cardiac events in patients with chronic coronary artery disease and angiographically visible (*solid line*) or invisible (*dashed line*) collateral vessels ($p = 0.002$)

1.4.4.2 Quantitative Collateral Assessment

In a small patient cohort of 120 individuals with chronic CAD who underwent PCI and followed-up for cardiovascular ischaemic events for 6–22 months, Pijls et al. performed a quantitative measurement of collateral relative to normal antegrade flow recruitable during a 2-minute PCI-related vessel occlusion.[117] In 90 of the 120 patients, ischaemia was present at balloon inflation, and in 82 of these patients, relative collateral flow was ≤23%. During the follow-up period, 16 patients had an ischaemic event (death, myocardial infarction or unstable angina pectoris). Fifteen of these 16 patients were in the group with insufficient collateral flow ($p < 0.05$).[117] This study would be irrelevant with regard to the question of prognostic significance of collaterals in chronic CAD because of its inferior statistical power. However, it illustrates that the introduction of a more precise measurement technique than angiography for assessing collaterals (coronary pressure-derived relative collateral flow) may partly compensate for small patient sample size and brief follow-up duration.

In 403 patients with stable angina pectoris who underwent PCI and quantitative collateral assessment, our laboratory monitored the occurrence of major adverse cardiac events (cardiac death, myocardial infarction, unstable angina pectoris) and stable angina pectoris during an average follow-up of 94±56 weeks.[118] Relative collateral flow was determined using intracoronary pressure or Doppler guide wires. The overall cardiac ischaemic event rate (above events and stable angina pectoris) during follow-up was 23% in patients with high collateral flow (≥0.25 relative to normal flow) and 20% in patients with low collateral flow ($p =$ not significant). However, only 2.2% of patients with good collateral flow suffered a major cardiac ischaemic event compared with 9.0% among patients with poorly developed collaterals ($p = 0.01$; Fig. 1.49). The incidence of stable angina pectoris was higher in patients with well than in those with poorly developed collaterals (21% vs. 12%; $p = 0.01$).[118] The latter finding of this study reflects the relevance of sufficient collaterals as indicator for CAD severity

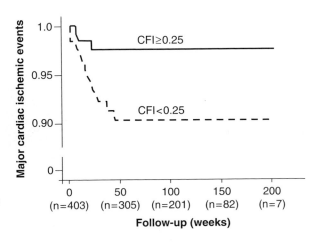

Fig. 1.49 Cumulative event rate of death, myocardial infarction or unstable angina pectoris in 403 patients with chronic stable coronary artery disease according to the presence (*solid line*) or absence (*dashed line*) of collateral relative to normal antegrade flow (collateral flow index, CFI) ≥0.25

in vessels not treated by PCI, whereas the former suggests their significance as prognostic factor. However, as several other investigations cited in this paragraph, the one by Billinger et al. was also insufficiently powered to answer the question whether collaterals are lifesaving in patients with chronic CAD.[118]

Analysis of our database on quantitative invasive collateral assessment provided clinical and haemodynamic data of 845 individuals (aged 62 ± 11 years), 106 patients without CAD and 739 patients with chronic stable CAD, who underwent a total of 1,053 quantitative, coronary pressure-derived collateral measurements between March 1996 and April 2006.[106] All patients were prospectively included in the CFI database containing information on recruitable collateral flow parameters obtained during a 1-minute coronary balloon occlusion. CFI was calculated as follows:

$CFI = (P_{occl}-CVP)/(P_{ao}-CVP)$, where P_{occl} is mean coronary occlusive pressure, P_{ao} is mean aortic pressure and CVP is central venous pressure (see also Chapter 2). The frequency distribution of CFI is depicted in Fig. 1.50, whereby it is evident that there are preformed functional collaterals in about one-fourth of individuals even in the absence of CAD (i.e. no coronary artery stenotic lesion) and that there is a rightward shift of CFI with increasing CAD severity (number of vessels with CAD). This illustrates the well-known observation of collateral flow being an indicator for CAD, which is further exemplified by the result that

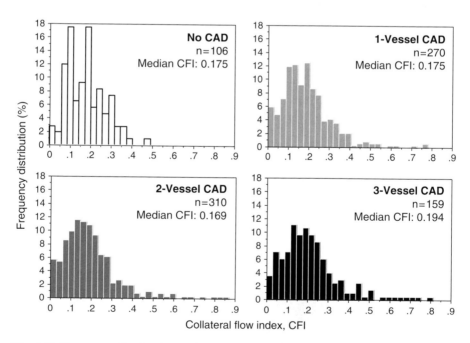

Fig. 1.50 Frequency distribution (*vertical axes* in percent) of collateral relative to normal antegrade coronary flow values (collateral flow index, CFI; *horizontal axes*) obtained in 106 individuals without angiographic evidence of coronary artery disease (CAD) and in 739 patients with one- to three-vessel CAD

Fig. 1.51 Box plot of collateral relative to normal antegrade coronary flow (collateral flow index, CFI; *vertical axis*) according to the presence or absence of chronic total coronary occlusion (*horizontal axis*). Box lines indicate mean values and 75% confidence interval, and error bars indicate 95% confidence interval

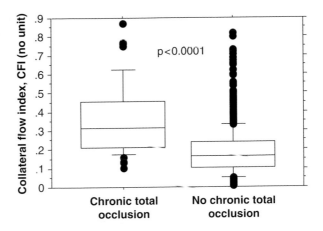

CAD patients with chronic total coronary occlusions have higher collateral flow than individuals without chronic total occlusion (Fig. 1.51). In the study by Meier et al.[106], patients were divided into groups with poorly developed (CFI < 0.25) or well-developed collateral vessels (CFI ≥ 0.25). Follow-up information on the occurrence of all-cause mortality and major adverse cardiac events after study inclusion was collected. Cumulative 10-year survival rates in relation to all-cause deaths and cardiac deaths were 71 and 88%, respectively, in patients with low CFI and 89 and 97% in patients with high CFI ($p = 0.0395$, $p = 0.0109$; Fig. 1.52). The cumulative survival rate free of cardiac death or infarct and free of cardiac death, infarct or unstable angina pectoris is shown in Fig. 1.53. As an alternative to the described quantitative measurement of CFI, an intracoronary ECG was

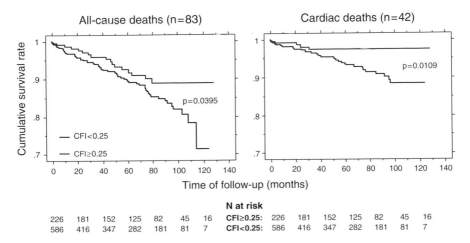

Fig. 1.52 Cumulative survival rates in patients with chronic stable coronary artery disease related to all-cause (*left side*) and cardiac (*right side*) mortality according to the presence of low and high collateral flow index (CFI, i.e. collateral relative to normal antegrade coronary flow)

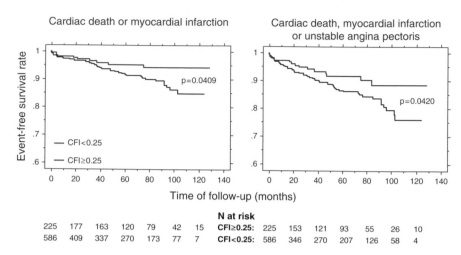

Fig. 1.53 Cumulative event-free survival rates related to major adverse cardiac events: cardiac death or myocardial infarction (*left side*), cardiac death, myocardial infarction or unstable angina pectoris (*right side*) according to the presence of low and high collateral flow index (CFI, i.e. collateral relative to normal antegrade coronary flow)

obtained during coronary occlusion in all patients from the angioplasty guide wire in addition to the surface leads (Fig. 1.54). For that purpose, an alligator clamp was attached close to the end of the wire and connected to ECG lead V1. Thus, coronary collaterals without or with intracoronary ECG signs of ischaemia

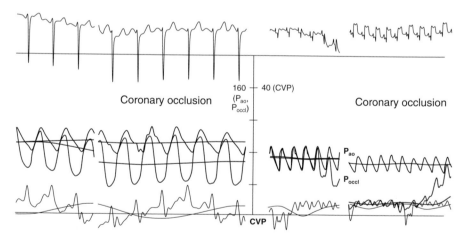

Fig. 1.54 Intracoronary ECG (*upper part*) and pressure tracings (*lower part*) in a patient without evidence of myocardial ischaemia during a 1-minute coronary balloon occlusion (*left side*; no ECG signs of ischaemia, i.e. sufficient collaterals), and in a patient with marked ECG ST-segment elevations during the 1-minute coronary occlusion (*right side*; insufficient collaterals). Concomitantly, mean and phasic distal coronary pressure decreased much less during coronary occlusion (P_{occl}, *red pressure curves*) in the patient with sufficient collaterals than in the patient with insufficient collaterals (*right side*). P_{ao} aortic pressure (*black pressure curve*), *CVP* central venous pressure (*black pressure curve*)

Fig. 1.55 Cumulative survival rates related to cardiac mortality in patients without and in those with ECG signs of myocardial ischemia on intracoronary ECG during a 1-minute coronary balloon occlusion. Myocardial ischemia defined as ECG ST segment elevation > 0.1mV (ST↑).[106]

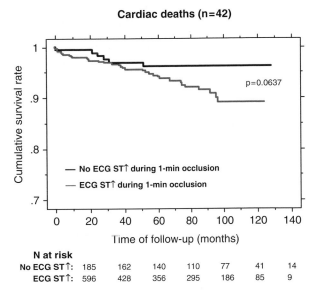

(i.e. ST-segment elevation of > 1 mm or > 0.1 mV) at the end of the 1-minute coronary occlusion were determined (Fig. 1.54). Employing this independent dichotomous method for collateral qualification, cumulative survival free of cardiac death at 10 years of follow-up was 96% in patients with sufficient collaterals to prevent signs of ischaemia during occlusion and 89% among patients with insufficient collaterals.[106] Using Cox proportional hazards analysis, the following variables independently predicted elevated cardiac mortality: age, low CFI (as continuous variable) and current smoking. This study provides firm evidence that a well-functioning coronary collateral circulation saves lives in patients with chronic stable CAD.

Abbreviations

CAD	coronary artery disease
CFI	collateral flow index (no unit)
CK	creatine kinase
CVP	central venous pressure (mmHg)
HOCM	hypertrophic obstructive cardiomyopathy
LAD	left anterior descending artery
LCX	left circumflex coronary artery
LV	left ventricle, left ventricular
P_{ao}	mean aortic pressure (mmHg)
PCI	percutaneous coronary intervention
P_{occl}	mean coronary occlusive or wedge pressure (mmHg)
RCA	right coronary artery
TASH	transcoronary ablation of septal hypertrophy

References

1. Proudfit W. Origin of concept of ischeamic heart disease. *Br Heart J.* 1983;50:209–212.
2. Michaels L. Aetiology of coronary artery disease: an historical approach. *Br Heart J.* 1966;1966:258–264.
3. Herrik J. Clinical features of sudden obstruction of the coronary arteries. *JAMA.* 1912;59:2015–2020.
4. Lower R. Tractatus de corde, item de motu et colore sanguinis, et chyli in eum transitu. *Amstelaedami.* 1669.
5. Heberden W. Commentaries on the history and cure of diseases. In: Wilius F, Kays T, eds. *Classics of Cardiology.* New York: Dover; 1961:220–224.
6. Lower R. *Early Science in Oxford.* Oxford: Oxford University Press; 1932.
7. Prinzmetal M, Simkin B, Bergman HC, Kruger HE. Studies on the coronary circulation. II. The collateral circulation of the normal human heart by coronary perfusion with radioactive erythrocytes and glass spheres. *Am Heart J.* 1947;33:420–442.
8. Thebesius A. Dissertatio de circulo sanguinis in corde. *Lugdunum Batavorum.* 1708.
9. von Haller A. Elementa physiologiae corporis humani. *Lausanne.* 1757:371.
10. Heberden W. A letter to Dr. Heberden, concerning the angina pectoris; and an account of the dissection of one who had been troubled with that disorder. Read at the college November 17, 1772. *Medical Transactions Published by the College of Physicians in London.* 1785;3:1–11.
11. Kobler J. *The Reluctant Surgeon. A Biography of John Hunter.* Garden City, NY: Doubleday and Co.; 1960.
12. Hunter J. *A treatise on the Blood, Inflammation, and Gun-Shot Wounds.* Philadelphia: Thomas Bradford; 1796.
13. West S. The anastomoses of the coronary arteries. *The Lancet.* 1883;1:945–946.
14. Hyrtl J. *Wien;* 1855.
15. Henle J. *Handbuch der Systematischen Anatomie des Menschen.* Braunschweig: Friedrich Vieweg und Sohn; 1866.
16. Cohnheim J, von Schulthess-Rechberg A. Ueber die Folgen der Kranzarterienverschliessung für das Herz. *Virchows Arch.* 1881;85:503–537.
17. Fulton W, van Royen N. Morphology of the collateral circulation in the human heart. In: Schaper W, Schaper J, eds. *Arteriogenesis.* Boston, Dirdrecht, London: Kluwer Academic Publishers; 2004:297–331.
18. Spalteholz W. Die Koronararterien des Herzens. *Verhandl Anat Gesell.* 1907;30:141.
19. Schlesinger M. New radiopaque mass for vascular injection. *Lab Invest.* 1957;6:1–11.
20. Seiler C, Kirkeeide R, Gould K. Measurement from arteriograms of regional myocardial bed size distal to any point in the coronary vascular tree for assessing anatomic area at risk. *J Am Coll Cardiol.* 1993;21:783–797.
21. Rodriguez F, Reiner L. A new method of dissection of the heart. *Arch Pathol.* 1957;63:160–163.
22. Schlesinger M. An injection plus dissection study of coronary artery occlusions and anastomoses. *Am Heart J.* 1938;15:528–568.
23. Langer D. Anastomosen der Kranzarterien des Herzens. *Sitzungsbericht der Wiener Akad. Math.-Naturwiss.* 1880;81.
24. Hirsch C, Spalteholz W. Koronararterien und Herzmuskel. *Deutsche medizinische Wochenschrift.* 1907;33:790–795.
25. Zoll PM, Wessler S, Schlesinger MJ. Interarterial coronary anastomoses in the heart, with particular reference to anemia and relative cardiac anoxia. *Circulation.* 1951;4:797–815.
26. Blumgart HL, Schlesinger MJ, Davis D. Studies on the relation of the clinical manifestations of angina pectoris, coronary thrombosis and myocardial infarction to the pathological findings. *Am Heart J.* 1940;19:1–91.

27. Baroldi G. The collaterals of the coronary arteries in normal and pathologic hearts. *Circ Res.* 1956;4:223–229.
28. Pitt B. Interarterial coronary anastomoses. Occurence in normal hearts and in certain pathologic conditions. *Circulation.* 1959;20:816–822.
29. Pepler W, Meyer B. .Interarterial coronary anastomoses and coronary arterial pattern. A comparative study of South African Bantu and European hearts. *Circulation.* 1960;22:14–24.
30. Bloor C, Keefe J, Browne M. Intercoronary anastomoses in congenital heart disease. *Circulation.* 1966;33:227–231.
31. Reiner L, Molnar J, Jimenez F, Freudenthal R. Interarterial coronary anastomoses in neonates. *Arch Pathol.* 1961;71:103–112.
32. Crainicianu A. Anatomische Studien über die Koronararterien und experimentelle Untersuchungen über ihre Durchgängigkeit. *Virchows Arch Path Anat.* 1922;238:1.
33. Gross L. *The Blood Supply of the Heart.* Oxford: Oxford University Press; 1921.
34. Fulton WFM. Arterial anastomoses in the coronary circulation. I. Anatomical features in normal and diseased hearts demonstrated by stereoarteriography. *Scottish Med J.* 1963; 8:420–434.
35. Fulton WFM. Arterial anastomoses in the coronary circulation. II. Distribution, enumeration and measurement of coronary arterial anastomoses in health and disease. *Scott Med J.* 1963;8:466–474.
36. Fulton WFM. Immersion radiography of injected specimens. *Brit J Radiol.* 1963;36:685–688.
37. Wall J. A letter from Dr. Wall to Dr. Heberden, on the same subject (angina pectoris). *Medical Transactions Published by the College of Physicians in London.* 1785;3:12–24.
38. MacAlpin R, Weidner W, Kattus AJ, Hanafee W. Electrocardiographic changes during selective coronary cineangiography. *Circulation.* 1966;34:627–637.
39. Osler W. Lectures on angina pectoris and allied states. In. New York: D. Appleton and Company; 1897:52.
40. Wenckebach K. Toter Punkt, "second wind", und Angina pectoris. *Wien. klin. Wchschr.* 1928;41:1.
41. Paulin S. Interarterial coronary anastomoses in relation to arterial obstruction demonstrated in coronary arteriography. *Invest Radiol.* 1967;2:147–159.
42. Gensini GG, Bruto da Costa BC. The coronary collateral circulation in living man. *Am J Cardiol.* 1969;24:393–400.
43. Helfant RH, Vokonas PS, Gorlin R. Functional importance of the human coronary collateral circulation. *N Engl J Med.* 1971;284:1277–1281.
44. Hamby R, Aintablian A, Schwartz A. Reappraisal of the functional significance of the coronary collateral circulation. *Am J Cardiol.* 1976;38:304–309.
45. Rowe G. An angiographic and clinical study of coronary collateral circulation. *Basic Res Cardiol.* 1979;74:131–141.
46. Eng C, Patterson R, Horowitz S, et al. Coronary collateral function during exercise. *Circulation.* 1982;66:309–316.
47. Goldstein R, Stinson E, Scherer J, Seningen R, Grehl T, Epstein SE. Intraoperative coronary collateral function in patients with coronary occlusive disease. Nitroglycerin responsiveness and angiographic correlations. *Circulation.* 1974;49:298–308.
48. Goldstein RE, Michaelis LL, Morrow AG, Epstein SE. Coronary collateral function in patients without occlusive coronary artery disease. *Circulation.* 1975;51:118–125.
49. Smith SJ, Gorlin R, Herman M, Taylor W, Collins JJ. Myocardial blood flow in man: effects of coronary collateral circulation and coronary artery bypass surgery. *J Clin Invest.* 1972;51:2556–2565.
50. Grüntzig A, Senning A, Siegenthaler W. Nonoperative dilatation of coronary-artery stenosis: percutaneous transluminal coronary angioplasty. *N Engl J Med.* 1979; 301:61–68.

51. Feldman R, Pepine C. Evaluation of coronary collateral circulation in conscious humans. *Am J Cardiol.* 1984;53:1233–1238.
52. Ofili E, Kern M, Tatineni S, et al. Detection of coronary collateral flow by a Doppler-tipped guide wire during coronary angioplasty. *Am Heart J.* 1991;122: 221–225.
53. Pijls NHJ, van Son JAM, Kirkeeide RL, de Bruyne B, Gould KL. Experimental basis of determining maximum coronary, myocardial, and collateral blood flow by pressure measurements for assessing functional stenosis severity before and after percutaneous coronary angioplasty. *Circulation.* 1993;86:1354–1367.
54. Seiler C, Fleisch M, Garachemani A, Meier B. Coronary collateral quantitation in patients with coronary artery disease using intravascular flow velocity or pressure measurements. *J Am Coll Cardiol.* 1998;32:1272–1279.
55. Wustmann K, Zbinden S, Windecker S, Meier B, Seiler C. Is there functional collateral flow during vascular occlusion in angiographically normal coronary arteries? *Circulation.* 2003;108:2213–2220.
56. Schaper W. Comparative arteriography of the collateral circulation of the heart. In: Schaper W, ed. *The Collateral Circulation of the Heart.* Amsterdam: North Holland Publishing Co.; 1971:39–50.
57. Schaper W, Flameng W, De Brabander M. Comparative aspects of coronary collateral circulation. *Adv Exp Med Biol.* 1972;22:267–276.
58. Schaper W, Flameng W, Wusten B, Palmowski J. The distribution of coronary and of coronary collateral flow in normal hearts and after chronic coronary occlusion. *Adv Exp Med Biol.* 1973;39:151–60.
59. Schaper W, Jageneau A, Xhonneux R. The development of collateral circulation in the pig and dog heart. *Cardiologia.* 1967;51:321–325.
60. Gregg D. The natural history of coronary collateral development. *Circ Res.* 1974;35:335–344.
61. Weaver M, Pantely G, Bristow J, Ladley H. A quantitative study of the anatomy and distribution of coronary arteries in swine in comparison with other animals and man. *Cardiovasc Res.* 1986;20:907–917.
62. Campbell C, Takanashi Y, Laas J, Meus P, Pick R, Replogle R. Effect of coronary artery reperfusion on infarct size in swine. *J Thorac Cardiovasc Surg.* 1981;81:288–296.
63. Blumgart H, Zoll P. The experimental production of intercoronary arterial anastomoses and their functional significance. *Circulation.* 1950;1:10–27.
64. Eckstein R. Coronary interarterial anastomoses in young pigs and mongrel dogs. *Circ Res.* 1954;2:460–465.
65. Lumb D, Hardy L. Collateral circulation and survival related to gradual occlusion of the right coronary artery in the pig. *Circulation.* 1963;27:717–725.
66. Vastesaeger M, Van der Straeten P, Friart J, Candaele G, Ghys A, Bernard R. Intercoronary anastomoses like those seen in postmortem coronarography. *Acta Cardiol.* 1957;12:365–401.
67. Lumb G, Hardy L. Collaterals and coronary artery narrowing. I. The effect of coronary artery narrowing on collateral channels in swine. *Lab Invest.* 1964;13:1530–1540.
68. Ramo B, Peter R, Ratliff N, Kong Y, McIntosh H, Morris JJ. The natural history of right coronary arterial occlusion in the pig. Comparison with left anterior descending arterial occlusion. *Am J Cardiol.* 1970;26:156–161.
69. Spalteholz W. *Die Arterien der Herzwand. Anatomische Untersuchungen an Menschen- und Tierherzen. Nebst Erörterung der Voraussetzung für die Herstellung eines Kollateralkreislaufes.* Leipzig: S. Hirzel; 1924.
70. Lumb G, Hardy L. Collateral circulation and survival related to gradual occlusion of the right coronary artery in the pig. *Circulation.* 1963;27:717–721.
71. Bloor C. Functional significance of the coronary collateral circulation. *Am J Pathol.* 1974;76:562–586.

72. Sjöquist P, Duker G, Almgren O. Distribution of the collateral blood flow at the lateral border of the ischemic myocardium after acute coronary occlusion in the pig and the dog. *Basic Res Cardiol.* 1984;79:164–175.
73. Maxwell M, Hearse D, Yellon D. Species variation in the coronary collateral circulation during regional myocardial ischaemia: a critical determinant of the rate of evolution and extent of myocardial infarction. *Cardiovasc Res.* 1987;21:737–746.
74. Rasmussen M, Reimer K, Kloner R, Jennings R. Infarct size reduction by propranolol before and after coronary ligation in dogs. *Circulation.* 1977;56:794–798.
75. Yellon D, Hearse D, Maxwell M, Chambers D, Downey J. Sustained limitation of myocardial necrosis 24 hours after coronary artery occlusion: verapamil infusion in dogs with small myocardial infarcts. *Am J Cardiol.* 1983;51:1409–1413.
76. Smith E, Lefer A. Stabilization of cardiac lysosomal and cellular membranes in protection of ischemic myocardium due to coronary occlusion: efficacy of the nonsteroidal anti-inflammatory agent, naproxen. *Am Heart J.* 1981;101:394–402.
77. Burke S, DiCola G, Lefer A. Protection of ischemic cat myocardium by CGS-13080, a selective potent thromboxane A2 synthesis inhibitor. *J Cardiovasc Pharmacol.* 1983;5:842–847.
78. Maclean D, Fishbein M, Braunwald E, Maroko P. Long-term preservation of ischemic myocardium after experimental coronary artery occlusion. *J Clin Invest.* 1978;61:541–551.
79. Evans R, Val-Mejias J, Kulevich J, Fischer V, Mueller HS. Evaluation of a rat model for assessing interventions to salvage ischaemic myocardium: effects of ibuprofen and verapamil. *Cardiovasc Res.* 1985;19:132–138.
80. Connelly C, Vogel W, Hernandez Y, Apstein C. Movement of necrotic wavefront after coronary artery occlusion in rabbit.Movement of necrotic wavefront after coronary artery occlusion in rabbit. *Am J Physiol.* 1982;243:H682–690.
81. Fiedler V. Reduction of acute myocardial ischemia in rabbit hearts by nafazatrom. *J Cardiovasc Pharmacol.* 1984;6:318–324.
82. Rösen R, Marsen A, Klaus W. Local myocardial perfusion and epicardial NADH-fluorescence after coronary artery ligation in the isolated guinea pig heart. *Basic Res Cardiol.* 1984;79:59–67.
83. Gaide M, Cameron J, Altman C, Myerburg R, Bassett A. Myocardial infarction in the guinea pig: cellular electrophysiology. *Life Sci.* 1985;36:2391–2401.
84. Smith G, Geary G, Ruf W, Fore F, Oyama M, McNamara J. Quantitative effect of a single large dose of methylprednisolone on infarct size in baboons. *Cardiovasc Res.* 1980;14:408–418.
85. Geary G, Smith G, McNamara J. Quantitative effect of early coronary artery reperfusion in baboons. Extent of salvage of the perfusion bed of an occluded artery. *Circulation.* 1982;66:391–396.
86. Reimer KA, Ideker RE, Jennings RB. Effect of coronary occlusion site on ischemic bed size and collateral blood flow in dogs. *Cardiovasc Res.* 1981;15:668–674.
87. Nienaber C, Gottwik M, Winkler B, Schaper W. The relationship between the perfusion deficit, infarct size and time after experimental coronary artery occlusion. *Basic Res Cardiol.* 1983;78:210–226.
88. Sigwart U. Non-surgical myocardial reduction for hypertrophic obstructive cardiomyopathy. *Lancet.* 1995;346:211–214.
89. Durand E, Mousseaux E, Coste P, et al. Non-surgical septal myocardial reduction by coil embolization for hypertrophic obstructive cardiomyopathy: early and 6 months follow-up. *Eur Heart J.* 2008;29:348–355.
90. Werner G, Ferrari M, Heinke S, et al. Angiographic assessment of collateral connections in comparison with invasively determined collateral function in chronic coronary occlusions. *Circulation.* 2003;107:1972–1977.
91. Wani S, Seiler C. Transcoronary ablation of septal hypertrophy in HOCM: septal collaterals may cause unwanted inferior myocardial infarction. *Kardiovask Med.* 2007;10:401–402.

92. Rowe G. Inequalities of myocardial perfusion in coronary artery disease ("coronary steal"). *Circulation*. 1970;42:193–194.
93. Schaper W, Lewi P, Flameng W, Gijpen L. Myocardial steal produced by coronary vasocilation in chronic coronary artery occlusion. *Basic Res Cardiol*. 1973;68:3–20.
94. Seiler C, Fleisch M, Meier B. Direct intracoronary evidence of collateral steal in humans. *Circulation*. 1997;96:4261–4267.
95. Werner GS, Fritzenwanger M, Prochnau D, et al. Determinants of coronary steal in chronic total coronary occlusions donor artery, collateral, and microvascular resistance. *J Am Coll Cardiol*. 2006;48:51–58.
96. Gould KL. Coronary steal. Is it clinically important? *Chest*. 1989;96:227–228.
97. Urban P, Meier B, Finci L, de Bruyne B, Steffenino G, Rutishauser W. Coronary wedge pressure: a predictor of restenosis after coronary balloon angioplasty. *J Am Coll Cardiol*. 1987;10:504–509.
98. Wahl A, Billinger M, Fleisch M, Meier B, Seiler C. Quantitatively assessed coronary collateral circulation and restenosis following percutaneous revascularization. *Eur Heart J*. 2000;21:1776–1784.
99. Jensen L, Thayssen P, Lassen J, et al. Recruitable collateral blood flow index predicts coronary instent restenosis after percutaneous coronary intervention. *Eur Heart J*. 2007;28:1820–1826.
100. Kern MJ. Collateral flow and restenosis: appreciating hydraulics and outcomes of percutanous coronary intervention. *Eur Heart J*. 2000;21:1730–1732.
101. Spaan J, Piek J, Hoffman J, Siebes M. Physiological basis of clinically used coronary hemodynamic indices. *Circulation*. 2006;113:446–455.
102. Nathoe HM, Buskens E, Jansen EW, et al. Role of coronary collaterals in off-pump and on-pump coronary bypass surgery. *Circulation*. 2004;110:1738–1742.
103. Nathoe HM, Koerselman J, Buskens E, et al. Determinants and prognostic significance of collaterals in patients undergoing coronary revascularization. *Am J Cardiol*. 2006;98:31–35.
104. Koerselman J, de Jaegere PP, Verhaar MC, Grobbee DE, van der Graaf Y, Group SS. Prognostic significance of coronary collaterals in patients with coronary heart disease having percutaneous transluminal coronary angioplasty. *Am J Cardiol*. 2005;96:390–394.
105. Hjemdahl P, Eriksson SV, Held C, Forslund L, Nasman P, Rehnqvist N. Favourable long term prognosis in stable angina pectoris: an extended follow up of the angina prognosis study in Stockholm (APSIS). *Heart*. 2006;92:177–182.
106. Meier P, Gloekler S, Zbinden R, et al. Beneficial effect of recruitable collaterals: a 10-year follow-up study in patients with stable coronary artery disease undergoing quantitative collateral measurements. *Circulation*. 2007;116:975–983.
107. Abbott JD, Choi EJ, Selzer F, et al. Impact of coronary collaterals on outcome following percutaneous coronary intervention (from the National Heart, Lung, and Blood Institute Dynamic Registry). *Am J Cardiol*. 2005;96:676–680.
108. Antoniucci D, Valenti R, Moschi G, et al. Relation between preintervention angiographic evidence of coronary collateral circulation and clinical and angiographic outcomes after primary angioplasty or stenting for acute myocardial infarction. *Am J Cardiol*. 2002;89:121–125.
109. Hansen JF. Coronary collateral circulation: clinical significance and influence on survival in patients with coronary artery occlusion. *Am Heart J*. 1989;117:290–295.
110. Gohlke H, Heim E, Roskamm H. Prognostic importance of collateral flow and residual coronary stenosis of the myocardial infarct artery after anterior wall Q-wave acute myocardial infarction. *Am J Cardiol*. 1991;67:1165–1169.
111. Boehrer JD, Lange RA, Willard JE, Hillis LD. Influence of collateral filling of the occluded infarct-related coronary artery on prognosis after acute myocardial infarction. *Am J Cardiol*. 1992;69:10–12.

112. Clements IP, Christian TF, Higano ST, Gibbons RJ, Gersh BJ. Residual flow to the infarct zone as a determinant of infarct size after direct angioplasty. *Circulation.* 1993;88:1527–1533.

113. Kodama K, Kusuoka H, Sakai A, et al. Collateral channels that develop after an acute myocardial infarction prevent subsequent left ventricular dilation. *J Am Coll Cardiol.* 1996;27:1133–1139.

114. Nicolau JC, Nogueira PR, Pinto MA, Serrano CVJ, Garzon SA. Early infarct artery collateral flow does not improve long-term survival following thrombolytic therapy for acute myocardial infarction. *Am J Cardiol.* 1999;83:21–26.

115. Elsman P, van 't Hof AW, de Boer MJ, et al. Role of collateral circulation in the acute phase of ST-segment-elevation myocardial infarction treated with primary coronary intervention. *Eur Heart J.* 2004;25:854–858.

116. Ishihara M, Inoue I, Kawagoe T, et al. Comparison of the cardioprotective effect of prodromal angina pectoris and collateral circulation in patients with a first anterior wall acute myocardial infarction. *Am J Cardiol.* 2005;95:622–625.

117. Pijls NHJ, Bech GJW, El Gamal MIH, et al. Quantification of recruitable coronary collateral blood flow in conscious humans and its potential to predict future ischemic events. *J Am Coll Cardiol.* 1995;25:1522–1528.

118. Billinger M, Kloos P, Eberli FR, Windecker S, Meier B, Seiler C. Physiologically assessed coronary collateral flow and adverse cardiac ischemic events: a follow-up study in 403 patients with coronary artery disease. *J Am Coll Cardiol.* 2002;40:1545–1550.

119. Werner G, Surber R, Kuethe F, et al. Collaterals and the recovery of left ventricular function after recanalization of a chronic total coronary occlusion. *Am Heart J.* 2005;149:129–317.

120. Sobel B, Bresnahan G, Shell W, Yoder R. Estimation of infarct size in man and its relation to prognosis. *Circulation.* 1972;46:640–647.

121. Roberts R, Henry P, Sobel B. An improved basis for enzymatic estimation of infarct size. *Circulation.* 1975;52:743–754.

122. Hirai T, Fujita M, Nakajima H, et al. Importance of collateral circulation for prevention of left ventricular aneurysm formation in acute myocardial infarction. *Circulation.* 1989;79:791–796.

123. Habib GB, Heibig J, Forman SA, et al. Influence of coronary collateral vessels on myocardial infarct size in humans. Results of phase I thrombolysis in myocardial infarction (TIMI) trial. The TIMI Investigators. *Circulation.* 1991;83:739–746.

124. Sabia P, Powers E, Ragosta M, Sarembock I, Burwell L, Kaul S. An association beween collateral blood flow and myocardial viability in patients with recent myocardial infraction. *N Engl J Med.* 1992;327:1825–1831.

125. Christian T, Schwartz R, Gibbons R. Determinants of infarct size in reperfusion therapy for acute myocardial infarction. *Circulation.* 1992;86:81–90.

126. Sorajja P, Gersh B, Mehran R, Lansky A, Krucoff M, Webb J, Cox D, Brodie B, Stone G. Impact of collateral flow on myocardial reperfusion and infarct size in patients undergoing primary angioplasty for acute myocardial infarction. *Am Heart J.* 2007;154:379–384.

127. Elhendy A, Cornel J, Roelandt J, et al. Impact of severity of coronary artery stenosis and the collateral circulation on the functional outcome of dyssynergic myocardium after revascularization in patients with healed myocardial infarction and chronic left ventricular dysfunction. *Am J Cardiol.* 1997;79:883–888.

128. Waldecker B, Waas W, Haberbosch W, Voss R, Wiecha J, Tillmanns H. Prevalence and significance of coronary collateral circulation in patients with acute myocardial infarct. *Z Kardiol.* 2002;91:243–248.

129. de Boer M, Reiber J, Suryapranata H, van den Brand M, Hoorntje J, F Z. Angiographic findings and catheterization laboratory events in patients with primary coronary

angioplasty or streptokinase therapy for acute myocardial infarction. *Eur Heart J.* 1995;16:1347–1355.
130. Schwartz H, Leiboff R, Bren G, et al. Temporal evolution of the human coronary collateral circulation after myocardial infarction. *J Am Coll Cardiol.* 1984;4:1088–1093.
131. Pérez-Castellano N, Garcia E, Abeytua M, et al. Influence of collateral circulation on in-hospital death from anterior acute myocardial infarction. *J Am Coll Cardiol.* 1998;31:512–518.
132. Regieli J, Jukema J, Nathoe H, et al. Coronary collaterals improve prognosis in patients with ischemic heart disease. *Int J Cardiol.* 2008;31:Epub ahead of print.

Chapter 2
Assessment of the Human Coronary Collateral Circulation

2.1 Theoretical Aspects in the Assessment of the Coronary Collateral Circulation

The reference method for coronary blood flow measurements in the experimental animal model is the microsphere indicator deposition method. The principle of deposition methods is that the microsphere deposition is proportional to the flow per unit mass of tissue. Using microsphere methods and small myocardial pieces, regional flow values vary considerably between one-third and twice the average flow. This fractal vascular tree geometry is present throughout the plant and animal world, and its conservation across species is thought to be due to evolutionary advantages conferred through efficient distribution of nutrients. In that context, the coronary artery tree is structured according to the law of minimum viscous energy loss during the transport of blood, a design which principally accounts also for the option of intercoronary anastomoses. The collateral circulation is a major determinant of myocardial infarct size (IS) reduction in case of a coronary occlusion.

Coronary arterial vasomotion allows the adaptation of blood supply to the myocardium under different conditions of demand. In the assumed absence of coronary collateral flow, a brief coronary occlusion normally induces a four- to fivefold increase in blood flow above resting level immediately after release of the occlusion. Analogous to the structural option of intercoronary anastomoses crossing the boundaries of vascular territories, there is the possibility of a vasomotor response of collateral vessels to hyperaemic stimuli. The clinical equivalent of such functional collateral response can be the development of tolerance to repetitive bouts of myocardial ischaemia, manifesting as relief of angina pectoris or diminishing electrocardiogram (ECG) signs of ischaemia. Assuming a constant myocardial oxygen utilization, the only determinants of ECG signs of ischaemia or IS are time of coronary artery occlusion, collateral supply and myocardial preconditioning, the protagonists in the list of contributors to the development of myocardial tolerance to repetitive ischaemia. The variable response of ECG signs of myocardial ischaemic adaptation to collateral recruitment points to ischaemic preconditioning as another relevant factor responsible for ischaemia attenuation following repetitive coronary occlusions.

C. Seiler, *Collateral Circulation of the Heart*, DOI 10.1007/978-1-84882-342-6_2,

2.1.1 Introduction

The functional relevance of coronary collateral vessels in humans had been a matter of debate for many years.[1] Much of this controversy was likely due to inadequate means for gauging human coronary collaterals,[2,3] and to the investigation of populations too small to be representative for all the patients with coronary artery disease (CAD). Mostly for ethical reasons, assessment of the coronary collateral circulation in man is different from the methods employed in the experimental animal model. Yet, knowledge of the gold standard for coronary perfusion measurement is mandatory for understanding the assessment of the human coronary collateral circulation, such as is insight into the structural design principles of the coronary artery tree and into the relationship between signs of myocardial ischaemia and its determinants.

2.1.2 Coronary Blood Flow Measurements in the Animal Model

In the experimental animal model, the measurement of coronary flow can be performed using a number of widely differing methods, such as washout of radioactive inert gases, uptake of radioisotopes of potassium and its analogues, thermoelectrical flow probes, electromagnetic and Doppler flow meters and angiography. However, measurement of blood flow and its distribution to small myocardial regions cannot be made with the flow meters or the direct Fick technique, since the vascular inflow to and outflow from these areas cannot be isolated. It is, therefore, necessary to use the techniques involving an indicator which is distributed to various myocardial territories proportional to the regional blood flows. The amounts of indicator entering the area, retained in it, and leaving it must be determined. This prerequisite of regional flow measurement is fulfilled by the microsphere deposition method.[4] It is obvious that, for ethical reasons, microsphere deposition methods, i.e. capillary embolization with particles 5–25 μm in size cannot be used in humans. The basic principle of all deposition methods for regional flow measurement is that the deposition is proportional to the flow per unit mass of tissue, i.e. that the fraction of the cardiac output going to a particular region is defined by the fractional deposition of a marker in that region. Hence, deposited markers give a measure of flow per unit mass of tissue at the level of capillaries.

Regional myocardial blood flow (ml/min)

$$= \quad \text{cardiac output} \quad \times \quad \text{regional} \quad \# \quad \text{microspheres/total} \quad \#$$
$$\text{microspheres}$$

In the case of *radiolabelled* microspheres, the number (#) of microspheres is derived from the measured radioactivity of the tissue sample and of the arterial reference sample injected into the left atrium. If in addition, the coronary sinus is sampled at a certain flow rate and if coronary venous radioactivity is obtained, total myocardial blood flow can be corrected for incomplete microsphere trapping,[5] which may occur using very small microspheres between 5 and 10 μm. Absolute flow per unit mass of tissue (i.e. perfusion in ml/min/g, the reference parameter for coronary blood flow) is calculated by weighing the tissue sample. Following the advent of radiolabelled microspheres,[6] they have become the gold standard for blood flow measurements.[4] Because the use of radioactivity has turned out to be increasingly problematic due to restrictive legislation and high costs of storage and disposal as well as due to the desire of reducing radiation load to personnel, non-radioactive coloured and fluorescent microspheres have been developed.[4] The principles of microsphere deposition methods just described also apply in the case of coloured and fluorescent microspheres. Hale et al. introduced the method for obtaining blood flow with coloured microspheres,[7] whereby blood and tissue samples were digested and the spheres isolated by centrifugation and then counted in a haemocytometer. Fluorescent microspheres were introduced 2 years later.[8] Using five or six different fluorescent labels in the same experiment, good correlations were demonstrated between radioactive and fluorescent microspheres for blood flow in heart, ischaemic and non-ischaemic myocardium, kidneys and lungs and a variety of other organs.[8]

Employing microsphere deposition techniques, it has also been shown very consistently that regional myocardial perfusion is spatially heterogeneous.[9] Using myocardial pieces less than 1% of the ventricular mass, it has been found that local flow values range between one-third and twice the average flow.[9] Furthermore, a mathematical relationship between the size of the pieces and the heterogeneity of flow values has been documented, to the effect that the finer the myocardium is cut, the broader the distributions of regional flows become. Such behaviour of increasing variability or dispersion of the observed parameter with growing resolution of the observational method is a fractal phenomenon when the changes are proportional (dispersion is related to size of myocardial pieces by a non-integer power function).[9] Fractal vascular tree geometry is found throughout the plant and animal world, and the conservation of these structures across species is thought to be due to evolutionary advantages conferred through efficient distribution of nutrients.[10–14] Although the *functional* consequences of the coronary tree structure as observed by the mentioned microsphere studies are biologically more important than its underlying geometry, grasping the design principles of the coronary circulation is crucial for understanding several concepts of assessing coronary collateral pathways.

2.1.3   Structural Design and Function of the Coronary Circulation

The structure of the coronary arterial circulation can be described on the basis of the above-mentioned ubiquitous principle of efficient nutrient distribution. One of the principal nutrients for the myocardium is oxygen. Normally, there is a match between the myocardial oxygen requirements and coronary supply, the reason for which lies not only in the unique structural design but also in the functional adaptability of the coronary artery circulation and the interrelationship between the two.[15] Myocardial oxygen demand is mostly determined by ventricular wall stress, heart rate and myocardial contractility.[16] Additionally, it is directly determined by the *amount* of myocardium requiring oxygen. Oxygen supply meets the respective demand by the capacity of the blood to carry oxygen and by the rate of coronary blood volume flow (in ml/min). Since the oxygen-carrying capacity remains quite constant in the coronary circulation, varying oxygen demands by the myocardium are predominantly satisfied by altering coronary flow rates (Q). Delivering blood volume at a certain rate Q is an energy-consuming process. In the context of the above-mentioned fractal vascular tree structures omnipresent in nature, energy-efficiency in the fluid distribution appears to be the underlying axiom. Illustration of this principle was indirectly provided by Murray as early as 1926, when he investigated nine kinds of botanical trees for the relationship between the circumference of stems and branches and the weight of all the parts peripheral to those points.[17,18] A non-integer power law was found: cross-sectional area of the stems and branches = $k \times$ weight$^{2/5}$ (k being a constant; Fig. 2.1).

In a circulatory system built by connecting and branching tubes, the perfusion pressure drop along increasingly smaller tubes is an indicator for the energy consumed or dissipated during the transport of fluid within the circulation. According to Ohm's law, the perfusion pressure drop can be described as the product of the vascular resistance (R) to flow and the flow rate Q:

$$\Delta P = R \times Q$$

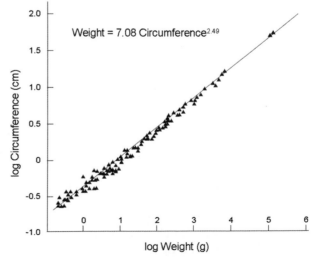

Fig. 2.1 Power law relation between the weight of nine different kinds of trees (*horizontal axis*; logarithmic scale) and the stem circumference (*vertical axis*; logarithmic scale). Range of circumference of branch stems to the main stem of the tree: 0.25–56.4 cm; range of weight of leaves to the entire tree: 0.18 g to 120 kg. Number of measurements: 116[17,18]

In the systemic circulation, ΔP is the difference between aortic perfusion pressure (P_{ao}, mmHg) and central venous pressure (CVP, mmHg). In the normal blood circulation, vascular resistance R is mainly due to viscous friction between the blood and the vascular wall. Based on Ohm's law, pressure drop along the vascular path is further described by Hagen-Poiseuille's law, which specifies the components of vascular geometry contributing to its resistance against flow (Fig. 2.2). If the principle of energy efficiency for the transport of blood in the coronary circulation governs its structural design as it is demon-

$$P_{ao} - CVP = \underbrace{R}_{8\mu\pi^{-1}\,L/r^4} \times Q$$

Fig. 2.2 Ohm's law (*black figures*) of the relationship between the perfusion pressure drop (P_{ao}–CVP) in the systemic circulation and the product of vascular resistance and volume flow. Vascular resistance to flow (R) is specified by Hagen-Poiseuille's law (*red figures*). Abbreviations: CVP = central venous pressure (mmHg); L = vascular branch length (cm); P_{ao} = aortic pressure (mmHg); Q = volume flow rate of blood (ml/min or cm^3/min); R = vascular resistance to flow (dyn s cm^{-5}); r = vascular radius (cm); μ = blood viscosity (0.03 dyne s cm^{-2}); π = 3.14159 26535 89793...

strated for a multitude of different organs and species,[14] then the law of minimum energy dissipation applies. The term 'minimum energy dissipation' is defined by the balance between two energy-consuming factors related to the transport of blood[15,17,18]: the Hagen-Poiseuille law on one hand (the bigger the tubes, the less energy is dissipated), and the energy delivered by the organism for the building and maintenance of the tubing and its content on the other hand (called energy content of blood; the bigger the tubes, the more energy is necessary). Energy loss or dissipation is optimal with regard to vessel size in case of a balance between viscous friction energy loss and the energy content of blood (Fig. 2.3). Mathematically, optimal vessel radius for a given blood flow rate Q at any point of interest in the vascular tree is equal to the first derivative of the two energy components being zero. Consequently, the following non-integer power law can be derived describing the relationship between cross-sectional vascular area (A, mm^2) at any point in the coronary artery tree and the respective flow rate Q:

$$A = 0.4 \times Q^{2/3}$$

Using various measurement techniques, normal myocardial perfusion under resting conditions has been documented to be close to 1 ml/min/g of tissue (Fig. 2.4).[19–21] Thus numerically, Q can be replaced by regional myocardial mass M, supplied by blood at any point of interest in the coronary tree. The regional myocardial mass M located downstream of a certain point in the

Design of the coronary artery tree structure

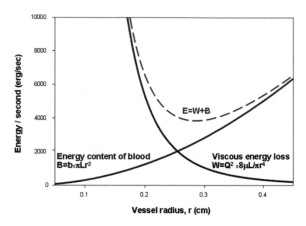

Fig. 2.3 Principle of minimum viscous energy loss during the transport of blood. Relationship between energy loss per second (*vertical axis*) due to viscous friction (W; black line) and the radius of a coronary artery (r; *horizontal axis*) at an assumed flow rate of 250 cm^3/min (perfusion of a left ventricle with a mass of 250 g). On the same scale, the energy content of blood plus the vascular structure (B; *blue line*) and the sum of both (E; *red line*) are plotted. Total energy loss (W + B; *red line*) becomes minimal when the first derivative d(W + B)/dr is equal to zero, indicating the least energy loss per unit of time at the lowest point of the curve. The corresponding vessel radius of the theoretical coronary artery (left main coronary artery) carrying the mentioned flow would be 0.27 cm[15]. Abbreviations: see Fig. 2.2

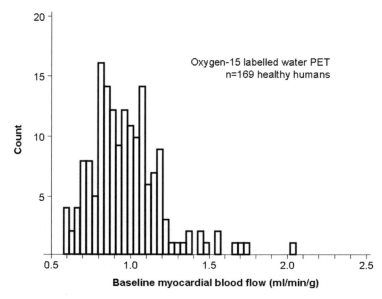

Fig. 2.4 Frequency distribution of uncorrected baseline myocardial blood flow values (*horizontal axis*) at rest as obtained by positron emission tomography (PET) using oxygen-15 labelled water in 169 healthy human individuals[20]

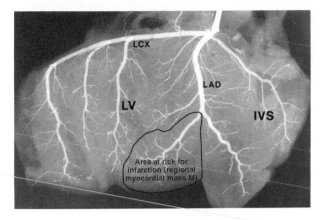

Fig. 2.5 Post-mortem coronary angiography of a canine left ventricle. The left coronary artery circulation is filled with barium-sulfate–gelatine mass and dissected according to the method of the 'unrolled heart', whereby the right ventricle was separated from the left ventricle (LV). The red perimeter indicates the area at risk for myocardial infarction or the ischaemic territory in case of an occlusion of the large diagonal branch of the left anterior descending coronary artery (LAD), and in the absence of inter-arterial anastomoses from the left circumflex coronary artery (LCX). Abbreviations: IVS = inter-ventricular septum; LV = left ventricle

coronary artery tree is equal to the anatomic area of risk (AR) for myocardial infarction (Fig. 2.5). The robustness of the power law describing the coronary artery tree structure in terms of vessel size and M has been confirmed using echocardiographic measures of left main coronary artery size and total left ventricular (LV) mass (Figs. 2.6 and 2.7[22]), as well as endurance exercise-induced change of left main coronary artery size relative to the corresponding, physiologic LV hypertrophy (Fig. 2.8[23]).

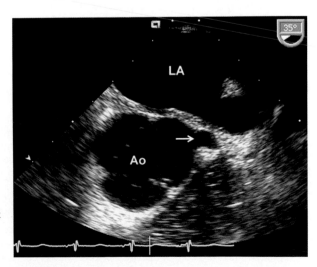

Fig. 2.6 Trans-oesophageal short-axis view of the aortic root (Ao) showing the proximal segment of the left main coronary artery (→). Abbreviation: LA = left atrium

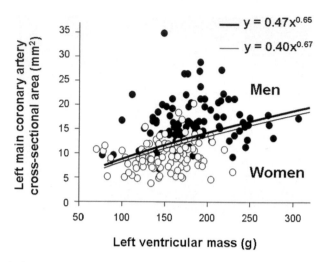

Fig. 2.7 Correlation between the left main coronary artery cross-sectional area (*vertical axis*) as obtained by trans-oesophageal echocardiography (see Fig. 2.6) and left ventricular mass as obtained by M-mode echocardiography in 200 individuals (100 women) without cardiac disease. The thick line represents the actual regression line fitted to a power equation; the thin line represents the theoretical power law equation according to minimum viscous energy dissipation

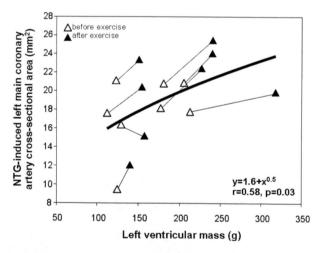

Fig. 2.8 Correlation between nitroglycerin (NTG)-induced left main coronary artery cross-sectional area (*vertical axis*) and left ventricular mass before and after an endurance exercise programme (*horizontal axis*). The bold line indicates the significant curvilinear regression between the two parameters. The thin lines connect individual ventricular mass-coronary calibre values before and after the exercise programme

The AR for myocardial infarction or regional myocardial mass M can be defined angiographically in terms of summed coronary artery branch lengths distal to any point in the coronary tree (L, cm) relative to the entire coronary artery tree length (L_{tot})[24]:

$$M/M_{\text{tot}} = L/L_{\text{tot}},$$

whereby M_{tot} corresponds to LV mass. Semiquantitatively, AR or M can also be estimated on the basis of the number of vascular branching points distal to the site of interest (Fig. 2.5). With regard to the absence or presence of (epicardial) anastomoses within the coronary tree, the traditionally hold view of the normal human coronary circulation as an *end-arterial* system[25,26] would have no adjacent myocardial regions with overlapping supply (Fig. 2.9), and thus, AR ($\equiv M$) would correspond to the summed coronary artery branch lengths distal to any point within the coronary tree.[24] In comparison, an *anastomotic* system[27] would be built with overlapping risk areas by epicardial collateral arteries or arterioles extending beyond the vascular territorial borders (Figs. 2.9, 2.10 and 2.11).

Since the heart can hardly increase oxygen extraction from haemoglobin on demand, increased acute requirements have to be fulfilled by instantaneous augmentation of coronary blood flow. Thus, 'on top' of the structure of coronary blood supply described above, there is *functional* adaptability of the coronary circulation. Coronary blood flow regulation including autoregulation occurs via coronary micro-vascular resistance changes (R_{m}; Fig. 2.12). Autoregulation refers to the intrinsic mechanism that maintains blood flow constant at varying aortic perfusion pressures between 60 and 130 mmHg.[28] Acute regulation of myocardial blood flow is mediated by extrinsic, but mainly by

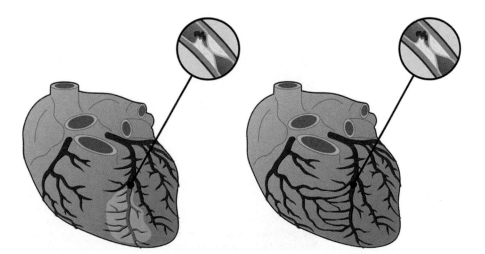

Fig. 2.9 Schematic drawing of the coronary artery circulation without (*left panel*) and with inter-arterial anastomoses (*right panel*) between the right coronary artery and the occluded left anterior descending artery (LAD; occluded beyond the third diagonal branch). The grey area indicates the area at risk for myocardial infarction (AR) in case of the LAD occlusion and in the absence of collaterals (corresponding to the infarct size in the example on the *left side*). The AR in the example on the right side is equal to zero because of the extended collaterals

Fig. 2.10 Right coronary
artery (RCA) angiogram
(left anterior oblique, cranial
view) in an individual
without coronary
atherosclerotic lesions
showing collateral arteries
(→) between the RCA and
left circumflex coronary
artery (LCX)

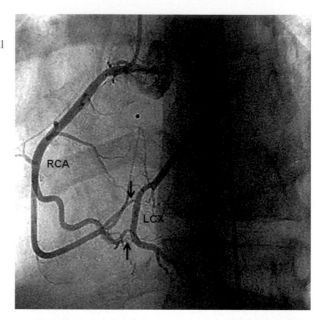

Fig. 2.11 Right coronary
artery (RCA) angiogram
(left anterior oblique, cranial
view) in an individual with
agenesis of the left main
coronary artery. The left
coronary artery system is
filled with contrast medium
via collateral arteries (→)
originating from the RCA.
Abbreviation: LAD = left
anterior descending artery

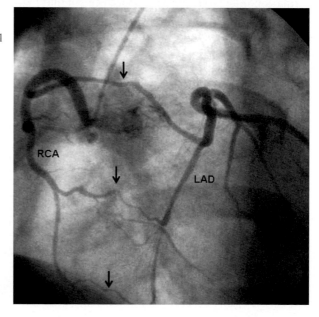

the following intrinsic factors: accumulation of local metabolites (mostly adenosine), neural innervation (sympathetic stimulation) and endothelium-derived
substances (nitric oxide, endothelin and acetylcholine). In the absence of collateral flow, a brief coronary occlusion of 1 minute normally induces a four- to

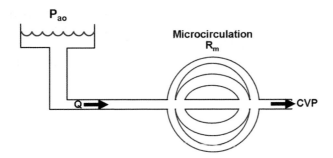

Fig. 2.12 Schematic drawing of the coronary epicardial, microcirculatory (*red part*) and venous system with the fluid mechanical components relevant for the description of coronary flow: aortic pressure (P_{ao}), central venous or right atrial pressure (CVP), coronary flow rate (Q) and microcirculatory resistance (R_m)

fivefold increase in blood flow or flow velocity above resting level immediately after release of the occlusion (Fig. 2.13). Initially, it was thought that short-lasting myocardial ischaemia is the most potent stimulus to achieve maximum flow or minimal myocardial resistance.[29] However, in animals, it appears that

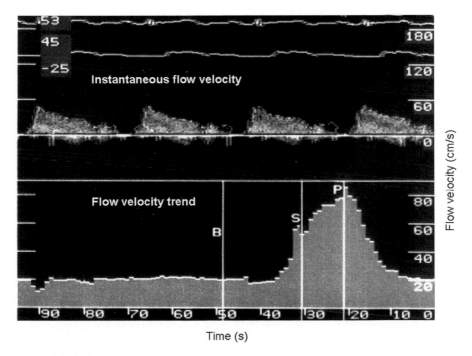

Time (s)

Fig. 2.13 Instantaneous coronary Doppler flow velocity spectrum (*upper part*) during four cardiac cycles, and average peak flow velocity trend (*lower part*) at baseline (B) and during hyperaemia (P) induced by intracoronary injection of adenosine. The coronary flow velocity reserve (maximum-to-baseline average peak flow velocity) in this case is equal to 4.1

even during low-flow ischaemia the resistance vessels retain some degree of vasomotor tone.[30] Analogous to the just-mentioned structural possibility of coronary arterial or arteriolar anastomoses (collateral arteries or arterioles) crossing the boundaries of vascular territories, there is, principally, the possibility of a functional or vasomotor response of collateral vessels to hyperaemic stimuli such as brief vascular occlusion. The clinical equivalent of such functional collateral response or collateral recruitment would be the development of tolerance to repetitive bouts of myocardial ischaemia, e.g. a relief of angina pectoris or warm-up angina pectoris.

2.1.4 Signs of Developing Tolerance to Myocardial Ischaemia

In 1802, William Heberden wrote in the context of the topic 'pectoris dolor'[31]: 'With respect to the treatment of this complaint, I have little or nothing to advance: nor indeed is it to be expected we should have made much progress in the cure of a disease, which has hitherto hardly had a place, or a name in medical books. . . .Opium taken at bed-time will prevent the attacks at night. I know one who set himself a task of sawing wood for half an hour every day, and was nearly cured'. The last sentence cited is regarded as the first description of the symptom of developing tolerance to recurring episodes of myocardial ischaemia (i.e. warm-up or walking through angina pectoris). However, collateral recruitment in response to multiple episodes of ischaemia is just one of the three possible explanations for the description by Heberden. The second is that of a cardiac mechanism different from collateral recruitment responsible for myocardial tolerance to ischaemia (ischaemic preconditioning; see below) and the third is exercise-induced permanent structural growth of coronary anastomoses (the latter would actually be less ischaemia). Fourthly, a combination of all could confer the perceived tolerance to ischaemia. As an alternative to angina pectoris, the degree of ECG ST elevation in response to a brief coronary artery occlusion is a more precise and robust means for the measurement of myocardial ischaemia (Fig. 2.14). As a surrogate for IS, clinical studies on the effect of various procedures of myocardial salvage have ubiquitously employed the magnitude of electrocardiographic changes during artificial coronary occlusion.[32] For example, during acute myocardial infarction, 'tombstone' ECG ST segment elevation (Fig. 2.14) is tightly associated with a large infarct in the left anterior descending coronary artery (LAD) region, the fact of which can be explained in part by the large area at risk of this territory, by site-specific myocardial vulnerability to ischaemia or both[33,34] (see also below).

In CAD patients, the *size* of myocardial infarction most importantly determines outcome after such an event.[35] Accordingly, it is the primary therapeutic goal to reduce cardiovascular mortality by shrinking IS (Fig. 2.15). The IS increases with coronary arterial occlusion time (t), myocardial AR, the lack of collateral supply, absence of preconditioning and myocardial oxygen demand

Fig. 2.14 ECG P-wave,
QRS-, T-wave curve with
marked ST-elevation
('tombstone' ECG with
defining criteria) indicating
very severe myocardial
ischaemia

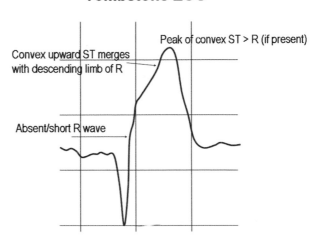

"Tombstone ECG"

Peak of convex ST > R (if present)

Convex upward ST merges
with descending limb of R

Absent/short R wave

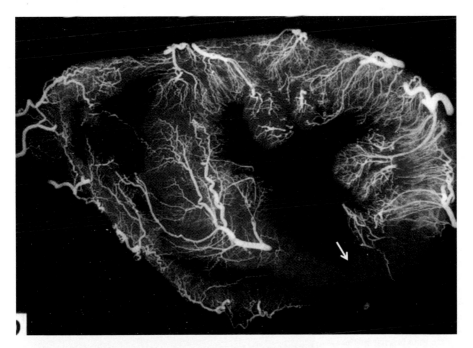

Fig. 2.15 Post-mortem coronary angiogram (*short axis view*) in a patient with infero-posterior myocardial infarction involving the left as well as the right ventricular wall. The infarct size (IS) is indicated by the extension of the myocardial area without contrast-filled coronary arteries. As an additional feature of the infarct area, the left ventricular posterior wall is thinned (→)

(i.e. the product of contractility, heart rate and ventricular wall stress)[36,37]; this can be expressed as follows:

$$IS \approx t \times AR \times coll^{-1} \times preconditioning^{-1} \times O_2 \text{ consumption}$$

According to the above-mentioned design principles of the coronary artery circulation, regional myocardial mass M or AR is equal to $M_{tot} \times L/L_{tot}$.[24] In the presence of collateral arteries supplied by an adjacent vascular area to an occluded coronary artery, L of the collateral supplying or contralateral artery is extended across regional boundaries toward the collateral receiving or ipsilateral artery, thereby diminishing or replacing AR of the occluded vessel and preventing infarction, i.e. reducing IS to zero (Figs. 2.16 and 2.17). As a consequence, AR is inversely related to the collateral flow (i.e. AR is a function of $coll^{-1}$), the fact of which has recently also been confirmed using cardiac magnetic resonance imaging (MR).[38] Thus, the mentioned equation describing IS can be simplified as follows:

$$IS \approx t \times coll^{-1} \times preconditioning^{-1} \times O_2 \text{ consumption}$$

Furthermore, if L of the collateral supplying artery is 'shrinking' AR of the collateral receiving artery, then L of collateral vessels may be employed as a measure of collateral supply. This can be regarded as the theoretical basis for the angiographic method of collateral grading according to the retrograde filling of the occluded ipsilateral artery (see below).[39]

Traditionally, therapeutic strategies for IS reduction consist of lowering O_2 consumption (heart rate reduction), and, above all, of minimizing coronary artery

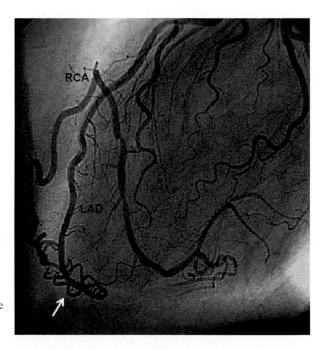

Fig. 2.16 Left coronary angiogram (*lateral view*) with extensive collateral supply of the chronically occluded right coronary artery (RCA) by a branch collateral artery ($\rightarrow$) originating from the left anterior descending coronary artery (LAD) and connecting to a right ventricular branch of the RCA. The summed coronary branch length of the LAD is, thereby, stretched by the length of the collateral artery plus the length of the RCA

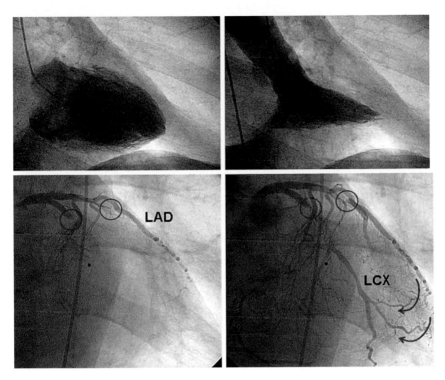

Fig. 2.17 Normal left ventricular angiogram (*upper panels*; right anterior oblique view) in a patient with three-vessel coronary artery occlusion (*red circles*; imaging of the right coronary artery during left coronary contrast injection; →; *lower panels*). The occluded left circumflex coronary artery (LCX) is filled by contrast via collaterals originating from the intermediary branch. Abbreviation: LAD = left anterior descending coronary artery

occlusion time until revascularization. However, in the presence of a chronic proximal total coronary occlusion with normal systolic LV function (Fig. 2.17), the duration of the occlusion is, obviously, irrelevant for IS. It is estimated that in patients undergoing coronary angiography, such a situation is encountered in up to one-third.[40,41] Similarly, it has been found in patients with acute myocardial infarction undergoing a brief coronary balloon occlusion with invasive collateral measurement that, in the presence of high collateral flow, the time to vascular reperfusion is not related to a functional measure of IS (ventricular wall motion recovery index) (Fig. 2.18[42]). In the settings described and assuming a constant O_2 utilization, the only determinants of IS are collateral supply and myocardial preconditioning, i.e. the protagonists in the list of contributors to the development of myocardial tolerance to repetitive ischaemia. In humans, the question, whether it is collateral recruitment, preconditioning or both which are responsible for reduced ECG ST elevation (surrogate for reduced IS) upon repetitive coronary occlusions, has been studied using the coronary angioplasty model with repetitive 1- to 3-minutes vascular occlusions[43] (Fig. 2.19).

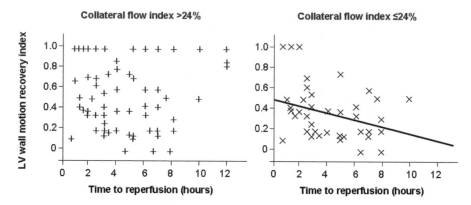

Fig. 2.18 Left ventricular wall-motion recovery index at 30-day after acute myocardial infarction (*vertical axis*) in relation to time to coronary reperfusion by primary percutaneous coronary intervention (*horizontal axis*). Wall-motion recovery index is independent of time to reperfusion among patients with well-developed coronary collaterals (*left panel*). There is an inverse correlation between wall-motion recovery index and time to reperfusion in patients with insufficient collaterals (*right panel*)

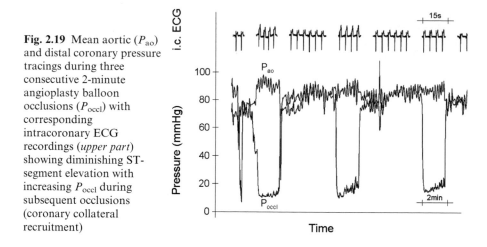

Fig. 2.19 Mean aortic (P_{ao}) and distal coronary pressure tracings during three consecutive 2-minute angioplasty balloon occlusions (P_{occl}) with corresponding intracoronary ECG recordings (*upper part*) showing diminishing ST-segment elevation with increasing P_{occl} during subsequent occlusions (coronary collateral recruitment)

In 1986, Murry et al. introduced the term 'ischaemic preconditioning', and referred to it as myocardial adaptation to ischaemic stress induced by recurring short periods of ischaemia and reperfusion.[44] The results of that study in dogs have been that, irrespective of collateral flow to the AR, four repetitive 5-minutes coronary occlusions followed by a 40-minutes permanent occlusion limits IS to one-fourth when compared to the situation without ischaemic preconditioning. However, what routinely remains concealed during citation of this landmark study is that its second protocol (identical preconditioning procedure followed by a more realistic 3-hours occlusion) has *not* documented myocardial protection by preconditioning but exclusively by collateral flow at a

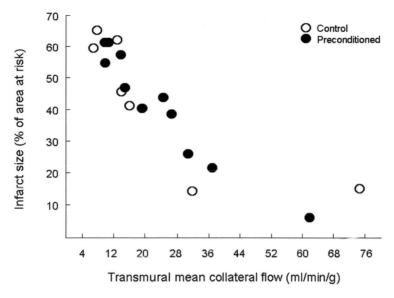

Fig. 2.20 Relationship between infarct size (*vertical axis*) and collateral flow to the occluded left circumflex coronary artery (LCX) region (*horizontal axis*). Preconditioned animals (n = 9 dogs) were treated by four 5-minute LCX occlusions (separated by 5 minutes of reperfusion) and then a sustained 3-hour occlusion. Control animals (n = 7) received a single 3-hour LCX occlusion. There is no difference in infarct size between preconditioned and control animals[44]

level above ∼0.3 ml/min/g (Fig. 2.20).[44] All the same, warm-up and walking through angina pectoris, traditionally ascribed to coronary vasodilation with opening of collateral channels, have recently been attributed more often to preconditioning, a biochemical process triggered and mediated by the release of adenosine from ischaemic myocytes, and by the subsequent activation of adenosine A1 receptors.[45,46] Ischaemic preconditioning has been extensively studied and yet the exact mechanism of protection remains unclear.[47] The earlier, biomechanical interpretation for the development of ischaemic toler- ance has been even temporarily abandoned because the presence of collateral vessels on angiography could not be shown to predict warm-up angina.[48] However, Rentrop et al. in 1985 demonstrated augmented filling of collateral channels during coronary angiography (contralateral dye injection) in response to angioplasty balloon occlusion when compared to the situation before occlusion.[39] Similarly as in many studies focusing on the effect of ischaemic preconditioning,[49-52] Rentrop et al. investigated only one of the potential contributors to the development of myocardial ischaemia tolerance, i.e. collateral recruitment without assessing the degree of ischaemia. Billinger et al. performed a study with simultaneous measurement of intracoronary ECG ST elevation and quantitative collateral assessment during 120 seconds of coronary balloon occlusion in 30 patients undergoing percutaneous cor- onary intervention (PCI).[43] The results of that study in patients with poorly

Fig. 2.21 Mean aortic (P_{ao}) and distal coronary pressure tracings during three consecutive 2-minute angioplasty balloon occlusions (P_{occl}) with corresponding intracoronary ECG recordings (*upper part*) showing no change in ST-segment elevation and no change of P_{occl} during subsequent occlusions

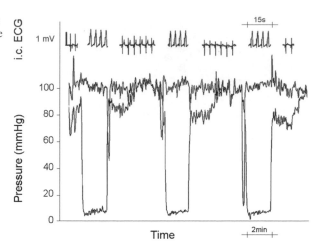

developed collaterals revealed a majority of patients (23 of 30) with collateral recruitment between the first and third coronary balloon occlusions (Fig. 2.19); a minority showed no change (Fig. 2.21) or even a decrease in collateral flow. In association with collateral recruitment, ECG ST signs of developing tolerance to repetitive bouts of myocardial ischaemia have been observed (Fig. 2.22). However, the variable response of ECG signs of

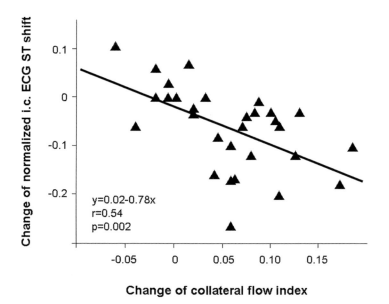

Change of collateral flow index

Fig. 2.22 Relationship between change of ECG ST segment shift during three subsequent 2-minute coronary occlusions (*vertical axis*; ST shift normalized for QRS amplitude) and change of collateral flow index (*horizontal axis*; collateral flow index during the third minus that during the first occlusion). Abbreviation: i.c. = intracoronary

myocardial ischaemic adaptation to collateral recruitment (the latter accounting for only about one-third of the association) has indicated ischaemic preconditioning as another relevant factor responsible for ischaemia attenuation following repetitive coronary occlusions.[43]

Therefore, the phenomenon of warm-up angina pectoris first described by Heberden[31] is most likely related to both ischaemic preconditioning and collateral recruitment. For the non-invasive coronary collateral characterization in humans, the search for signs of developing tolerance to myocardial ischaemia is quite suitable though not entirely specific.

2.2 Non-invasive Characterization of Collaterals

The factors related to the extent of collateralization are the duration of myocardial ischaemic symptoms and the severity of coronary artery stenoses. Thus, non-invasively detectable factors indicative of severe coronary artery stenoses point towards a well-developed collateral circulation, whereby the large variability of collateral flow for a given stenosis severity suggests low accuracy of such indicators. The following ECG parameters have been employed for characterizing the human coronary collateral circulation: sinus bradycardia, ventricular ectopic beats, the presence of a U wave and the amount of QT-dispersion. Using exercise-induced ECG U wave alterations, complete absence of myocardial ischaemia during coronary balloon occlusion has been predicted with a sensitivity of 69% and a specificity of 72%.

In comparison to non-occlusive chronic CAD, the setting of acute ECG ST segment elevation myocardial infarction is more distinctive for the purpose of non-invasive collateral assessment, since the total coronary occlusion allows the interpretation of the extent and the degree of ST elevation on the basis of its contributing factors, area at risk and collateral circulation. However, infarct location by ECG may no longer identify the coronary artery responsible for the event when abundant collaterals are present.

2.2.1 Indicators for the Coronary Collateral Circulation

As mentioned, the patient's history does not provide a high likelihood of detecting a well-developed coronary collateral circulation. In the positive event, warm-up or walking through angina pectoris may indicate best the existence of functionally relevant collateral arteries. The question is whether there are clinical symptoms and signs *indirectly* pointing to a competent collateral circulation, i.e. whether certain clinical variables are associated with well-developed collaterals. Well-established factors positively determining the extent of collateralization are the duration of myocardial ischaemic symptoms and the severity of coronary artery stenoses, i.e. indicators for the severity of CAD.[53,54] Thus, non-invasively detectable factors indicative of severe coronary artery stenoses could point towards a well-developed collateral circulation, whereby

Fig. 2.23 Correlation between coronary collateral function (*vertical axis*; collateral relative to normal antegrade flow) and degree of coronary artery narrowing (*horizontal axis*)

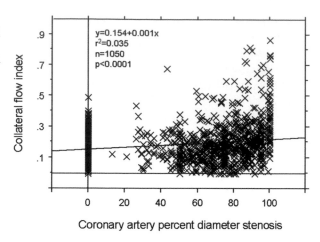

the known large variability of collateral flow for a given stenosis severity suggests low accuracy of such indicators in detecting conductive collaterals (Fig. 2.23). In chronic stable CAD, indicators for severely narrowed coronary arteries are the degree of angina pectoris, the level of physical effort at which ECG signs of ischaemia or chest pain occur and the incidence of specific ECG signs during exercise (see below). In the event of an acute myocardial infarction, the 'model' for non-invasive collateral assessment becomes more distinctive as compared to chronic non-occlusive CAD, because the coronary artery is occluded, and the signs of ischaemia, e.g. on the surface ECG, can be related solely to collateral supply and ischaemic preconditioning and not to varying degrees of stenoses.

In both chronic CAD and the acute coronary syndrome, to use the ECG for non-invasive collateral assessment is reasonable because of the tight relationship between ECG signs of ischaemia and the status of the collateral circulation, and because it reflects the degree of ischaemia as well as the subsequent IS much more precisely than the symptomatic status of the patient.

2.2.2 The Surface Lead ECG for Estimation of the Collateral Circulation

2.2.2.1 Chronic CAD

Except for the situation with a chronic total coronary occlusion, the contribution to net myocardial perfusion of antegrade flow via the stenotic native coronary artery and collateral flow cannot be differentiated non-invasively (see also Section 2.3). Conversely and theoretically, it can be expected that in a collateral supplying artery there is more flow or a higher flow velocity during resting conditions than in the situation without collaterals, the fact of which has been confirmed in the literature.[55,56] As a consequence, the capacity to increase flow (coronary flow reserve) in the collateral supplying artery may be impaired, but no exact conclusions can be drawn from that on the amount of collateral perfusion taking off the vessel of interest. Accordingly, it is not feasible to decide whether signs of myocardial ischaemia are caused by the stenosis of the native vessel, by insufficiently conductive collaterals or both. Nevertheless, the following ECG parameters have been employed more or less usefully for characterizing the human coronary collateral circulation: sinus bradycardia, ventricular ectopic beats, the presence of a U wave and the amount of QT-dispersion. In general, all of these ECG signs are indicators of myocardial electrical stability (bradycardia) or instability in response to ischaemia, i.e. heterogeneity of repolarization or variable regional repolarization delay. In this context, early experimental work in dogs has elegantly documented that the electrical current required to induce ventricular fibrillation is lowered from approximately 6 milliampère during coronary artery patency to 3.5 milliampère immediately after coronary occlusion.[57] During the course of that study, the ventricular fibrillation threshold increased relative to the development of coronary collateral anastomoses (Fig. 2.24).[57]

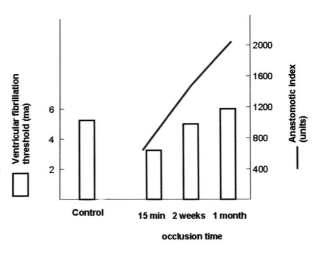

Fig. 2.24 Relationship between anastomotic index and ventricular fibrillation threshold (*vertical axes*) before ('control'), 15 minutes, 2 weeks and 1 month after coronary occlusion in open-chest dogs. The current in milliampère (ma) required to induce ventricular fibrillation was obtained by passing constant current pulses through left ventricular myocardium[57]

Bradycardia has been described to be a particularly good model of coronary angiogenesis in the experimental animal model,[58,59] and in rats it has been found to be dependent on vascular endothelial growth factor activation.[60] Slowing the heart rate results in augmented coronary blood flow due to over-proportional diastolic prolongation leading to increased tangential vascular shear stress. Such mechanical factors have been hypothesized to induce angiogenesis.[61] Alternatively, resting bradycardia as a marker of a physically well-conditioned organism could just *indicate* the angiogenic or arteriogenic effect of regular physical exercise. It is in part due to this conceptual uncertainty that in humans there has not been much evidence of bradycardia being associated with coronary collateral development.[62] Even to a lesser extent, the presence of bradycardia is feasible to serve as a diagnostic tool for the detection of a well-developed coronary collateral circulation.

Ventricular arrhythmias precipitated by myocardial ischaemia due to acute coronary occlusion are the cause of a majority of sudden cardiac deaths.[63] In the context of the above-mentioned direct relationship between ventricular fibrillation threshold in response to acute coronary occlusion and the state of the collateral circulation in animals,[57] studies in humans on this topic have focused on coronary stenosis severity and the occurrence of ventricular ectopic activity during balloon angioplasty,[64] or they have looked for angiographic or clinical determinants for out-of-hospital ventricular fibrillation in patients with acute myocardial infarction.[65,66] While Airaksinen et al. did find an association between the presence of ischaemia-induced ventricular arrhythmia and the lack of angiographic collaterals,[64] Gheeraert et al. showed that the frequency of collateral vessels to the infarct-related artery did not differ among patients with and without ventricular fibrillation.[65] However, in a meta-analysis on risk factors for primary ventricular fibrillation during acute myocardial infarction performed subsequently, the same group found absence of a history of angina pectoris (vaguely indicative of poorly developed collaterals) to be related to ventricular fibrillation.[66] In accordance with these controversial results, the use of ventricular ectopic beats for the non-invasive characterization of collaterals is likely not feasible. However, indicators of repolarization heterogeneity have been documented to be more promising for the non-invasive assessment of the collateral circulation.

Appearance of *ECG U wave* (Fig. 2.25) at rest or during exercise is known to point to significant CAD with critical arterial narrowing.[67] Miwa et al. specifically investigated whether exercise-induced U wave alterations in patients with angina pectoris occur in the context of well-functioning collateral vessels.[68] In 125 patients with stable effort angina pectoris who underwent a 1-minute coronary balloon occlusion during their PCI, the authors have found less ischaemic ECG ST changes and chest pain during coronary occlusion in those with (n = 46) versus those without (n = 79) exercise-induced U wave changes.[68] In predicting complete absence of myocardial ischaemia during balloon inflation by the presence of U wave alterations, the sensitivity has been 69% and the specificity 72%.[68] It has been speculated that U waves are related to regional heterogeneity of recovery from transient severe transmural myocardial ischaemia or regional repolarization delay in ischaemic but viable myocardium. It is, however, not entirely plausible that absence of signs of myocardial ischaemia during a brief coronary occlusion due to well-developed collaterals should then manifest as pronounced U waves, i.e. an indicator of severe ischaemia.

The ECG *QT interval* dispersion (maximal minus minimal QT interval on a 12-lead ECG) has become a non-invasive measure for assessing the degree of myocardial repolarization heterogeneity, which itself has been interpreted as a

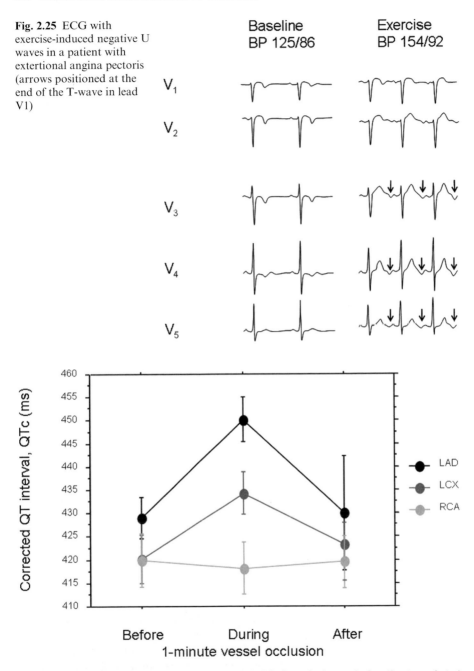

Fig. 2.25 ECG with exercise-induced negative U waves in a patient with extertional angina pectoris (arrows positioned at the end of the T-wave in lead V1)

Fig. 2.26 Corrected QT interval (QTc; *vertical axis*) before, during and after (*horizontal aixs*) a 1-minute angioplasty balloon occlusion in 150 patients with chronic stable CAD at a proximal site of the left anterior descending coronary artery (LAD), the left circumflex (LCX) and the right coronary artery (RCA). There is no significant change in QTc during occlusion of the RCA

substrate supporting the development of serious ventricular arrhythmias and sudden cardiac death.[69] There has been an almost complete lack of clinical studies investigating the relationship between QT interval and the status of the collateral circulation. Tandogan et al. examined 100 patients with chronic CAD who had at least an 85% stenosis in the left anterior descending artery (LAD) or in the proximal right coronary artery (RCA).[70] The surprising main result of that study has been that the patients without angiographic collaterals revealed a shorter QTc dispersion (corrected QT dispersion = 47 ms) than the patients with collateral vessels (QTc dispersion = 64 ms; p = 0.003). Conversely, preliminary data from our laboratory indicate that the QTc extension observed during a 1-minute coronary balloon occlusion in the left (but not in the right) coronary artery (Fig. 2.26) is absent or even manifests as an abbreviation among patients with a well versus poorly developed coronary collateral circulation (Fig. 2.27).

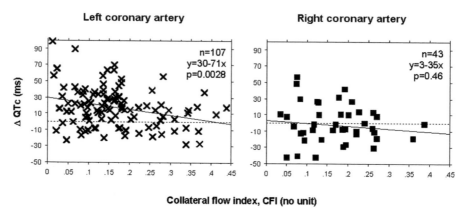

Fig. 2.27 Correlation between change of corrected QT interval (ΔQTc, i.e. QTc during minus QTc before occlusion; *vertical axis*) in response to a 1-minute coronary occlusion of the left (*left panel*) and the right coronary arteries (*right panel*) and the simultaneously obtained coronary collateral function (collateral flow index; *horizontal axis*). There is an inverse relationship between the two parameters in the left but not the right coronary artery territory

2.2.2.2 Acute Myocardial Infarction

In comparison to chronic CAD and except for chronic total coronary occlusion, the setting of acute ECG ST elevation myocardial infarction is much more distinctive for the purpose of non-invasive collateral assessment, since the total coronary occlusion allows the interpretation of the extent and the degree of ST elevation on the basis of its contributing factors, i.e. duration of occlusion (symptoms of continuous chest pain), collateral supply to the occluded vascular territory and myocardial area at risk for infarction, which itself is inversely related to collateral supply (see above). In this context, Christian et al.

investigated the relationship between an ECG ST segment elevation score and radionuclide ([99m]technetium sestamibi) measures of myocardial AR (= perfusion defect size) and collateral flow (= perfusion defect severity) in 67 patients with acute myocardial infarction who underwent primary PCI.[71] The principal results of this study have been that the initial standard 12-lead ECG provides insight into AR, and, even more so, collateral flow, and can estimate subsequent IS. The ECG score employed for the estimation of ST segment elevation is calculated as follows:

For anterior myocardial infarction,

$$AR = 4.5 \text{ (number of leads with ST elevation} \geq 1 \text{ mm)} - 1.2;$$

for inferior myocardial infarction,

$$IS/AR = 1.8 \text{ (mm of ST elevation in leads II, III, aVF)} + 6.0$$

These formulas have been developed to predict the extent of jeopardized myocardium at admission with an acute myocardial infarction.[72,73] Christian et al. also demonstrated that using an ECG multivariate model, the following factors independently determined final IS as measured by [99m]technetium sestamibi: infarct location as a measure of area at risk (p < 0.0001), ST segment elevation score as a measure of residual blood flow via collaterals (p = 0.003) and time elapsed from chest pain onset (p = 0.06).[71] Figure 2.28 provides an example for the calculation of ST segment elevation score in a patient with acute anteroseptal myocardial infarction according to the ECG (symptom onset 8.5 hours before admission): AR = 4.5 (three leads with ST elevation ≥ 1 mm) – 1.2 = 12.3 (i.e. AR = 12.3% of LV myocardium). The suspected lesion in this case was the subtotal proximal stenosis of the RCA which supplied collateral flow to the chronically occluded LAD (Fig. 2.29). Due to an additional, severe stenotic lesion of the mid-LAD, the first diagonal-branch-area as the 'last meadow' supplied by the collateral-spending RCA became severely ischaemic (Fig. 2.29; no infarction according to normal creatine kinase and troponin I levels immediately before coronary intervention). The LV angiography revealed no wall motion abnormalities of the anterolateral wall and an ejection fraction of 60%. This case illustrates several aspects with regard to the ECG use for collateral characterization in acute coronary syndrome and are as follows: (a) As in the univariate analysis of Christian et al.'s study,[71] the presence of well-developed collaterals most strongly predicts the lack of ST segment elevation, whereas time to presentation in the catheterization laboratory only weakly relates to ST elevation. (b) AR is less tightly associated with ST segment elevation than collateral supply, because AR 'shrinks' with collateral supply, and, thus, is dependent on collateral supply. AR in the sense of infarct location may no longer identify the coronary artery responsible for the event when abundant collaterals are present. (c) In the individual case, final IS may not be foretold by ST segment elevation.

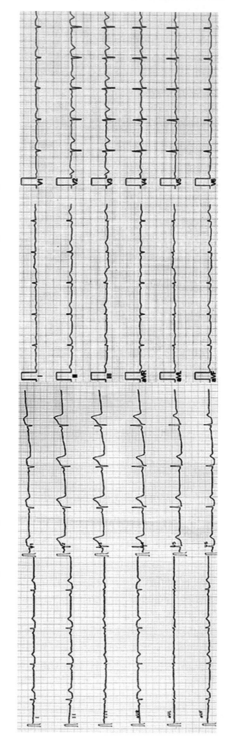

Fig. 2.28 12-Lead ECG in a patient with acute anteroseptal myocardial infarction before (*left panel*) and after (*right panel*) primary percutaneous coronary intervention (PCI). Following the intervention, there is no evidence of a transmural myocardial infarction

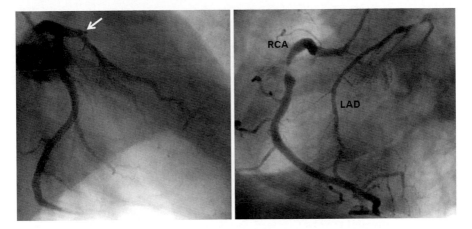

Fig. 2.29 Left (*left panel*) and right coronary angiography (*right panel*) of the same patient as in Fig. 2.28 showing a chronic total occlusion (→) of the left anterior descending coronary artery (LAD) and a subtotal occlusion of the proximal right coronary artery (RCA), the collateral-supplying artery of the LAD (*right panel*)

2.3 The Coronary Occlusion Model

Coronary collateral quantification requires occlusion of the collateral receiving artery.

Investigating collateral-dependent myocardium downstream of a natural occlusion is attractive for several reasons, despite not being representative for all patients with CAD: once the diagnosis of a chronic total occlusion has been established angiographically, the collateralized region can be examined *non-invasively*; high collateral perfusion values are easier to detect and less prone to measurement errors than low flow; studies of dynamic collateral perfusion changes are technically less demanding in the non-invasive than in the invasive setting. However, studying collateral-dependent myocardium requires selection of patients with *viable* collateralized myocardium.

The following issues with regard to the artificial occlusion model have to be considered: occlusion site, number of occlusions and occlusion duration. The contribution of all collateral vessels to a collateral recipient artery is best obtainable using a proximal occlusion site. This is not feasible in case of the left main coronary artery. Low-inflation pressure, 1-minute balloon occlusion at other proximal, non-stenotic sites has proven to be a safe procedure. In studies focusing on one single value of collateral flow, there is just one occlusion lasting 1 minute, and the measurement is obtained at the end of the occlusion. If the focus is on ischaemic preconditioning and collateral recruitment, then 1 minute for each of three to four repetitive occlusions is likely not sufficient and ought to be 2 minutes.

The simplest but imprecise way to qualify collaterals is to ask the patient about the presence of angina pectoris during2 balloon occlusion. Yet, chest pain developed during coronary occlusion is dependent on the duration of ischae-mia, the degree of collaterals, prior myocardial infarction, autonomic nerve dysfunction, psychological and neurobiological characteristics of the patient and the degree of stretching of the coronary arterial wall by the occluding angioplasty balloon.

A dichotomous definition of coronary collateral vessels that are insufficient and sufficient, respectively, to prevent myocardial ischaemia is given by the presence and absence of ECG ST segment elevation >0.1 mV. The presence or absence of ST segment elevation on intracoronary ECG allows accurate differ-entiation between quantitatively obtained poor and good collateral function. ECG ST segment qualification of coronary collaterals is helpful in predicting long-term survival in patients with chronic CAD.

Despite the presence of chronic total coronary occlusion, systolic LV func-tion may be normal thanks to a well-developed collateral circulation. Conver-sely, despite the occurrence of coronary collaterals, a substantial number of patients with chronic total occlusions reveal various degrees of systolic LV dysfunction. Recovery of LV systolic dysfunction in a myocardial area sub-tended by chronic total occlusion and supplied by collaterals occurs in 40–50% following recanalization of the occlusion. Simultaneous assessment of regional LV function using tissue Doppler imaging and invasive collateral function measurement has revealed a statistically relevant association between LV func-tion and collateral function.

2.3.1 Introduction

In the case example just described (Figs. 2.28 and 2.29), it becomes *intuitively* evident that a natural or artificial occlusion of the ipsilateral, i.e. collateral receiving artery is indispensable for precise assessment of coronary flow via anastomoses. Conversely, without occlusion of the ipsilateral artery, the con-tribution of antegrade flow (via the patent native coronary artery) and collat-eral flow to net myocardial perfusion remains indistinguishable. This concept can also be derived *theoretically* using basic hydromechanic principles (Fig. 2.30). The coronary circulation can be reduced to a two-branch arterial tree with one anastomotic path in-between. Each of the vascular pathways to the myocardium (i.e. the 'antegrade' via a stenotic coronary artery and the collateral pathway) is expressed as its conductance (C), which is the inverse of vascular resistance. According to Ohm's law, conductance is defined as the blood volume flow rate per time for a given perfusion pressure drop along the path. Vascular conductance is chosen as the key parameter of interest on physiological grounds, because supply of blood to the myocardial cell accord-ing to its demand for oxygen and nutrient exchange within a certain range of perfusion pressures is the most important variable for organ function. Aside from the 'antegrade' (C_s) and the collateral conductance (C_{coll}), there is the

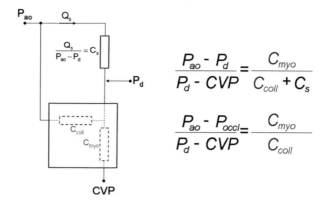

$$\frac{P_{ao} - P_d}{P_d - CVP} = \frac{C_{myo}}{C_{coll} + C_s}$$

$$\frac{P_{ao} - P_{occl}}{P_d - CVP} = \frac{C_{myo}}{C_{coll}}$$

Fig. 2.30 Schematic of an electrical analogue model of the coronary circulation with its perfusion pressure source (mean aortic pressure, P_{ao}), one bifurcation, whereby one branch is obstructed by a stenotic lesion (flow conductance in the stenotic branch, C_s), and the other branch is connected to the stenotic branch via an anastomosis (collateral flow conductance, C_{coll}). C_s is calculated by Ohm's law on the basis of flow in (Q_s) and pressure drop across the stenotic vessel. The composite of collateral and downstream myocardial conductance (C_{myo}) is indicated by the square. Pressure values directly obtainable aside from P_{ao} are distal coronary pressure (P_d) and central venous pressure (CVP)

terminal, myocardial or microcirculatory pathway with its conductance (C_{myo}). From a morphological point of view, this simplified coronary circulation consists of two systems: the stenotic epicardial artery is a lumped system, and can, therefore, be assessed by the measurement of localized parameters. In contrast, the coronary collateral pathway and the myocardial microcirculation form a distributed system, and they are, therefore, not accessible to selective measurements. In the absence of a coronary intrusion and with patent human epicardial coronary arteries, it is feasible to obtain the following localized parameters using invasive measurement techniques: aortic pressure (P_{ao}), epicardial ('antegrade') coronary artery flow rate (Q_s; using coronary cross-sectional area and Doppler-derived blood flow velocity measurements), coronary pressure distal to the stenotic lesion (P_d), and CVP (which acts as the back pressure in the coronary circulation). The question to be answered for the system is which interference or manipulation has to be performed in order to derive the three separate conductance values of interest. C_s can be calculated on the basis of Q_s, P_{ao} and P_d. The two unknown values of C_{coll} and C_{myo} have to be determined on the basis of two equations (Fig. 2.30). However, only one of them can be obtained by 'disturbing' or interfering with the system using a well-defined manipulation and by assessing the response to such an action. The most obvious manipulation consists of occluding the 'antegrade' epicardial coronary artery, and thus, to measure P_{occl}, the necessary parameter for computing the ratio of C_{myo} to C_{coll}.

2.3.2 Natural Occlusion Model

Approximately one-third of all coronary angiograms in patients with CAD show a chronic total occlusion of a coronary artery, and its presence often excludes patients from treatment by PCI.[40] Chronic total coronary occlusions are one of the commonest reasons for referral for coronary artery bypass surgery, and many are left untreated because of ambiguity regarding procedural success and long-term benefit. However, clinical data suggest that, if successful, revascularizing a chronic total occlusion provides a survival benefit.[74] It has been shown that only about 1 of 10 PCI procedures are for single vessel chronic total occlusions, and this has changed little over the last decade.[75] Since collateral development does not depend on the presence of viable myocardium but on a pressure gradient along preformed interarterial connections,[76] well-developed collateral arteries may also be observed with infarcted myocardium. Recanalizing chronic total occlusions to well-collateralized but non-viable myocardium is not reasonable and carries a high risk of reocclusion of up to 19% using bare metal stents.[77] Restenosis and reocclusion may be related to the generally high collateral flow supplied to vascular territories downstream of chronic occlusions, which act as competitor against the antegrade flow through the recanalized artery.[78] If the coronary occlusion occurs not abruptly but gradually, then there might be time for steady collateral growth leading to prevention of transmural myocardial infarction. In a series of our own laboratory that included 50 patients with chronic total occlusion, 27 had suffered a myocardial infarction in the region of interest, whereas 23 had not. Average collateral flow relative to normal flow among patients with collateral-dependent infarcted myocardium was significantly lower (0.280 ± 0.142) when compared to patients without infarction in the collateralized area (0.471 ± 0.206, $p = 0.0004$), but the former was higher than the average collateral flow in patients without chronic occlusion (Fig. 2.31).

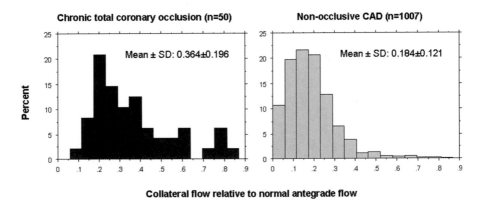

Fig. 2.31 Frequency distribution of collateral relative to normal antegrade coronary flow (collateral flow index) in patients with chronic total occlusion (*left panel*) and in those with non-obstructive coronary artery disease (CAD; *right panel*)

Based on the above information, it is evident that investigating collateral-dependent myocardium downstream of a natural chronic total occlusion is attractive for several reasons, while, at the same time, it is not representative for the entire group of CAD patients, and even less so for healthy individuals. (a) Once coronary angiography has established the diagnosis of a chronic total occlusion, the viable collateralized myocardial region can be examined *non-invasively* by an array of different techniques, which potentially can even measure absolute tissue perfusion in ml/min/g, i.e. the reference parameter for assessing coronary blood supply: by echocardiography with wall motion analysis and contrast imaging, by nuclear cardiology techniques such as [99m]technetium sestamibi single photon emission computed tomography imaging, by positron emission tomography (PET) or by MR. (b) Generally high collateral perfusion values are technically easier to detect and less prone to measurement errors than low-flow values. (c) Studies of dynamic changes of collateral perfusion in response to different physiological or pharmacological actions are technically less demanding and, thus, more feasible in the non-invasive than in the invasive setting. (d) However, studying collateral-dependent myocardium requires a meticulous selection of patients with *viable* collateralized myocardium (i.e. the patients without a history of infarction). (e) The fact that one-third of coronary angiographies reveal a chronic occlusion and that only about half of these patients have viable myocardium in the collateralized area constitutes a substantial selection bias of CAD patients (about 16% of the entire CAD population). (f) Additionally, there is a selection bias even with regard to the population with chronic total occlusions, in that those patients without symptoms despite a chronic occlusion may not be referred to coronary angiography in the first place.

Notwithstanding the limitations of the natural occlusion model, it is a well-established model for pathophysiological studies on collateral flow and its response to hyperaemic stimuli, on contractile dysfunction of viable but dysfunctional myocardium and on novel techniques for the non-invasive detection of collateralized myocardial territories. Except for some particular aspects of collateral perfusion, the function or (patho-)physiology of the collateral circulation is focused on in Chapter 4. In relative terms of antegrade coronary flow, collateral flow to a chronically occluded, non-infarcted region amounts to almost half the normal value (see above). Collateral-dependent and collateral-independent *absolute* myocardial blood flow or perfusion is of high interest (Table 2.1) and can be determined in patients using PET, myocardial contrast echocardiography (MCE), and, possibly, newer techniques such as contrast MR imaging. Using ^{13}N-ammonia PET in 26 patients with collateral-dependent myocardium, Vanoverschelde et al. found that blood flow at rest to collateralized versus remote segments was similar in patients without regional wall motion abnormalities (0.85 and 0.83 ml/min/g respectively); in patients with dysfunctional myocardium, collateral perfusion was lower than remote perfusion (0.77 and 0.96 ml/min/g respectively, p < 0.001).[79] It is, however, evident that the average collateral to normal perfusion ratio in that study was close to 1 and not just 0.5. Uren et al. employed PET with ^{15}O-labelled water

Table 2.1 Perfusion of collateral dependent myocardium* at rest in patients with chronic total occlusion

First author of study	Method	n	Collateral-dependent blood flow (ml/min/g)	Remote area blood flow (ml/min/g)	Normal myocardial blood flow (ml/min/g)
McFalls	PET, $^{15}O_2$ water	5	0.86±0.14	0.99±0.10	0.86±0.10
Uren	PET, $^{115}O_2$ water	9	0.91±0.20	0.99±0.26	–
Vanoverschelde	PET, ^{13}N-ammonia	26	0.81±0.20	0.88±0.21	–
Sambuceti	PET, ^{13}N-ammonia	19	0.61±0.11	0.63±0.17	1.0±0.20
Own data	Quantitative MCE	6	0.57±0.29	1.25±0.25	0.83±0.32
Muehling	First-pass contrast MR	30	0.98±0.28	1.12±0.11	1.14±0.21
Total		95	0.79	0.98	0.96

*Cases of viable and non-viable myocardium.
Abbreviations: MCE = myocardial contrast echocardiography; MR = magnetic resonance imaging; PET = positron emission tomography; n = number of study participants.

and observed in nine patients with an entirely collateralized but normally functioning myocardial region that absolute perfusion in the collateral dependent area at rest was 0.91 ml/min/g and 0.99 ml/min/g in the remote region.[80] In comparison, Sambuceti et al. documented absolute flow at rest of 0.61 ml/min/g in the collateralized region of 19 patients with chronic total occlusion and without a history of myocardial infarction (^{13}N-ammonia PET), whereas in the remote area it was 0.63 ml/min/g, both values of which were lower than myocardial perfusion in 13 normal control individuals (1.00 ml/min/g).[81] McFalls et al., using similar techniques (^{15}O-labelled water PET) and by examining five patients with normal ventricular function and who had an occluded major epicardial artery, observed a collateral dependent flow of 0.86 ml/min/g and a remote flow of 0.99 ml/min/g.[82] Data from our own laboratory obtained by quantitative MCE (see below for details about the technique) in a very similar patient population reveal a trend to lower collateral-dependent absolute perfusion of approximately 0.6 and 1.2 ml/min/g in the remote myocardial region (Table 2.1). Quantitative MR first-pass perfusion imaging using gadolinium-diethylene triamine pentaacetic acid as contrast medium has been used to detect angiographically proven chronic total coronary occlusion (time delay of hyperaemic contrast arrival versus LV >0.6 seconds; Fig. 2.32; sensitivity of 90%, specificity of 83%) and to obtain

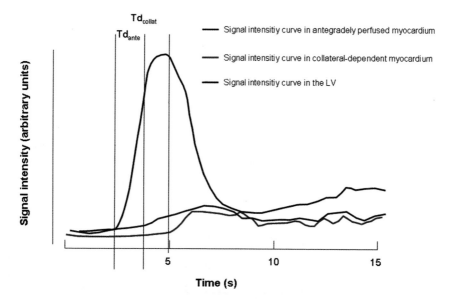

Fig. 2.32 Magnetic resonance imaging contrast signal intensity curves (*vertical axis*) recorded over time (*horizontal axis*) in a patient with chronic total coronary occlusion. The signal intensity curve for the left ventricle (LV) serves as arterial input and is depicted with tissue curves of antegradely perfused and collateralized myocardium. Td$_{ante}$ is the delay of contrast appearance in the antegradely perfused myocardium in comparison to the LV; Td$_{coll}$ is the delay of contrast appearance in the collateralized myocardium in comparison to the LV[83]

collateral-dependent myocardial blood flow (on average 0.98 ml/min/g; Table 2.1).[83] However, this potentially non-invasive technique for collateral assessment has to be validated in comparison with established techniques, and in particular, the following issues have to addressed: measurement precision of determining contrast arrival in collateralized territories (which may be difficult to discern from background noise; Fig. 2.32) and the biological influence of coronary steal on the perfusion distribution during pharmacological stress.[84]

2.3.3 *Artificial Occlusion Model*

At present, invasive cardiac examination is a prerequisite for reliable quantitative assessment of the human coronary collateral circulation. In the natural occlusion model, it is needed to confirm total coronary obstruction, and in the artificial occlusion model, it is essential for briefly blocking the vessel using an angioplasty balloon catheter. Additionally and as theoretically derived above, coherent and *exclusive* collateral characterization (Fig. 2.33) necessitates the permanent or temporary occlusion of the epicardial collateral receiving or ipsilateral artery, yielding the so called recruitable- as opposed to spontaneously visible-collateral flow.

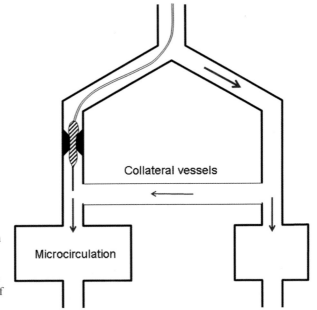

Fig. 2.33 Schematic of a two-branch coronary circulation with a stenotic, balloon-occluded vessel (*left*) and a non-stenotic vessel (*right*), both connected via a collateral vessel. The microcirculation is indicated by two rectangles. The red arrows show the direction and give an estimate of the amount of flow

In general, the following issues with regard to the coronary angioplasty model have to be considered: occlusion site, number of occlusions and occlusion duration.

2.3.3.1 Occlusion Site

It is most reasonable to perform the angioplasty balloon occlusion at the site of the stenosis to be treated, the fact of which may seem obvious. However theoretically, it would be most advantageous to assess the collateral circulation in an area at risk as large as possible, because then the sum of all supplying collateral vessels would be accounted for. Since in the absence of a chronic total occlusion, the epicardial coronary system is a widely communicating system, the lumped contribution of all collateral vessels could be obtained using a most proximal occlusion site. The most proximal site of the left coronary artery (LCA) is the left main coronary artery. Except for the situation of an indicated left main coronary artery PCI, we have not used the angioplasty model in this setting for collateral assessment. Yet, the proximal balloon occlusion site in the absence of a stenotic lesion is being chosen routinely at our laboratory. To perform a low-pressure balloon occlusion in a normal coronary artery segment has proven to be a safe procedure.[27,85] Normal coronary artery balloon occlusions have been performed at our institution in over 200 cases, and no adverse clinical events have been observed related to the procedure. More than 100 of these patients underwent a follow-up coronary angiography without evidence of a stenotic lesion at the (normal) site of the balloon occlusion. Thus, to choose the most proximal occlusion site (except for the left main coronary artery) is safe, but should be performed in a normal segment only in case of the absence of a stenotic lesion to be treated in this vessel. At our institution, the normal segment occlusion is performed using a slightly oversized angioplasty balloon (in vessels ≥ 3 mm in diameter, 0.5 mm oversize) at very low-inflation pressure. The balloon is inflated very slowly and under repeated angiographic control of the occurrence of coronary occlusion (inflation pressure mostly close to 1 atmosphere). Furthermore, the site of the balloon occlusion should be selected remote from a side branch, because the side branch could be a supplying collateral artery not accounted for collateral assessment in case of its blockage. A short balloon length may have to be chosen in order to exclude side branches from being occluded. The issue of side-branch exclusion is particularly relevant with regard to septal branches of the LAD, because septal collateral arteries are quite prevalent accounting for almost half the collateral pathways.[86]

2.3.3.2 Occlusion Duration

The coronary artery balloon occlusion model or PCI model has become popular as a tool for investigating the development of tolerance to repetitive bouts of myocardial ischaemia, because it provides the opportunity of applying exactly defined ischaemic periods. The definition is based on the number and duration of balloon occlusions. The development of myocardial tolerance to ischaemia is likely due to the biochemical mechanism of ischaemic preconditioning and to the biophysical action of collateral recruitment.[32] However, the individual as well as the net contribution of both mechanisms has been controversial, which may be related to the lack of studies with simultaneous assessment of preconditioning and collateral recruitment, and to the diversity of balloon occlusion protocols. Irrespective of the protocol's purpose (assessment of myocardial tolerance to ischaemia or 'one-time' collateral measurement), it ought to be defined and systematically applied. The terms of definition consist of the number and duration of balloon occlusions, and of the specification when the measurements are taken. In studies focusing on one single value of collateral degree or flow, there is just one occlusion lasting exactly 1 minute, and the measurement is obtained at the end (i.e. within the last 10 seconds) of the occlusion. If the focus is on ischaemic preconditioning and collateral recruitment, the duration of 1 minute for each of the repetitive occlusions is very likely not sufficient to initiate protection from ischaemia.[87] It appears that the duration of ischaemia needed to initiate myocardial adaptation in patients' lies between 60 and 180 seconds, and probably even closer to 180 than to 120 seconds.[88] However, the rate of symptoms and of ventricular arrhythmias increases with the occlusion duration, which raises ethical problems in the context of long lasting balloon occlusion protocols.

Employing the angioplasty model, following are the qualitative and quantitative methods subsequently described for the characterization of the collateral circulation: degree of angina pectoris and ECG changes, LV function abnormalities, angiographic collateral score using the contralateral coronary injection technique, angiographic washout collaterometry, coronary occlusive guidewire sensor measurements and myocardial contrast echocardiographic perfusion measurement of the temporarily collateralized region.

2.3.4 Angina Pectoris and ECG During Coronary Occlusion

2.3.4.1 Angina Pectoris

The simplest but rather imprecise way to qualify collateral vessels is to ask the patient about the presence of angina pectoris shortly before the end of arterial balloon occlusion. The predictive value of chest pain, if absent or present, for the distinction between high- and low-quantitative collateral function is low (Fig. 2.34). In 845 individuals with (n = 739) and without CAD (n = 106) who underwent a total of 988 invasive quantitative collateral measurements at our institution, the discordance between angina pectoris during coronary balloon occlusion and the occurrence of ECG ST segment elevation >0.1 mV was substantial: 180 individuals among 315 without ECG signs of ischaemia experienced chest pain, and conversely, 57 patients among 673 with ECG signs of ischaemia had no angina pectoris, i.e. silent myocardial ischaemia. In this context, it should be remembered that the severity of chest pain developed during myocardial ischaemia is dependent on several factors, such as the duration of ischaemia, the degree of recruitment of collaterals, prior transmural myocardial infarction, autonomic nerve dysfunction,[89] psychological and neurobiological characteristics of the patient and even the degree of stretching of the coronary arterial wall by the occluding angioplasty balloon. Thus, estimates

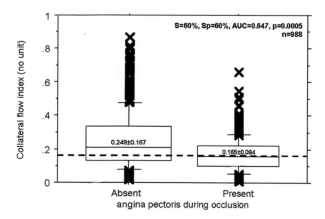

Fig. 2.34 Distinction of collateral relative to normal antegrade coronary flow (*vertical axis*; collateral flow index) at a level of 0.183 (best cutoff; *dashed line*) by the absence or presence of angina pectoris during a 1-minute coronary occlusion. Abbreviations: AUC = area under the curve (receiver operating characteristics analysis); s = sensitivity; sp = specificity. The margins of the box plots indicate mean values, 75 and 95% confidence limits

of the severity of angina pectoris should ideally be made in studies in which the inflation pressure of the balloon is kept constant. For the detection of myocardial ischaemia, ECG ST segment changes are much more reliable than the awareness of angina pectoris (see below). Therefore, the definition of silent myocardial ischaemia is based on the presence of ECG signs of ischaemia in the absence of chest pain. It is a common belief that patients with diabetes mellitus suffer from silent myocardial ischaemia more frequently than non-diabetic patients.[90] In order to accurately detect the prevalence of silent myocardial ischaemia among, e.g. diabetic patients, coronary collateral flow should be accounted for, because it is one of the most important factors influencing the occurrence of chest pain despite the above-mentioned discordance between ECG signs of ischaemia and angina pectoris. Among 452 patients with CAD who underwent invasive collateral assessment at our institution (113 individuals with diabetes mellitus and 339 non-diabetic patients matched at a ratio of 1:3 for age, gender and quantitative collateral flow), a total of 77 had silent myocardial ischaemia (17%). The occurrence of ECG signs of ischaemia during a 1-minute coronary balloon occlusion was not different between diabetic and non-diabetic patients, but that there was a trend towards more prevalent silent ischaemia in diabetic patients (Fig. 2.35).

2.3.4.2 ECG Signs of Ischaemia

In comparison to angina pectoris during coronary balloon occlusion (Fig. 2.34), the presence or absence of ST segment elevation on intracoronary ECG allows more accurate differentiation between quantitatively obtained poor and good

Fig. 2.35 Frequency (*vertical axis*) of the occurrence of ECG signs of myocardial ischaemia (intracoronary ECG ST-segment elevation $\geq$0.1 mV) and of silent ischaemia (absence of angina pectoris in the presence of ECG signs of ischaemia; *horizontal axis*) in patients with and without diabetes mellitus

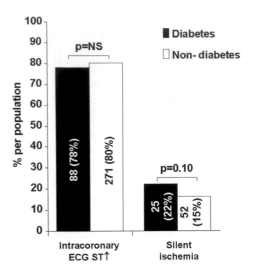

collateral function (Fig. 2.36). Irrespective of simultaneous quantitative collateral measurement, the intracoronary ECG at a threshold of ST elevation >0.1 mV is widely accepted as a sensitive tool for the detection of ischaemia.[91] Accordingly, an independent dichotomous definition of coronary collateral vessels that are insufficient and sufficient, respectively, to prevent myocardial ischaemia of a briefly occluded vascular area is given by the presence and absence of intracoronary ECG ST segment elevation >0.1 mV. Nevertheless, the following issues in the context of intracoronary ECG ST changes as a gauge

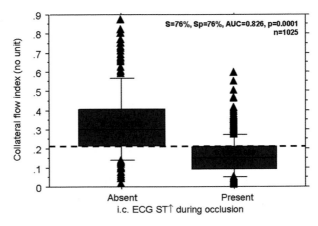

Fig. 2.36 Distinction of collateral relative to normal antegrade coronary flow (*vertical axis*; collateral flow index) at a level of 0.215 (best cutoff; *dashed line*) by the absence or presence of intracoronary (i.c.) ECG ST-segment elevation $\geq$0.1 mV (i.e. myocardial ischaemia) during a 1-minute coronary occlusion. Abbreviations: AUC = area under the curve (receiver operating characteristics analysis); s = sensitivity; sp = specificity. The margins of the box plots indicate mean values, 75 and 95% confidence limits

for ischaemia have to be considered: (a) Does ECG ST segment elevation reflect potential IS (i.e. *the* parameter determined by coronary occlusion time, collateral supply, AR for infarct, myocardial preconditioning and oxygen consumption)? Experimental studies in rabbits documented that a reduction in normalized ECG ST elevation by ischaemic preconditioning from 1 to 0.625 is associated with diminished IS from 38 to 8% of the ischaemic AR.[92] (b) Is the ECG electrode location representative for the myocardial area of interest? Friedman et al. demonstrated that myocardial ischaemia during PCI can be detected by intracoronary ECG with greater sensitivity than by surface ECG.[91] (c) Is the time of coronary occlusion sufficient to fully manifest ischaemia? As indicated above, in human studies on ischaemic preconditioning, 90–120 seconds of vascular occlusion would be more reliable than 60 seconds for detecting its effect on decreasing ST deviation during subsequent bouts of ischaemia.[32] In the same sense, a number of patients with poor collateral function by invasive quantitative means and false negative ECG signs of ischaemia would probably reveal ST elevation only after 60 seconds of occlusion (Fig. 2.37), and thus, an extended occlusion would render the intracoronary ECG assessment of collaterals more sensitive. Figure 2.37 illustrates that in cases of RCA balloon occlusions and in the absence of well-developed collaterals, the intracoronary ST segment elevation crosses the 0.1 mv threshold only after 60 seconds.[93] Despite this limitation of a 1- compared to a 2-minute balloon occlusion, the intracoronary ECG ST segment qualification of coronary collaterals is helpful in predicting long-term survival in patients with chronic CAD (Fig. 2.38). (d) Are there determinants of ECG ST elevation other than coronary occlusion time, collateral supply, AR for infarct, myocardial preconditioning and oxygen consumption, such as variable sensitivity to ischaemia depending on coronary arterial supply areas (Figs. 2.39 and 2.40)? The left panel of Fig. 2.37 documents

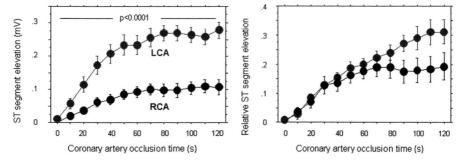

Fig. 2.37 Intra-individual ECG ST segment changes before and during 120 seconds of coronary balloon occlusion as obtained via the angioplasty guide wire positioned distal to the occlusion site. The *left panel* shows absolute ST segment elevation measured in the LCA- (*blue symbols*) and RCA-group (*black symbols*). The *right panel* depicts ST segment elevation relative to the respective R wave amplitude as obtained in the LCA- (*blue symbols*) and RCA-group (*black symbols*)

Fig. 2.38 Cumulative survival rates related to cardiac mortality in patients without and in those with ECG signs of myocardial ischaemia on intracoronary ECG during a 1-minute coronary balloon occlusion. Myocardial ischaemia defined as ECG ST segment elevation >0.1 mV (ST↑)

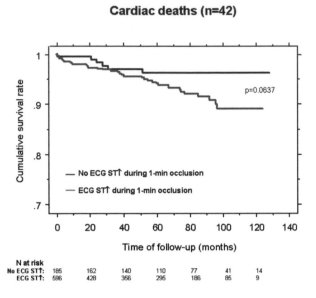

Cardiac deaths (n=42)

p=0.0637

Cumulative survival rate

— No ECG ST↑ during 1-min occlusion

— ECG ST↑ during 1-min occlusion

Time of follow-up (months)

N at risk							
No ECG ST↑:	185	162	140	110	77	41	14
ECG ST↑:	596	428	356	295	186	85	9

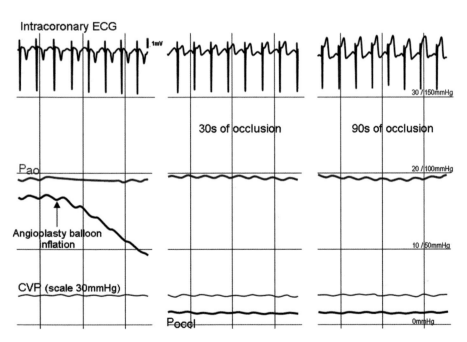

Intracoronary ECG

1mV

30s of occlusion   90s of occlusion

30 / 150mmHg

Pao

20 / 100mmHg

Angioplasty balloon inflation

10 / 50mmHg

CVP (scale 30mmHg)

Poccl

0mmHg

Fig. 2.39 Simultaneous recordings of mean aortic (P_{ao}), distal coronary (P_{occl}) and central venous pressure (CVP) as well as an intracoronary ECG (*upper part*) shortly before and during coronary angioplasty balloon occlusion of a left coronary artery. The amount of ECG ST elevation at 90 seconds of occlusion is more pronounced than in the right coronary artery (see Fig. 2.40)

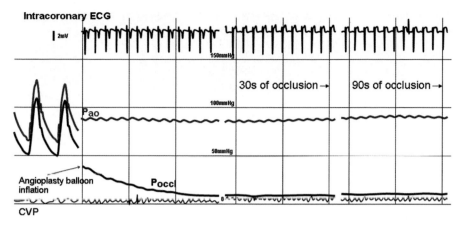

Fig. 2.40 Simultaneous recordings of phasic (before occlusion) and mean aortic (P_{ao}), distal coronary (P_{occl}) and central venous pressure (CVP) as well as an intracoronary ECG (*upper part*) before and during coronary angioplasty balloon occlusion of a right coronary artery. The amount of ECG ST elevation at 90 seconds of occlusion is less pronounced than in the left coronary artery (see Fig. 2.39)

that the more extended supply area of the LCA versus the RCA (with similar occlusion sites in both groups) is related to more pronounced intracoronary ST segment elevations in response to a 2-minute balloon occlusion, i.e. myocardial area at risk is related to the amount of ST elevation.[93] After normalizing the degree of ST elevation for area at risk (division by the R-amplitude), signs of ischaemia at the end of the 2-minute occlusion still differ between LCA and RCA territories, indicating a higher vulnerability to ischaemia in the LCA than the RCA region. One possible explanation for this finding is a lower oxygen consumption during RCA than during LCA occlusion caused by a lower ischaemia-induced heart rate.[93]

2.3.5 LV Function During Coronary Occlusion

Despite the presence of several chronic total coronary occlusions, there may be an entirely normal systolic LV function thanks to a well-developed collateral circulation (Fig. 2.41). Conversely, despite the occurrence of coronary collateral channels, a substantial number of patients with chronic total occlusions reveals various degrees of systolic LV dysfunction. In this context, systolic LV function can be related to necrotic or viable myocardium. It is pathophyiologically controversial whether the latter is due to metabolic hibernation or to repetitive bouts of ischaemia with subsequent events of stunning.[79,81] The possibility of LV functional recovery with its beneficial effect on survival provides the rationale for the technically demanding attempt to recanalize a chronic total occlusion.[94] The extent of functional improvement depends on the presence of viable

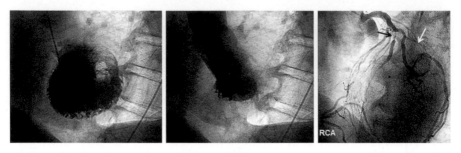

Fig. 2.41 Normal left ventricular angiogram (60° left anterior oblique view; *left and middle panel*) in a patient with chronic three-vessel coronary artery occlusion (→; *right panel*, left anterior oblique cranial view). Abbreviation: RCA = right coronary artery

myocardium, which itself is a function of collateral supply to provide at least a minimum of metabolic support. It has been controversial whether the extent of collaterals is directly related to LV functional recovery after successful treatment of a chronic total occlusion.[95,96] Using quantitative means for collateral assessment, Werner et al. found that the recovery of impaired systolic LV function after revascularization of a chronic occlusion does not depend on the quality of collateral function.[97] This can be interpreted that collateral development does not depend on the presence of viable myocardium. However, Werner et al. also obtained the result that collateral function in patients with normal global systolic LV function was better than in those with reduced LV ejection fraction <60% (53/126 = 42%).[97] Of the 53 patients with global and the 20 patients with regional LV dysfunction, follow-up LV angiography on average 4.9 months after successful treatment of the chronic occlusion has shown improvement in 29 patients (= 40%, i.e. 60% unchanged).[97] The elegant aspect of the investigation just described is its application of both the natural and the artificial model of coronary occlusion allowing to discern between the contribution of collaterals to the primarily normal global systolic LV function (collateral relative to normal flow = 0.48), and the effect of recanalization of the chronic occlusion on LV recovery (lower collateral to normal flow ratio = 0.39).[97] By employing a slightly different methodology with the information of absence or presence of infarction in the area subtended by a chronic total occlusion and with subsequent quantitative collateral assessment during recanalization, an optimal cutoff value of collateral to normal flow of ≥0.30 was determined at our institution to predict accurately the absence of myocardial infarction (Fig. 2.42).

Alternatively to the combined natural and artificial occlusion model, regional systolic and diastolic LV function can be compared with simultaneously obtained collateral function by the transient artificial coronary occlusion model. While cross-sectional studies performed at least hours after the occurrence of coronary occlusion have unequivocally shown the preserving effect of collaterals on ventricular pump function,[98–101] only very few investigations have elucidated the relationship between LV function and concurrent collateral

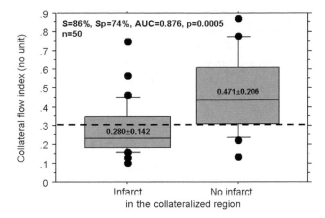

Fig. 2.42 Distinction of collateral relative to normal antegrade coronary flow (*vertical axis*; collateral flow index) at a level of 0.30 (best cutoff; *dashed line*) by the presence (n = 27) or absence (n = 23) of myocardial infarction in the collateralized region of a chronic total coronary occlusion (identical with region of collateral assessment). Abbreviations: AUC = area under the curve (receiver operating characteristics analysis); s = sensitivity; sp = specificity. The margins of the box plots indicate mean values, 75 and 95% confidence limits

flow at the start of events, thus allowing insight into the evolving interdependence of these factors. Rentrop et al. determined the ratio between coronary wedge and mean aortic pressure (during the second balloon occlusion) and compared it non-simultaneously to LV ejection fraction (during the third

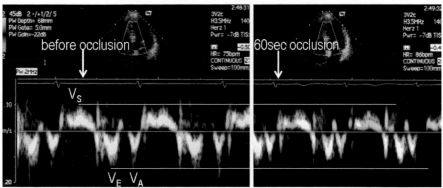

Fig. 2.43 Tissue Doppler imaging for the assessment of left ventricular long-axis function (septal region) as obtained before (*left panel*) and during (*right panel*) a 1-minute proximal left anterior descending coronary artery occlusion with measurement of collateral function (collateral flow index, CFI). In this patient with insufficient collateral function to prevent signs of ischaemia during occlusion, systolic (V_s) and diastolic (V_E and V_A) tissue velocities decreased during as compared to before occlusion

balloon occlusion) in 29 patients with CAD.[102] By stratifying the patients according to stenosis location, the fact that only global and not regional systolic function was obtained was accounted for; the correlation between LV ejection fraction and collateral function was better among patients with large than with small areas at risk. Simultaneous assessment of regional LV function using transthoracic tissue Doppler imaging and invasive collateral function measurement in 50 patients with CAD at our institution has revealed a statistically relevant association between systolic as well as diastolic LV function and collateral function (Figs. 2.43 and 2.44).[103] In particular, mid-ventricular myocardial velocity as obtained from apical four- and two-chambered echocardiographic views has correlated during systole (isovolumetric contraction velocity and peak systolic excursion velocity) and during diastole (early diastolic excursion velocity) with collateral function.[103]

Sufficient collaterals (CFI=0.55)

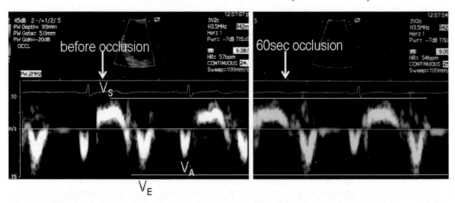

Fig. 2.44 Tissue Doppler imaging for the assessment of left ventricular long-axis function as obtained before (*left panel*) and during (*right panel*) a 1-minute proximal left anterior descending coronary artery occlusion with measurement of collateral function (collateral flow index, CFI). In this patient with sufficient collateral function to prevent signs of ischaemia during occlusion, systolic (V_s) and diastolic (V_E and V_A) tissue velocities did not change during as compared to before occlusion

2.4 Angiographic Collateral Assessment

The most widely used method for assessing the coronary collateral circulation is contrast angiography because of its availability and the superior imaging quality regarding the often small-sized collateral vessels. In the majority of coronary angiographies, collateral vessels are, however, estimated using the inferior non-occlusion model. The predominant angiographic collateral pathway in the presence of chronic total occlusion is via septal collaterals in more than two-fifths, via distal branch collaterals in one-fifth and via atrial collaterals with proximal take-off in approximately one-third. Traditional angiographic criteria for presence of collateral vessels are opacification of an artery or its branches after injection of the contralateral artery, opacification of an arterial segment distal to its complete occlusion after contrast injection proximal to the occlusion and visualization of a vessel joining the segments of the same artery proximal and distal to an occlusion. The most widely used angiographic grading system is that originally described by Rentrop et al.: grade 0 = no collaterals; grade 1 = side-branch filling of the recipient artery without filling of the main epicardial artery; grade 2 = partial filling of the main epicardial recipient artery and grade 3 = complete filling of the main epicardial recipient artery. Natural or artificial occlusion of the collateral receiving artery augments the sensitivity of detecting and grading collateral vessels using angiography. A semiquantitative grading method of collateral connections validated in chronic total occlusions defines three different connection grades: grade 0 = no continuous connection between collateral supplying and receiving vessel; grade 1 = threadlike continuous connection and grade 2 = side-branch like connection. Washout of contrast distal to a balloon-occluded collateral recipient vessel at a threshold of 11 heart beats accurately distinguishes between sufficient and insufficient collateral supplies.

2.4.1 Introduction

The most widely used method for assessing the coronary collateral circulation is contrast angiography because of its availability and the relatively superior imaging quality regarding the often small-sized collateral vessels. In the majority of coronary angiographies, collateral vessels are not assessed using the occlusion model. Obviously, this is not the case in the one-third of CAD patients with chronic total occlusion encountered during coronary angiography, and in individuals with acute myocardial infarction who underwent primary PCI. However, the artificial occlusion model with a double intubation of the LCA and RCA using angioplasty balloon or guidewire occlusion of the collateral receiving artery of interest is performed only rarely, because this procedure is technically more demanding (Fig. 2.45). As opposed to the coronary patency method employed during single vessel intubation with assessment of *spontaneously visible* collateral vessels, the coronary occlusion model images *recruitable* collaterals. The coronary occlusion technique renders the angiographic method for collateral qualification more sensitive when compared to the coronary patency technique.

The normal human heart and that affected by CAD contain numerous anastomotic vessels ranging between 40 and 200 μm.[104,105] However, the size of the majority of these vessels is beyond the spatial resolution even of analogue angiographic imaging chains. With modern-day digital storage media and a resolution of >0.2 mm, quantitative coronary angiography of collaterals, which would be ideal, is not applicable.[106] In principle, a semi-quantitative or

Fig. 2.45 Right coronary
angiogram (RCA;
anteroposterior view) with
double-intubation technique
in a patient with chronic
total occlusion of the
proximal left anterior
descending coronary artery
(LAD). During RCA
contrast injection, the
recanalized LAD occlusion
is re-obstructed by the non-
inflated angioplasty balloon
(*opaque marker*). The LAD
is filled entirely via a large
branch collateral artery ($\rightarrow$)

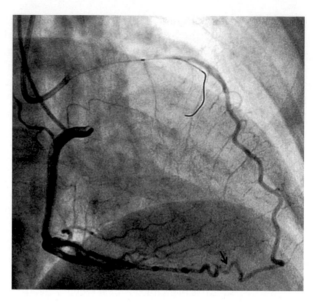

qualitative angiographic method for collateral assessment should account for
potential intraindividual changes of collateral flow over time, collateral-recipi-
ent vessel filling (ipsilateral vessel), the number of collateral vessels, the branching patterns and lengths of collaterals.[107] The ability to fulfil these criteria is
dependent on maintaining consistency in the filming technique as well as in the
catheterization laboratory methods as subsequently described.

2.4.2 Angiographic Collateral Pathways

In 200 coronary angiograms of 200 patients with severe CAD, Levin observed
collaterals only in cases with arterial narrowing exceeding 90% in diameter
(105 with that degree of RCA obstruction, 127 with LAD obstruction and 48
with LCX obstruction).[108] Among patients with RCA obstruction, there were
10 different collateral pathways (Fig. 2.46), in those with LAD obstruction,
seven pathways were noted (Fig. 2.47) and in patients with LCX obstruction,
five pathways were observed (Fig. 2.48), whereby more than one pathway could
be present in one individual. Conversely, a substantial fraction of patients did
not reveal collaterals, despite the presence of a severe or complete coronary
obstruction: 31 of 105 (30%) in case of the RCA, 57 of 127 (45%) in case of the
LAD and 27 of 48 (56%) in case of the LCX.[108] Recently, Rockstroh and
Brown as well as Werner et al.[86,106] categorized Levin's 22 collateral pathways
into septal, intra-arterial (bridging collaterals), epicardial with proximal take-
off (atrial collaterals) and epicardial with distal take-off (branch collaterals)
(Fig. 2.49). In 100 patients with total chronic occlusion of a major coronary
artery, Werner et al. documented at least one collateral path in all individuals (a
total of211 pathways with 86% of the patients having >1). The predominant

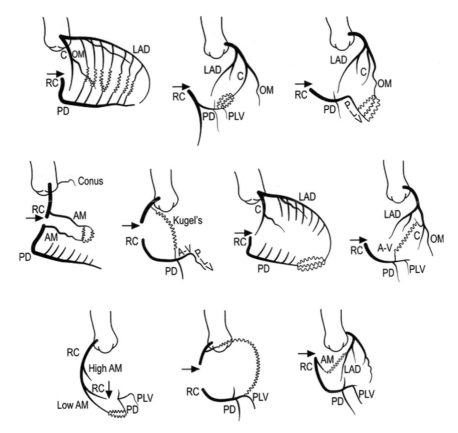

Fig. 2.46 Angiographic collateral pathways in right coronary artery (RCA) occlusion as described by Levin.[108] Abbreviations: AM = acute marginal branch of the RCA; A-V = artery to atrioventricular node; C = left circumflex coronary artery; LAD = left anterior descending coronary artery; LC = left circumflex coronary artery (LCX); LAO = left anterior oblique view; OM = obtuse marginal branch of the LCX; PD = posterior descending branch of the RCA; PLV = posterior left ventricular branch of the RCA (posterolateral branch); RAO – - right anterior oblique view

angiographic collateral pathway was in more than 2/5 septal collaterals, close to 1/5 had distal branch collaterals, and approximately 1/3 had atrial collaterals with proximal take-off (Fig. 2.49).[86] In comparison, Levin documented a prevalence of septal collaterals in only 20%, distal branch collaterals in 52%, epicardial collaterals with proximal take-off in 42% and bridging collaterals in 9%.[108] The different distributions of collateral pathways between the cited works are likely related to the dissimilar populations examined with exclusively chronic total occlusions and a mixture of differently severe degrees of CAD respectively. Figure 2.11 gives an example of a patient with congenital agenesis of the left main coronary artery and epicardial collateral arteries with proximal take-off (atrial branches). The RCA angiography of the patient with proximal

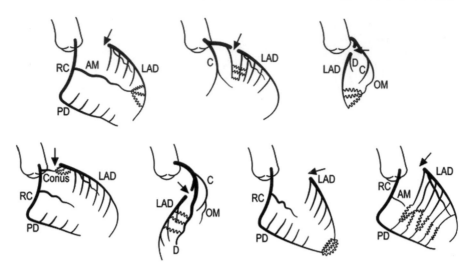

Fig. 2.47 Angiographic collateral pathways in left anterior descending coronary artery occlusion as described by Levin.[108] Abbreviations: AM = acute marginal branch of the right coronary artery (RCA); C = left circumflex coronary artery; D = diagonal branch of the LAD; LAD = left anterior descending coronary artery; LC = left circumflex coronary artery (LCX); LAO = left anterior oblique view; OM = obtuse marginal branch of the LCX; PD = posterior descending branch of the RCA; RAO = right anterior oblique view

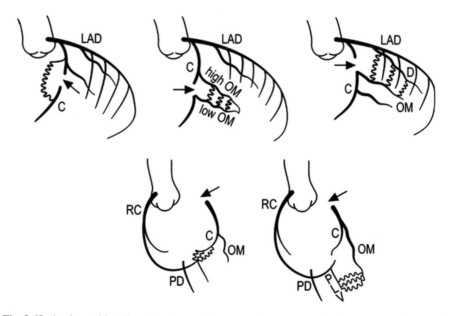

Fig. 2.48 Angiographic collateral pathways in left circumflex coronary artery occlusion as described by Levin.[108] Abbreviations: C = left circumflex coronary artery; D = diagonal branch of the LAD; LAD = left anterior descending coronary artery; LC = left circumflex coronary artery (LCX); LAO = left anterior oblique view; OM = obtuse marginal branch of the LCX; PD = posterior descending branch of the RCA; RC(A) = right coronary artery; RAO = right anterior oblique view

Fig. 2.49 Schematic drawing of four principal angiographic coronary collateral pathways according to Rockstroh and Brown.[106] See text for description

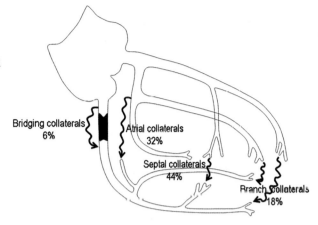

Fig. 2.50 Right coronary angiogram (right anterior oblique cranial view) in a patient with chronic total occlusions (→) of the proximal and mid-left anterior descending coronary artery (LAD). There are numerous collateral arteries from the right coronary artery to the LAD including an apical branch collateral vessel, septal and atrial (also RCA conus branch) collaterals

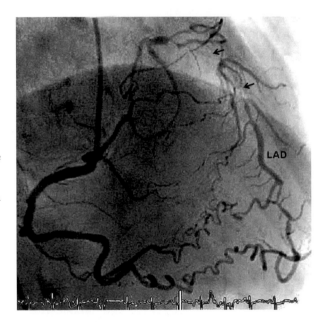

and mid-LAD occlusion shown in Fig. 2.50 illustrates that atrial, septal and distal branch collaterals supplied by the RCA may be present side by side in the same individual.

2.4.3 Qualitative Angiographic Methods

Initial angiographic methods to classify collateral vessels in living patients have employed a dichotomous system of present or absent collaterals.[1,109] The criteria of Gensini and da Costa[109] for the presence of collateral vessels were as follows: (a) opacification of an artery or its branches after injection of the contralateral artery; (b) opacification of an arterial segment distal to its complete occlusion after contrast injection proximal to the occlusion and (c) distinct visualization of a vessel joining the segments of the same artery proximal and distal to an occlusion. Current qualitative methods consider further aspects of coronary collateral angiographic appearance, such as collateral flow grade, frame count, bifurcation count, collateral length grade, the relationship between the area at risk for myocardial infarction and collaterals, and collateral recipient vessel filling.[107] Assessment of those aspects requires correct identification of collateral as compared to parent epicardial vessels. If a vessel meets one of the following criteria, then it is considered a collateral artery or arteriole rather than an epicardial parent artery: (a) The vessel connects to a distal segment of the same epicardial artery. (b) The vessel connects to another vessel classified as a collateral vessel. (c) The vessel has a mean diameter of <0.7 mm (vessels with a diameter <0.3 mm may not be angiographically visible). However, a collateral artery can often have a diameter ≥0.7 mm (Fig. 2.50). (d) The vessel extends beyond half the distance between its parent artery and the adjacent epicardial territory (Fig. 2.50). (e) The vessel takes off at a branch angle <135° with respect to the upstream vessel (Fig. 2.50). The mentioned angle is an empirical finding,[107] which, theoretically, reflects an average ratio of the vascular diameter of the parent to the collateral vessel. According to the law of minimum viscous energy loss for blood distribution,[15] the collateral and parent vessels approach a dividing angle of 90° as the size of the collateral vessel is <10% of the parent artery. Practically, the determination of branching angles at a bifurcation is dependent on the image projection, and it is the largest angle obtainable which is under discussion here. (f) The vessel is very tortuous (Fig. 2.50). This criterion for a collateral vessel is weak, because tortuosity just indicates previous or ongoing vascular remodelling in response to a chronically increased demand of the myocardium for blood flow. In the process of, for example, developing ventricular hypertrophy, blood flow demand is increased due to greater mass; according to the just-mentioned law,[15] the artery is becoming enlarged, which occurs not just cross-sectionally but also in length. Since the heart as a whole does not enlarge simultaneously (but much later in the process of hypertrophy), the lengthened vessel becomes convoluted or develops a corkscrew appearance (Fig. 2.50). (g) The vessel is a newly visible branch during follow-up coronary angiographies arising from a major epicardial artery.

2.4.3.1 Collateral Flow Grade

The angiographic aspect of collateral flow grade does not focus on a collateral recipient artery, which is often not visible, but on the anastomotic vessel itself. The grading is based on visibility of the radiographic contrast medium within the collateral. Grade 0 flow: No dye visible (only detectable in comparison to a different time point). Grade 1 flow: Dye is not visible throughout the cardiac cycle but in ≥3 consecutive frames. Grade 2 flow: The collateral is moderately opaque and visible during ≥$^3/_4$ of the cardiac cycle. Antegrade dye motion is visible. Grade 3 flow: The collateral is well opacified (<0.7 mm) and has clear antegrade dye motion. Grade 4 flow: Large collateral (>0.7 mm) with antegrade filling.

2.4.3.2 Collateral Frame Count

The collateral frame count is the number of cineframes required for contrast media to reach the recipient vessel (Fig. 2.51). Given the difficulty in defining where a collateral vessel begins and where the parent artery ends, the proximal part of the parent vessel is used for frame counting.[107] Frame 0 is that frame in which dye extends across ≥70% of the length of the left main or the RCA (Fig. 2.51). The last frame counted is the frame in which dye first enters the recipient epicardial artery (Fig. 2.51). Due to the different filming speeds used, frame count ought to be converted to seconds in order to be comparable. This crude index of collateral flow is not relevant in absolute terms, but rather for intraindividual comparison over time.

Frame 0   Frame 20   Frame 69

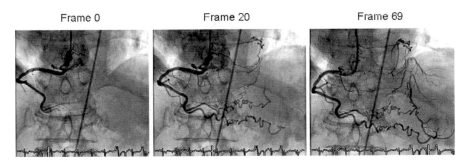

Fig. 2.51 Right coronary angiogram (anteroposterior cranial view) in the same patient as in Fig. 2.50 showing the dynamics of collateral filling of the occluded left anterior descending coronary artery (LAD). Frame 0 (*left panel*) is defined as the frame in which dye extends across ≥70% of the length of the collateral-supplying vessel, i.e. in this case the right coronary artery. The last frame counted is the frame in which dye first enters the recipient epicardial artery (frame 20; *middle panel*). *Filling* of the collateral-receiving vessel requires a number of further cineframes (*right panel*)

2.4.3.3 Bifurcation Count

The collateral bifurcation count is the number of terminating arms in a collateral system with a single origin. For example, a collateral vessel with two terminating arms originating from one bifurcation would have a bifurcation count of 2,[107] i.e. one bifurcation at the collateral separation from the parent artery and one bifurcation further downstream. Consequently, a collateral vessel that does not bifurcate has a bifurcation count of 1. Theoretically, such an estimation of the collateral supply area is reasonable, because the ratio between regional and total summed coronary (collateral) artery branch lengths is equal to the regional and total myocardial mass supplied by a certain point in the coronary artery tree.[24] The summed coronary artery branch lengths are substantially influenced by the number of bifurcations, i.e. the arterial length downstream of a bifurcation doubles in case of equally sized daughter vessels. For practical purposes and especially in the case of small collateral vessels, it may be very difficult to count terminating branches (Fig. 2.50). In order to detect differences in bifurcation counts over time, it is crucial to perform the counting using absolutely identical imaging projections at identical time points during the cardiac cycle.

2.4.3.4 Collateral Length Grade

Gibson et al. proposed a classification of the length of a collateral vessel as the number of eighths relative to the parent's artery length.[107] As the bifurcation count method, collateral length grading is reasonable to perform on theoretical grounds, since the length of a vascular network provides insight into the myocardial territory supplied by the system. However, considering factors influencing length assessment such as image resolution, image projection, volume and rate of contrast injection, duration of filming, vascular tortuosity, the practical value of collateral length grading is very limited.

2.4.3.5 Collateral Recipient Filling Grade

The most widely used angiographic grading system is that originally described by Rentrop et al.[39], which distinguishes between four degrees of collateral recipient artery filling by radiographic contrast medium: grade 0 = no collaterals; grade 1 = side branch filling of the recipient artery without filling of the main epicardial artery; grade 2 = partial filling of the main epicardial recipient artery; grade 3 = complete filling of the main epicardial recipient artery. Rentrop et al. focused on changes in collateral filling immediately before, during and after coronary balloon occlusion in 16 patients with CAD,[39] whereby spontaneously visible collateral grade before dilatation was 0 (n = 9) or 1 (n = 7) in all cases; recruitable collaterals during balloon occlusion revealed second- (n = 10) or third-degree (n = 3) recipient vessel filling, which disappeared entirely in all cases following percutaneous treatment of the stenotic lesions as illustrated in Fig. 2.52. Natural or artificial occlusion of the collateral receiving artery clearly augments the sensitivity of detecting collateral vessels using angiography (Fig. 2.52). Since one of the principal weaknesses of coronary angiography as an instrument for collateral assessment is its blunt quality, improving its ability to detect vascular detours is valuable. Figure 2.52 also exemplifies the difficulty of differentiating grade 0 from grade 1 recipient artery filling, because it is often impossible to discern the collateral from the epicardial recipient artery. Furthermore, it indicates that the duration of filming and the position of the field of view may

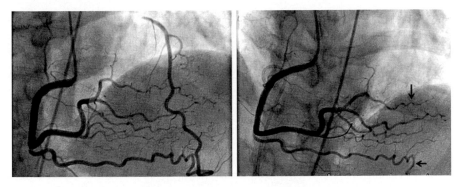

Fig. 2.52 Right coronary angiogram (cranial views) in a patient with chronic total occlusion of the left anterior descending coronary artery (LAD) before (*left panel*) and shortly after (*right panel*) recanalization with balloon angioplasty and stenting of the occlusion. Filling of the LAD via large branch and septal collaterals present during LAD occlusion disappears following coronary intervention, although the corkscrew-shaped branches previously constituting the collateral vessels are still present ($\rightarrow$)

substantially influence the assessment of retrograde recipient vessel filling, and thus, the distinction between second- and third-degree collaterals. In the presence of a third-degree recipient vessel filling, the concept of an inverse relation between area at risk for myocardial infarction and collateral supply can be nicely visualized to the effect that, e.g. the area at risk of a proximal LAD occlusion is equal to zero due to the complete retrograde filling of that vessel via collaterals (Fig. 2.11; agenesis of the left main coronary artery).

2.4.4 Semiquantitative Angiographic Methods

A recently reported quantitative angiographic analysis of collateral diameters on high-resolution cine films has underscored the relevance of the collateral diameter for its capacity to supply blood flow in relevant volume rates.[106] Rockstroh and Brown calculated the summed collateral flow capacity of three selected, well-visible collateral pathways in 13 patients. Collateral perfusion capacity was defined as the summed conductance in a parallel network of linear resistors, whereby the individual resistance values were computed by the Hagen-Poiseuille law.[106] An observed 16% increase in collateral diameter during 10 years of follow-up was related to a 214% augmentation in collateral flow capacity. Aside from the relative complexity of this approach, its applicability to modern digital storage standards with lower image resolution is limited. However, a semiquantitative assessment of the collateral diameters as originally suggested by Carroll et al.[110] has recently been refined and validated by Werner et al. in 100 patients who underwent recanalization of a chronic total coronary occlusion.[86] In that study, collaterals have been qualitatively characterized by recipient filling grade according to Rentrop et al.,[39] by their predominant anatomic location (see above) and by a new grading method of collateral connections (CC grade 0 = no continuous connection between collateral supplying and receiving vessel in 14%; CC1 = threadlike continuous connection in 51%; CC2 = side-branch like connection in 35%; Fig. 2.53). There was a direct and weak correlation between collateral connection grade and angiographic collateral degree of the recipient vessel according to Rentrop in that study (r = 0.32, p < 0.001). However, the principal result of the study by Werner et al. was that of a close association between CC grade and invasively determined parameters of collateral haemodynamics and function (see Chapter 5).[86]

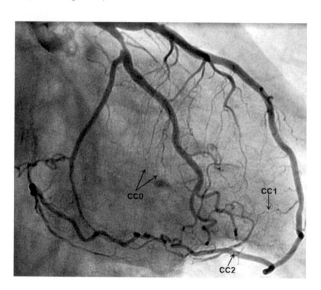

Fig. 2.53 Left coronary angiogram (anteroposterior view) in a patient with chronic total occlusion of the right coronary artery showing the different degrees of collateral connection (CC) grades. A large apical branch collateral artery originating from the left anterior descending coronary artery is a representative example of a CC2 collateral connection. See text for the definition of the different CC grades

2.4.5 Washout Collaterometry

The above-described qualitative angiographic method of collateral frame count is defined as the number of cineframes required for contrast media to reach the recipient vessel (see also Fig. 2.51). Similarly but without the difficulty of identifying collateral versus recipient vessels, the time or heart beat count or frame count to clearance or washout of radiographic contrast medium trapped distal to a balloon-occluded collateral receiving artery can be determined (Fig. 2.54). According to the principles of indicator dilution theory (flow = vascular volume/mean transit time of indicator),[111] the washout should be inversely related to the collateral flow entering the recipient vessel and being supplied by the contralateral vessel, i.e. the balloon-occluded artery should be cleared from contrast in less time in the presence of high collateral flow. With this background, it has been hypothesized that coronary collaterals sufficient to prevent ECG signs of myocardial ischaemia during a 1-minute balloon occlusion can be differentiated from insufficient collaterals by the contrast washout

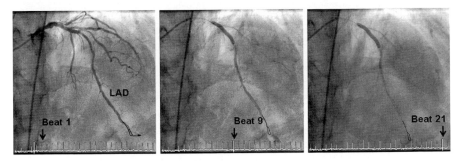

Fig. 2.54 Washout collaterometry during left coronary angiography (anteroposterior cranial view) in a patient immediately before proximal balloon occlusion of the left anterior descending coronary artery (LAD; *left panel*), 9 heart beats (*middle panel*) and 21 heart beats (*right panel*) after balloon occlusion. Even after 21 heart beats, the LAD and the also occluded diagonal branch are still filled with contrast medium indicating retarded washout due to poor collateral supply to the occluded LAD

heart beat count.[112] Figure 2.54 gives an example of a patient with high heart beat count until contrast washout; in fact, contrast-trapped distal to the LAD-occlusive balloon is not washed out until beat 22 counted from the time of balloon occlusion. Figure 2.55 provides an example of a patient with low heart

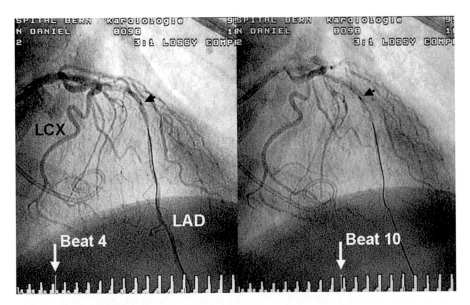

Fig. 2.55 Washout collaterometry during left coronary angiography (right anterior oblique cranial view) in a patient shortly after balloon occlusion of the mid-left anterior descending coronary artery (LAD; *left panel*) and 10 heart beats (*right panel*) after balloon occlusion. After 10 heart beats, the contrast trapped in the LAD distal to the occlusive balloon has practically disappeared

beat count of approximately 10 beats until contrast washout. Washout of contrast distal to the occluded vessel at a threshold of 11 heart beats accurately distinguishes between sufficient and insufficient collateral supply (sensitivity of 88%, specificity of 81%; Fig. 2.56).[112] Under the condition that coronary balloon occlusion still occurs during contrast injection into the collateral recipient vessel of interest, washout collaterometry is a widely practical semiquantitative method, because it does not require dual coronary catheterization or the use of intracoronary sensor wires. However, the above-mentioned indicator dilution theory points to a limitation inherent in washout collaterometry, i.e. the interindividually varying vascular volume downstream of the occlusion, which requires longer washout in case of large as compared to a small size irrespective of collateral supply.

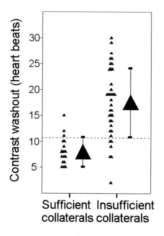

Fig. 2.56 Distinction between collaterals sufficient or insufficient to prevent ECG ST segment changes during a 1-minute coronary occlusion using occlusive radiographic contrast washout time. Sufficient and insufficient collaterals (*horizontal axis*; as defined at a collateral flow index of 0.30) using a threshold of 11 heart beats (*dashed line*) were identified with 88% sensitivity and 81% specificity (area under the curve = 0.89).[112] The large triangles with error bars indicate mean contrast washout time with standard deviations

2.5 Quantitative Coronary Pressure and Doppler Sensor Measurements

The ratio of distal coronary occlusive (P_{occl}) to aortic pressure (P_{ao}) after the subtraction of CVP ($[P_{occl}-CVP]/[P_{ao}-CVP]$), termed as pressure-derived collateral flow index (CFI_p), can be theoretically modelled by myocardial, stenotic and collateral conductance elements of the coronary circulation. CFI_p describes the occlusive collateral relative to the normal antegrade coronary flow during vascular patency. Velocity- or Doppler-derived CFI (CFI_v) is also used for the quantitative assessment of collateral relative to the normal antegrade coronary flow. CFI_p

and CFI_v are not 1:1 interchangeable because of biological/theoretical reasons. The distensibility of the coronary microcirculation renders vascular pressure theoretically unsuitable as a measure of flow. Since flow is the product of vascular cross-sectional area and spatially averaged flow velocity, the latter is not an exact measure of flow either. However, the quantitative effect of these considerations on the practicability of CFI_p is not important as demonstrated by simultaneous measurements of absolute collateral perfusion using MCE and CFI_p.

In chronic CAD, the implication of LV-filling pressure potentially influencing P_{occl} and CFI_p is that the pressure-derived quantitative collateral assessment should be replaced by Doppler-derived measurements in the presence of values beyond ~30 mmHg. In the setting of acute infarction, the effect of LV-filling pressure on CFI_p may become so important that CFI_p no longer reflects the collateral circulation but rather the IS. To actually measure CVP and not just assume a fixed value is important for preventing considerable errors in the calculation of CFI_p.

During collateral function assessment in normal coronary arteries, minimal occlusion pressure of 1–2 atmospheres ought to be reached very slowly by sensing imminent occlusion using the start of decline of distal coronary pressure and not primarily the angiographic detection of occlusion which only follows later. Using this protocol and a rather oversized, compliant angioplasty balloon, collateral assessment in normal coronary arteries is a safe technique.

2.5.1 Introduction

In Section 2.3 ('coronary occlusion model'), it has been theoretically derived that the three basic coronary arterial conductance elements (epicardial or stenosis conductance, C_s; microcirculatory or myocardial conductance, C_{myo}; collateral conductance, C_{coll}) can be derived by obtaining coronary volume flow rate per time (Q), averaged values of aortic pressure (P_{ao}), distal coronary pressure during vessel patency (P_d), CVP and distal coronary pressure during vessel occlusion (P_{occl}; Fig. 2.57). In the current context of quantitative collateral assessment, C_{coll} ($= Q_{coll}/[P_{ao}-P_{occl}]$) is the parameter of primary interest, and, as outlined above, occlusion of the collateral recipient artery allows best to determine it. Practically, ipislateral coronary occlusion is indispensable for quantitative collateral measurement. Some or even all of the variables of the above equation defining C_{coll} was obtained already during the advent of PCI. However, the number of individuals included in those early studies have been quite small, and, therefore, their results statistically questionable.[113,114] Rentrop et al. in their first description of the angioplasty balloon occlusion model reported in addition to the principal angiographic results also those of the ratio between distal coronary occlusive or wedge pressure, P_{occl} and P_{ao}, as obtained in 9 of 16 patients[39] (as exemplified in Fig. 2.58); there was a trend to a direct relationship between P_{occl}/P_{ao} and the angiographic collateral degree during coronary balloon occlusion. Probst et al. measured P_{ao} and the phasic distal occlusive pressure (defined

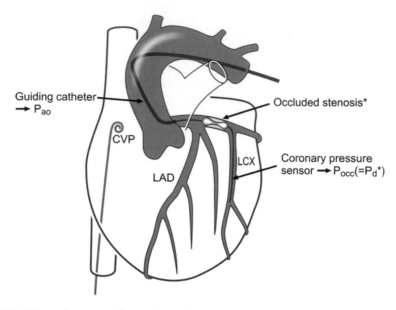

Fig. 2.57 Schematic drawing illustrating the haemodynamic parameters to obtain for quantitative collateral assessment. Pressure-derived collateral quantification requires coronary occlusion and measurement of mean aortic pressure (P_{ao}), mean distal coronary pressure (P_{occl}; coronary wedge pressure) and central venous, and respectively right atrial pressure (CVP). In addition, coronary volume flow rate Q for the calculation of coronary conductance can be obtained by Doppler-derived coronary flow velocity and the respective vascular calibre at the same site (combined coronary pressure/velocity measurement), or alternatively, by myocardial contrast echo-derived perfusion measurement

Fig. 2.58 Mean aortic (P_{ao}) and distal coronary pressure tracings before, during and shortly after a 2-minute angioplasty balloon occlusion (P_{occl}) with corresponding intracoronary ECG recordings (*upper part*; ST segment elevation during occlusion)

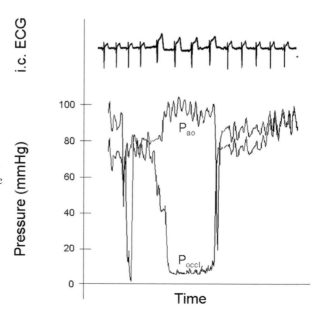

as the lowest distal systolic pressure following coronary occlusion) in 63 patients with one-vessel CAD and related those measurements to angiographically scored collateral vessels supplying the occluded artery (score 0–3, similar to the Rentrop score).[115] A direct and statistically relevant relationship between angiographic collateral score groups and P_{occl}/P_{ao} was found in that study, whereby even in the 35 patients without visible collaterals, P_{occl}/P_{ao} ranged high from 0.10 to 0.42, and the group average amounted to 0.25.[115] Macdonald et al. performed the first study (25 patients with proximal LAD CAD) with sophisticated collateral haemodynamic measurements in comparison to the ECG ST segment's response to a brief angioplasty balloon occlusion at the site of the stenosis.[116] Surface lead ECG ST segment elevation (n = 16) or depression (n = 9) during coronary occlusion indicated variably severe transmural or subendocardial ischaemia, and the following, simultaneously obtained haemodynamic parameters were related to the ECG changes: P_{occl}, P_{ao}, LV diastolic pressure and great cardiac vein flow.[116] According to the above considerations on collateral conductance C_{coll}, Ohm's law states that $C_{coll} = Q_{coll}/[P_{ao}-P_{occl}]$, where Q_{coll} is equal to great cardiac flow in case of a proximal LAD occlusion. In the study by Macdonald et al.[116], coronary wedge pressure (P_{occl}) normalized for P_{ao} was 0.236±0.070 in the group with more severe signs of myocardial ischaemia during coronary balloon occlusion (ST elevation) and it was 0.377±0.104 in the group with less severe ischaemia (p = 0.0005; Fig. 2.59). P_{occl}/P_{ao} directly and significantly correlated with collateral conductance C_{coll} (Fig. 2.60). Despite the extensive haemodynamic measurements performed in that investigation, it was limited by the fact that patients with even less signs of ischaemia than ST depression, i.e. those without ST segment changes, were excluded rendering the study population non-representative for a CAD population. In 1987, Meier et al. published their work in 49 CAD patients who underwent coronary wedge pressure measurements during PCI, whereby a $P_{occl} \geq 30$ mmHg was found to accurately predict the presence of spontaneously visible or recruitable collaterals.[117]

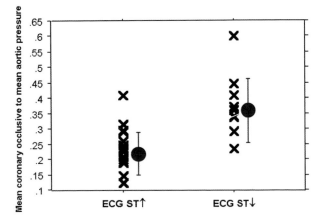

Fig. 2.59 Plot of individual values of mean coronary occlusive to mean aortic pressure (P_{occl}/P_{ao}; *vertical axis*) in relation to the presence of ECG ST-segment elevation (ECG ST↑) or depression (ECG ST↓; *horizontal axis*). Blue symbols with error lines indicate mean values ± standard deviation. Data from the study by Macdonald et al.[116]

Fig. 2.60 Correlation between coronary collateral conductance (*vertical axis*) and the ratio of mean coronary occlusive to mean aortic pressure (P_{occl}/P_{ao}; *horizontal axis*). Data from the study by Macdonald et al.[116]

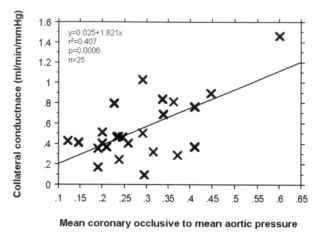

Mean coronary occlusive to mean aortic pressure

2.5.2 Determinants of Distal Coronary Occlusive Pressure

However, P_{occl} is not only dependent on the amount of collateral flow to the temporarily or permanently occluded vascular region. Potential determinants of P_{occl} are the driving pressure across a collateral pathway(s) (i.e. the pressure difference between the coronary pressure in the collateral supplying and receiving artery), the venous back pressure (central venous or right atrial pressure), but also extravascular pressure related to compression of intramural vessels by cardiac contraction and/or to transmission of diastolic LV pressure to the epicardial circulation.[118,119] The above-cited work by Macdonald et al. has already implicitly documented a possible influence of LV-filling pressure on P_{occl} by revealing a trend to a direct association between the two parameters.[116] In 1993, Pijls et al. provided the experimental basis for the determination of maximum coronary, myocardial and collateral blood flow by coronary pressure measurements,[120] whereby it was assumed that minimal microvascular resistance during pharmacologically induced hyperaemia is constant and independent of the presence or absence of an epicardial stenosis. Therefore, myocardial flow Q in the presence of a stenosis (the sum of flow through the stenotic vessel plus collateral flow) relative to myocardial flow without a stenosis Q_N (Q/Q_N = fractional flow reserve, FFR) could be calculated on the basis of distal coronary pressure and aortic pressure both after the subtraction of venous back pressure. The model was tested in dogs, whereby Doppler-derived measurements of stenotic coronary flow Q_s to normal flow Q_N was directly compared with $(P_d - CVP)/(P_{ao} - CVP)$ without, however, testing the situation of a complete coronary occlusion ($Q_s = 0$), i.e. the setting where $P_d = P_{occl}$.[120] Thus, the work of Pijls et al. did not validate their proposed concept of quantitative assessment of coronary collateral flow.[120] Furthermore, a number of assumptions in their model is probably incorrect without rendering it less applicable for practical purposes: the above-mentioned minimal micro-vascular resistance is likely not constant and differs with altering coronary pressures (particularly in the low-flow range)[119,121]; inducing pharmacological hyperaemia is often not maximal (i.e. 'minimal' resistance not minimal) and, therefore, varying interindividually[122]; zero-collateral-flow in the absence of a coronary stenosis may not be the case because of a more proximal origin of the collateral vessel in comparison to its more distal run off (Fig. 2.61) and collat-eral flow during repetitive coronary occlusions is not constant.[43] In 1995, Pijls et al. using the coronary angioplasty model in 120 patients with CAD performed a qualitative comparison between the ratio $(P_{occl}\text{–CVP})/P_{ao}\text{–CVP})$ and ECG ST segment changes during a 2-minute coronary occlusion, whereby in the 29 patients without signs of ischaemia, collateral relative to normal flow was always >24%.[123]

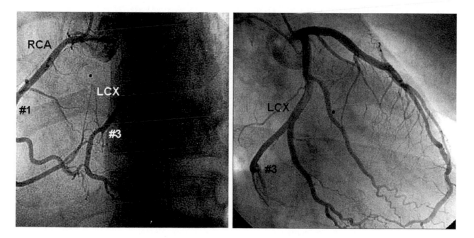

Fig. 2.61 Right coronary artery (RCA) angiogram (left anterior oblique, cranial view; *left panel*) in an individual without coronary atherosclerotic lesions showing collateral arteries (→) between the RCA and left circumflex coronary artery (LCX). *Right panel*: Left coronary angiogram (right anterior oblique, caudal view) of the same patient. The coronary angiogra-phy exemplifies the concept that due to a proximal origin (from the RCA) and a distal orifice (to the LCX) of a collateral artery, there may be collateral flow even in the absence of coronary artery stenoses. The origin of the collateral artery is located at the first major bifurcation of the RCA (#1); the orifice distal to the third bifurcation of the LCX (#3)

2.5.3 *Validation of Pressure-Derived Collateral Flow Index*

A direct and simultaneous evaluation of the coronary parameters possibly quantitative for collateral function $([P_{occl}\text{–CVP}]/[P_{ao}\text{–CVP}],$[120]$)$ in comparison to occlusive coronary flow or at least directly obtained flow velocity was not performed until 1998, when coronary Doppler- and pressure-derived ratios indicative of collateral flow during PCI were compared in 51 CAD patients.[124]

The ratio of coronary wedge or distal coronary occlusive to aortic pressure both after the subtraction of CVP ($[P_{occl}$–CVP$]/[P_{ao}$–CVP$]$) was termed pressure-derived CFI (CFI_p).[124] It can be theoretically derived on the basis of the above-described model of myocardial, stenotic and collateral conductance components of the coronary circulation (Fig. 2.62). Figure 2.63 shows two examples of CFI_p values sufficient and insufficient to prevent ECG signs of myocardial ischaemia (ST segment shift >0.1 mV) during coronary occlusion. The ratio between distal occlusive coronary flow velocity and the flow velocity at identical site as obtained after PCI of the upstream stenosis and following cessation of reactive hyperaemia was termed velocity- or Doppler-derived CFI (CFI_v) (Fig. 2.64).[124] Among the 11 of 51 patients without intracoronary ECG signs of ischaemia, CFI_p was 0.442 ± 0.160 and equal to 0.171 ± 0.094 in the 40 patients with insufficient collaterals (p = 0.0001).[124] There was a direct and statistically relevant association between CFI_p and CFI_v (Fig. 2.65), but CFI_p and angiographic collateral degree (score 0–3) as obtained during vessel patency were related weakly (Fig. 2.66). Using a threshold of $CFI_p = 0.30$, sufficient (i.e. no surface lead or intracoronary ST segment changes during occlusion >0.1 mV) and insufficient coronary collaterals could be correctly detected with 75% sensitivity and 92% specificity.[124] In comparison (see Fig. 2.36), over 1,000 pressure-derived CFI measurements using the definition of myocardial ischaemia just on the basis of intracoronary ECG ST elevation >0.1 mV provide a cutoff CFI_p of 0.215 for the most accurate detection of sufficient and insufficient collaterals (76% sensitivity and 76% specificity). This CFI_p-cutoff is in close

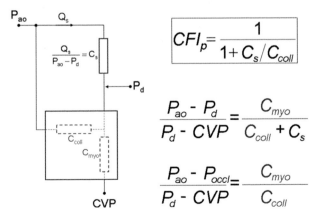

$$CFI_p = \frac{1}{1 + C_s/C_{coll}}$$

$$\frac{P_{ao} - P_d}{P_d - CVP} = \frac{C_{myo}}{C_{coll} + C_s}$$

$$\frac{P_{ao} - P_{occl}}{P_d - CVP} = \frac{C_{myo}}{C_{coll}}$$

Fig. 2.62 Same schematic as in Fig. 2.30 modelling the coronary circulation with mean aortic pressure (P_{ao}), one bifurcation, a stenotic lesion (flow conductance in the stenotic branch, C_s) and the other branch connected to the stenotic branch via a collateral vessel (collateral conductance, C_{coll}). Coronary pressure-derived collateral flow index (CFI_p; no unit) is related to coronary stenosis conductance (C_s) and coronary collateral conductance (C_{coll}; conductance = 1/resistance). Myocardial conductance C_{myo} and C_{coll} are obtainable by the measurement of P_{ao}, P_d (distal coronary pressure), P_{occl} (distal occlusive coronary pressure), CVP (central venous pressure) and Q_s (stenotic coronary flow)

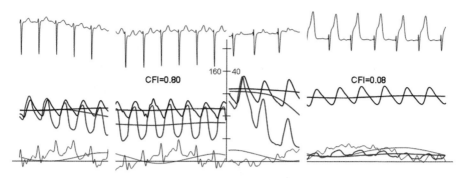

Fig. 2.63 Example of pressure/intracoronary ECG tracings from a patient with high collateral relative to normal antegrade flow (collateral flow index, CFI; left to the pressure scale) and without ECG signs of ischaemia during coronary occlusion. Right to the pressure scale: Example of pressure/ECG tracings from a patient with low CFI and marked ECG signs of ischaemia during coronary occlusion. Pressures are taken at two different scales: 160 mmHg for the phasic and mean aortic (*black thick curves*) and phasic and mean coronary (*red curves*) pressure, and 40 mmHg for phasic and mean central venous pressure (*black thin curves*). On the left side of each tracing, pressures and ECG are recorded before coronary occlusion; on the right side during occlusion. The distal coronary pressure (*red curve*) declines much less in response to the occlusion in the patient with high CFI as compared to that with low CFI. $CFI = (P_{occl}-CVP)/(P_{ao}-CVP)$; P_{occl} = coronary occlusive or wedge pressure; P_{ao} = aortic pressure; CVP = central venous pressure

agreement with a study among 61 patients with acute myocardial infarction who underwent [99m]technetium sestamibi before primary PCI andwho were investigated for collateral perfusion threshold values preserving myocardial viability.[125] A value of collateral relative to adjacent normal myocardial flow of 0.26 best separated the patients with and without subsequent infarction in

Fig. 2.64 Instantaneous coronary Doppler flow velocity spectrum obtained distal to a coronary occlusion (*upper part*) with bi-directional velocity profiles (*vertical axis*: velocity; *horizontal axis*: time). Coronary average peak flow velocity trend obtained distally (same site of Doppler sensor as above) during vessel patency ($V_{\emptyset-occl}$) and during vessel occlusion (V_{occl}; *lower part*). The ratio of $V_{occl}/V_{\emptyset-occl}$ is called Doppler- or velocity-derived collateral flow index (CFI$_v$)

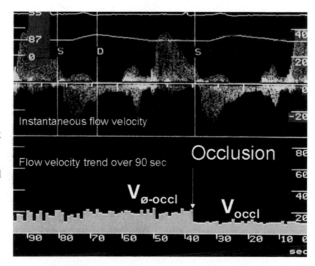

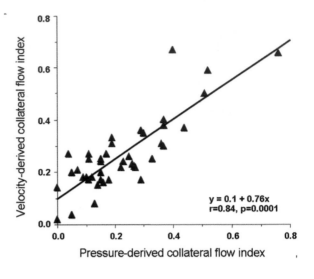

Fig. 2.65 Correlation between coronary Doppler- or velocity-derived collateral flow index (*vertical axis*) and pressure-derived collateral flow index (*horizontal axis*) as obtained simultaneously during a 1-minute coronary occlusion in 51 patients with CAD[124]

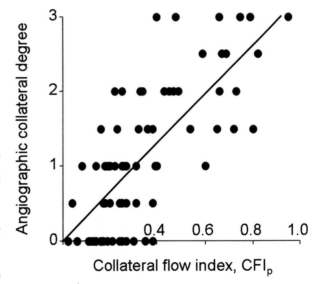

Fig. 2.66 Same patients as shown in Fig. 2.65. Relation between angiographic collateral degree as obtained during coronary artery patency (*vertical axis*) and pressure-derived collateral flow index (CFI$_p$; *horizontal axis*) as obtained simultaneously during a 1-minute coronary occlusion

that study (74% sensitivity and 74% specificity).[125] Figure 2.67 illustrates that in a larger than the initial population with simultaneous occlusive coronary sensor measurements, CFI$_p$ and CFI$_v$ are not exactly interchangeable, although they continue to correlate directly and significantly. In the lower range up to values around 0.2, CFI$_p$ underestimates CFI$_v$, whereas in the upper range >0.3, CFI$_p$ tends to overestimate CFI$_v$. There are theoretical as well as practical or technical reasons (see below) for the fact that CFI$_p$ and CFI$_v$ are not 1:1 transposable.

Fig. 2.67 Correlation between coronary Doppler- or velocity-derived collateral flow index (*vertical axis*) and pressure-derived collateral flow index (*horizontal axis*) as obtained simultaneously during a 1-minute coronary occlusion in a larger than the original population as described by Seiler et al.[124]

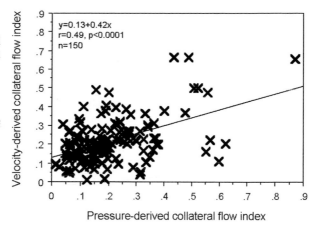

2.5.3.1 Theoretical Reason for a Difference Between CFI_p and CFI_v

Figure 2.68 illustrates a coronary circulation model with two equally sized myocardial regions and their respective minimal vascular resistances as obtained during hyperaemia, $Rmin_N$ and $Rmin_S$. The circulatory model shown earlier (Fig. 2.62) consists of just one myocardial resistance (respectively the inverse of

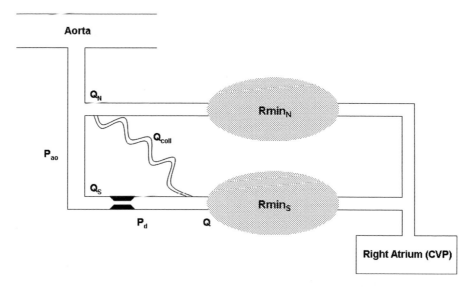

Fig. 2.68 Schematic drawing of the coronary circulation. The upper and the lower circuits are taken to supply the same amount of myocardial mass. Generally, it is assumed that in the absence of a stenosis (*lower circuit*) $P_{ao} = P_d$ (aortic and distal coronary pressure), $Q_N = Q_S$ (Q_N: hyperaemic flow without stenosis), $Rmin_N = Rmin_S$ (the microcirculatory resistances are equal), $Q_{coll} = 0$ (Q_{coll}: collateral flow). CVP: central venous (back) pressure. The oblique collateral path suggests that even in the absence of a stenosis, a small pressure difference between its origin and the orifice would render $Q_{coll} \neq 0$ (see Fig. 2.61 to illustrate the concept). See text with regarding the issue of $Rmin_N \neq Rmin_S$

Table 2.2 Determinants of the coronary pressure-flow relationship

Coronary pressure-flow (P–Q) determinants	Effect on the P–Q relation	Relevance for coronary functional measurements
Minimal vascular resistance R_{min} constant*	Linear P–Q relation	Correct at physiological pressures
Minimal vascular resistance R_{min} constant*	R = inverse of the slope of the P–Q relation	Coronary pressure = surrogate for Q
Distensibility of resistance vessels	Curvilinear relation in the low range of P–Q	$R_{minN} \neq R_{minS}$ at low coronary pressures
Elevated LV diastolic pressure	Rightward shift of P–Q relation	Divergence of FFR ($\uparrow$) and CFR ($\downarrow$)
Central venous pressure (back pressure)	Rightward shift in tamponade	To account for in the calculation of R
Cardiac arrest, respectively long diastole	Leftward shift of P–Q relation	P_{occl} dependent on heart rate
Collateral flow present	Determinant of P_{occl}; R_{min} lower	Minimal overestimation of Q_{coll} by CFI_p

*Minimal microvascular resistance independent of absence or presence of stenosis resistance or of collateral resistance ($R_{minN} = R_{minS} = R_{mincoll}$).
Abbreviations: CFI_p = pressure-derived collateral flow index; CFR = coronary flow reserve; FFR = fractional flow reserve; LV = left ventricular; P_{occl} = distal coronary occlusive or wedge pressure; Q_{coil} = collateral flow; R = vascular resistance.

it, the conductance), because it implicitly assumes equality of differently located minimal resistances. The theoretical reason for inequality of CFI_p and CFI_v is the possibility that $Rmin_N \neq Rmin_S$ (see also Table 2.2). If there is experimental evidence that $Rmin_N \neq Rmin_S$, then it is likely that $CFI_p \neq CFI_v$. According to Ohm's law, maximum myocardial flow in the presence of a stenosis (Q) relative to normal maximum myocardial flow without a stenosis (Q_N; Q/Q_N is the fractional myocardial flow reserve[120]) is written as follows:

$$Q/Q_N = ([P_d - CVP]/R\min_s)/([P_{ao} - CVP]/R\min_N)$$

This can be rearranged as follows:

$$Q/Q_N = (P_d - CVP)/(P_{ao} - CVP) \times R\min_N/R\min_S.$$

In case of a complete coronary occlusion, the part of Q coming from the stenotic coronary artery (Q_s) is equal to zero, and Q originates entirely from collateral flow Q_{coll}. In this situation, P_d is equal to P_{coll} and the above equation is written as follows:

$$Q_{coll}/Q_N = (P_{coll} - CVP)/(P_{ao} - CVP) \times R\min_N/R\min_{coll}.$$

Q_{coll}/Q_N is identical with CFI under the condition that $Rmin_N = Rmin_{coll}$. If this is the case, then the inverse of the slope of the above coronary pressure-to-flow fractions is equal to $Rmin_N$, $Rmin_S$ and $Rmin_{coll}$ respectively, and the fractional pressure intercept at zero flow is equal to CFI_p (Fig. 2.69). Q_{coll}/Q_N

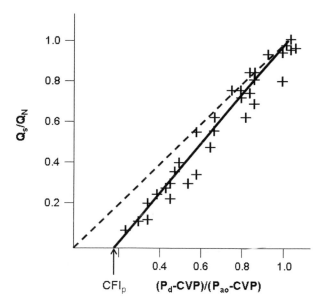

Fig. 2.69 Relationship between the ratio of hyperaemic flow in the presence (Q_S) to absence (Q_N) of variably severe coronary stenoses (*vertical axis*) and fractional flow reserve (FFR = $[P_d\text{–CVP}]/[P_{ao}\text{–CVP}]$). Assuming constant and equal minimal vascular resistances ($R\text{min}_N = R\text{min}_S$) and absence of collateral flow, the relation is represented by the identity line (*dashed line*), i.e. Q_S/Q_N can be obtained 1:1 by FFR. Pijls et al. observed that with increasing stenosis severity, Q_S/Q_N underestimated FFR, the fact of which was interpreted as the contribution of collateral flow to myocardial FFR.[120] In this case, FFR at zero flow = pressure-derived collateral flow index, CFI_p ($\rightarrow$). However, FFR at zero flow was not obtained in the study by Pijls et al.[120]. Alternatively or additionally, underestimation of FFR by Q_S/Q_N would also occur if microvascular resistance increased as distal perfusion fell ($R\text{min}_N < R\text{min}_S$; microvascular distensibility). Abbreviations: CFI_p = pressure-derived collateral flow index; CVP = central venous pressure; P_{ao} = mean aortic pressure; P_d = mean distal coronary pressure

can be expressed in terms of corresponding coronary flow velocities and main stem vascular cross-sectional areas at the site of velocity measurements:

$$A_{coll} \times V_{coll}/A_N \times V_N = (P_{coll} - CVP)/(P_{ao} - CVP) \times R\,\text{min}_N\,/R\,\text{min}_{coll}\,.$$

V_{coll}/V_N is the Doppler-derived CFI, CFI_v ($\equiv V_{occl}/V_{\emptyset\text{–occl}}$). Thus, CFI_p would be equal to CFI_v if $R\text{min}_N = R\text{min}_{coll}$ and if $A_{coll} = A_N$. That $A_{coll} = A_N$ is, intuitively, unlikely, although the ratio of the two under conditions of maximum vasodilation is probably constant. In that case, CFI_v would change at a constant rate with CFI_p under the condition that $R\text{min}_N = R\text{min}_{coll}$ as indicated by Pijls et al. [120]. Is there evidence that $R\text{min}_N \neq R\text{min}_{coll}$ or $R\text{min}_N \neq R\text{min}_S$? As described above, Pijls et al. in their conceptual work did not *prove* that $R\text{min}_N = R\text{min}_S$, because they did not obtain values of $(P_d\text{–CVP})/(P_{ao}\text{–CVP})$ during complete coronary occlusion in the absence of collateral flow ($Q_S/Q_N = 0$).[120] Under these conditions, the slope of the relationship between Q_s/Q_N and $(P_d-CVP)/(P_{ao}-CVP)$ should remain constant and should fall on the identity line (Fig. 2.69). However, at maximum vasodilation, diameters of all vessels depend on distending pressure, the fact of which is more pronounced at lower than at higher pressure.[126] According to Hagen-Poiseuille's law, vascular distensibility affects small resistance vessels more than large vessels. In 30 patients who underwent contrast echo-derived measurements of myocardial blood volume and coronary perfusion pressures during vascular occlusion and patency, it has been documented that the coronary microcirculation is distensible at a rate of 0.04 mL/100 g of myocardial blood volume per 1 mmHg of perfusion pressure change (Fig. 2.70). Therefore, $Rmin_N \neq Rmin_S$, since an epicardial stenosis not only adds resistance to coronary flow, but also additionally impedes myocardial perfusion by increasing microvascular resistance. Furthermore, $Rmin_N \neq Rmin_{coll}$, because collateral vessels variably facilitate myocardial perfusion relative to their size by lowering microvascular resistance via the passive elastic behaviour of the microvascular walls (Fig. 2.70). Despite the qualitative accuracy of these considerations, their quantitative effect on the practicability of pressure-derived CFI measurements is not important as a validation using MCE has documented (Fig. 2.71).[127] Furthermore, the assertion expressed by Spaan et al. that P_{occl}/P_{ao} in the absence of collaterals is on average equal to 0.2 cannot be confirmed,[119] since close to one-half of the over 900 invasive collateral measurements in our data base had a P_{occl}/P_{ao} value of <0.20.

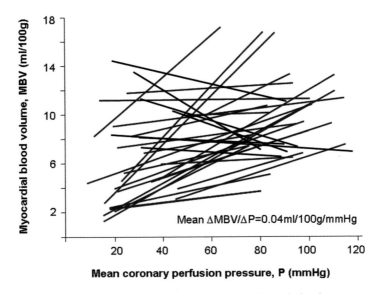

Fig. 2.70 Distensibility of the human coronary circulation. Correlation between myocardial blood volumes (*vertical axis*) and mean coronary perfusion pressures (*horizontal axis*) during coronary occlusion and following percutaneous coronary intervention (intra-individual changes shown as connecting lines). In 25 cases, there was a positive (*red lines*) and in seven cases a negative (*black lines*) relationship between the two parameters

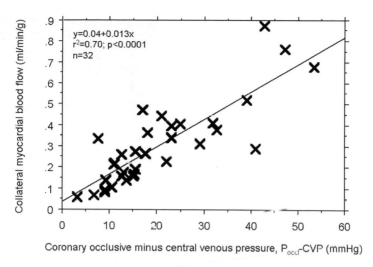

Fig. 2.71 Correlation between myocardial blood flow obtained in the collateralized region by contrast echocardiography (*vertical axis*; artificial coronary occlusion) and simultaneously measured coronary occlusive (wedge; P_{occl}) minus central venous pressure (CVP; *horizontal axis*)

Nevertheless, a practical consequence of the inequality of CFI_V and CFI_p should be that, ideally, simultaneous Doppler- and pressure-derived measurements are performed.

In 1999, Liebergen et al. published the results of a similar validation study as ours in 63 CAD patients who underwent PCI and haemodynamic quantification of recruitable collateral vessels.[128] The haemodyamic variables obtained included P_{coll}/P_{ao}, occlusive total, diastolic and systolic velocity time integral and occlusive diastolic maximum peak velocity. The absence or presence of ECG signs of ischaemia on a 12-lead surface ECG (cutoff 0.1 mV) was best detected by occlusive total and systolic velocity time integral and by P_{coll}/P_{ao}, the latter at a threshold of 0.30 (sensitivity = 70%, specificity = 94%).[128] Liebergen et al. also showed that P_{coll}/P_{ao} as well as occlusive total velocity time integral independently predicted the protective effect of collaterals with regard to the occurrence of ischaemia, which indicated that measurement of both parameters for the calculation of a coronary collateral resistance index might be more appropriate than either single parameter.[128]

2.5.3.2 Influence of LV Diastolic Pressure on CFI_p

Potentially, there is a transmission of LV cavity pressure via microcirculatory resistance increase or directly across an ischaemic and thin-walled ventricular wall to the epicardial coronary circulation including the collateral circulation. Figure 2.72 illustrates this concept in a patient with elevated LV-filling pressure of 30 mmHg in whom the brief end-diastolic LV pressure rise due to atrial contraction is visible in the coronary wedge pressure curve (P_{occl}, mean

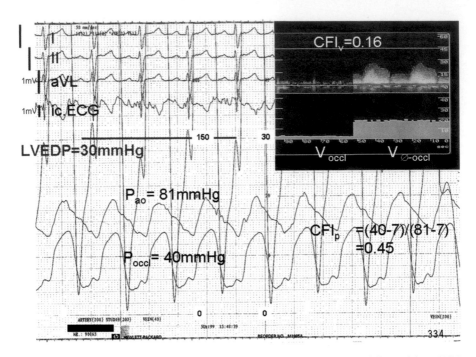

Fig. 2.72 Simultaneous recording in a patient with insufficient collateral flow of four ECG leads (surface leads and intracoronary, i.c., lead), left ventricular pressure (LVEDP = left ventricular end-diastolic pressure, scale 40 mmHg), phasic aortic pressure (P_{ao}, scale 200 mmHg), phasic coronary occlusive pressure (P_{occl}, scale 200 mmHg) and coronary occlusive flow velocity (V_{occl}, cm/s); non-occlusive flow velocity ($V_{\varnothing-occl}$, cm/s) is recorded sequentially. Pressure-derived collateral flow index (CFI$_p$, no unit) is calculated as mean coronary occlusive pressure (P_{occl}) minus central venous pressure (CVP = 7 mmHg) divided by mean aortic pressure (P_{ao}) minus CVP. CFI$_p$ overestimates CFI$_v$ which is probably due to high LVEDP

40 mmHg). Consequently, CFI$_p$ in such a case may not reflect collateral flow but elevated LV-filling pressure, as the simultaneously obtained Doppler-derived CFI$_v$ confirms (Fig. 2.72). Since coronary flow mainly occurs during diastole, LV diastolic pressure is more relevant with regard to its potential effect on microcirculatory resistance than LV systolic pressure. That LV diastolic pressure may not only influence P_{occl}, but conversely, the presence or absence of collateral flow sufficient to prevent ischaemia also diastolic LV pressure rise during coronary occlusion is illustrated in Fig. 2.73. In 50 CAD patients who underwent simultaneous measurements of P_{ao}, P_{occl}, CVP, LV pressure and intracoronary flow velocity, it has been found that the difference between pressure- and Doppler-derived CFI (CFI$_p$–CFI$_v$) remains constant up to an LV end-diastolic pressure of 27 mmHg, and beyond that it rises with increasing LV-filling pressure (Fig. 2.74).[118] However, such a transmission of LV cavity pressure to the epicardial collateral circulation occurs only in the presence of insufficient collaterals

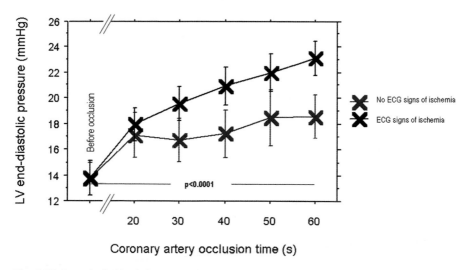

Fig. 2.73 Intra-individual changes before and during a 60-seconds coronary balloon occlusion over time (*horizontal axis*). Changes of left ventricular end-diastolic pressure are shown in patients with insufficient ($CFI_v < 0.25$, *black symbols*) and sufficient collaterals ($CFI_v \geq 0.25$, *blue symbols*); the p value is identical for both groups

(Fig. 2.74). These observations are consistent with those of Kattus and Gregg who reported an inhibition of collateral blood flow by LV distension in the open-chest dog.[129] Later, the reduction in collateral flow with increased LV preload has been found to be mediated by elongation of the collateral vessels as the ventricular size increases, and by augmented extravascular pressure tending to collapse the collaterals, a phenomenon called vascular waterfall mechanism.[130] The latter describes that the collective back-pressure-to-vascular-flow relationship remains constant over a certain range of back pressures, and at the 'waterfall

Fig. 2.74 Correlation between the difference of simultaneously obtained pressure- and Doppler-derived collateral flow index (CFI_p minus CFI_v; *vertical axis*) and left ventricular end-diastolic pressure (LVEDP; *horizontal axis*). Beyond an LVEDP of 30 mmHg, the divergence between the CFI_p and CFI_v increases in patients with low collateral flow

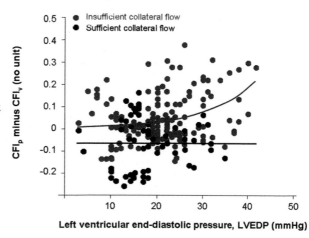

pressure' (around 24–30 mmHg for the collateral circulation[130]) experiences a break beyond which the flow depends inversely on back pressure.

2.5.4 Technical Considerations, Limitations, Pitfalls and Risks of Collateral Flow Index Measurements

2.5.4.1 Pressure-Derived CFI Measurements

The implication of LV-filling pressure potentially influencing P_{occl} and CFI_p is that pressure-derived quantitative collateral assessment should be replaced by Doppler-derived measurements in the presence of values beyond $\sim$30 mmHg during coronary occlusion and above 18 mmHg during vascular patency.[118] In chronic CAD, a relevant influence of such high LV-filling pressures on micro-circulatory resistance is present in less than 10% of patients (Fig. 2.76). In the setting of acute infarction with thinned myocardial wall, the effect of LV-filling pressure on CFI_p may become so important that CFI_p no longer reflects the collateral circulation but rather the IS, which is directly proportional to LV-filling pressure during the acute phase of infarct (Fig. 2.75). Thus, in acute myocardial infarction, only Doppler-derived collateral assessment should be used. Aside from this principal limitation of pressure-derived collateral quanti-tation in acute myocardial infarction, the robustness of coronary wedge pressure in comparison to occlusive velocity measurements using the current 0.014-inch guidewire sensors (RadiWire, Radi, Uppsala, Sweden; Volcano, Rancho Cordova, California, USA) outweighs by far the disadvantages in the setting of chronic CAD. Before positioning the pressure sensor downstream in the coronary artery, the calibrated sensor-derived pressure has to be electro-nically adjusted to the aortic pressure as derived from the fluid-filled guiding

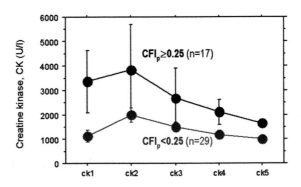

Fig. 2.75 Temporal changes of average ($\pm$standard error) creatine phosphokinase (CK; *vertical axis*) serum levels in patients with acute myocardial infarction and pressure-derived collateral flow index (CFI_p) $\geq$0.25 (*black symbols and lines*) and <0.25 (*red symbols and lines*). CK values were determined every 6 hours from the time of recanalization of the culprit lesion to 24 hours after the procedure (*horizontal axis*, ck1 to ck5)

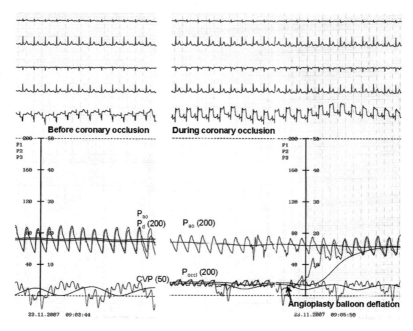

Fig. 2.76 Simultaneous ECG (*upper part*) and pressure tracings at a speed of 10 mm/s in a patient with low collateral flow before (*right side*) and during coronary balloon occlusion (*left side*). The intracoronary ECG lead shows marked ST-segment elevation during occlusion indicating collaterals insufficient to prevent myocardial ischaemia. Correspondingly, collateral flow index (CFI = [15–3]/ [68–3] = 0.185) is rather low. After pull-back of the pressure sensor wire, a pressure shift in comparison to the fluid-filled guiding catheter should be looked for routinely. In a non-stenotic vessel as it is the case here, both phasic aortic and distal coronary pressure curves should practically superimpose as it is depicted at the start and at the end of the tracing. Abbreviations: CVP = central venous pressure (scale 50 mmHg); P_{ao} = aortic pressure (scale 200 mmHg); P_d = distal coronary pressure (scale 200 mmHg); P_{occl} = distal coronary occlusive pressure (scale 200 mmHg)

catheter. For the purpose of actual mean aortic, coronary wedge and CVP gauging, a sweep of 10 mm/s is used (Fig. 2.76). CFI is derived from the average P_{ao}, P_{occl} and CVP of the last 7–10 beats before angioplasty balloon deflation. For the purpose of assessing the quality of the phasic pressure curve, the sweep is set at 25 mm/s (Fig. 2.77). Figure 2.77 shows an example of a patient with proximal LAD occlusion, no wall motion abnormalities of the LV, abundant angiographic collateral arteries from the RCA to the LAD, no ECG abnormalities indicative of myocardial ischaemia during coronary occlusion and a pressure-derived CFI of around 80% of normal antegrade flow following recanalization of the chronic occlusion. Technically, it is important to realize that the pressure sensor is located at the proximal end of the guidewire's opaque part in order to prevent gauging the balloon inflation pressure or the coronary pressure proximal to the occlusion site (Fig. 2.77). Figures 2.78 and 2.79 provide further pressure recordings of the just-mentioned patient illustrating the level of

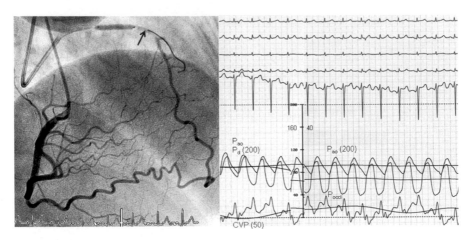

Fig. 2.77 Right coronary angiogram with double-intubation technique (*left panel*; anteroposterior cranial view) in a patient with normal systolic left ventricular function and chronic total occlusion of the proximal left anterior descending coronary artery (LAD). There are extensive angiographic coronary collateral arteries between the right coronary artery (RCA) and the LAD; angiographic collateral degree = 3. The ECG/pressure tracing recorded shortly afterwards is shown on the right side (paper speed = 25 mm/s). None of the ECG leads (intracoronary lead: lowest lead) reveals signs of myocardial ischaemia during as compared to before coronary balloon occlusion. Coronary distal occlusive pressure is obtained by the pressure sensor wire at the border between the opaque and the more transparent part ($\rightarrow$). Collateral flow index ~0.8. Abbreviations: CVP = central venous pressure (scale 50 mmHg); P_{ao} = aortic pressure (scale 200 mmHg); P_d = distal coronary pressure (scale 200 mmHg); P_{occl} = distal coronary occlusive pressure (scale 200 mmHg)

P_{occl} relative to P_{ao} in the balloon-occluded left and right coronary arteries. Biologically, Figs. 2.78 and 2.79 corroborate the notion that collateral arteries do function as bidirectional conduits (LAD collateral supply almost equal to RCA collateral supply), and that there is collateral recruitment during vascular occlusion. A technical aspect for optimizing the measurement of CVP is that it has to be recorded at a scale (0–40 mmHg) different from that for arterial pressures (0–200 mmHg). As a consequence, respiratory variations of CVP are more pronounced than in the case of arterial pressures (Fig. 2.79). Mean CVP should be obtained systematically as temporal average over several respiratory cycles. During pressure recordings, the patient should be asked to breath normally and not to speak in order to maintain physiological CVP variations. For example, the occurrence of chest pain during coronary occlusion as an additional feature of collateral supply should not be enquired during but immediately after angioplasty balloon occlusion. To actually measure CVP and not just to assume a fixed value between 0 and 10 mmHg is very important.[127,131] Perera et al. found mean errors in CFI of + 57, + 21, –3 and –20% using assumed values of 0, 5, 8 and 10 mmHg, respectively, as compared to directly obtained CVP.[131]

Left anterior descending coronary artery

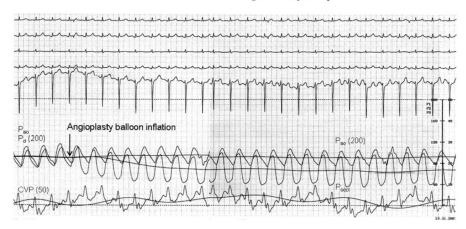

Fig. 2.78 Same patient as in Fig. 2.77. ECG/pressure tracing obtained in the proximal left anterior descending coronary artery with a much longer recording time than in Fig. 2.77. Abbreviations: CVP = central venous pressure (scale 50 mmHg); P_{ao} = aortic pressure (scale 200 mmHg); P_d = distal coronary pressure (scale 200 mmHg); P_{occl} = distal coronary occlusive pressure (scale 200 mmHg)

Right coronary artery

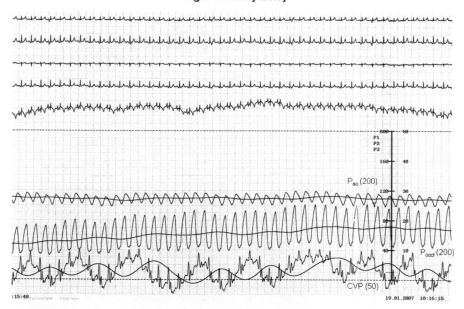

Fig. 2.79 Same patient as in Figs. 2.77 and 2.78. ECG/pressure tracing obtained in the proximal right coronary artery. Paper speed = 10 mm/s. The purpose of this and the last figure is to illustrate the bidirectional function of collaterals with a practically equal collateral flow index of approximately 0.8. Abbreviations: CVP = central venous pressure (scale 50 mmHg); P_{ao} = aortic pressure (scale 200 mmHg); P_d = distal coronary pressure (scale 200 mmHg); P_{occl} = distal coronary occlusive pressure (scale 200 mmHg)

As further technical aspects, P_d or P_{occl} pressure shifts due to leakage of electrical current and artificial systolic pressure peaks in relation to looping of the pressure guidewire have to be considered. Both problems occur more often during prolonged use and technically demanding manoeuvring of the wire, and it is more difficult to manage the former than the latter one. Straightening the pressure sensor guidewire by slight pullback resolves the problem of artificial pressure peaks dependably. Handling the problem of pressure shifts starts before positioning the wire downstream in the coronary artery with equalization of P_{ao} and P_d at the coronary ostium. A pressure difference between the fluid-filled guiding catheter and the distally positioned sensor in the absence of hyperaemia is indicative of a shift and not a biological difference, if the distal, sensor-derived pressure P_d is higher than the proximal, fluid-derived pressure P_{ao}, and if P_d is lower but its phasic curve is identical in shape as P_{ao}. Identification of a pressure shift also requires checking equality of P_{ao} and P_d after pullback of the pressure sensor wire to the ostium of the coronary artery. In case of inequality, coronary wedge pressure measurements obtained immediately before the pullback can be corrected by the amount of shift. However, in case of technical ease of positioning the sensor guidewire, a repeat CFI_p measurement should be considered.

2.5.4.2 Doppler-Derived CFI Measurements

Doppler- or velocity-derived collateral assessment by Doppler-tipped guidewires (20 MHz transducer frequency; Volcano) is much less robust than pressure-derived CFI measurement. This is mainly due to difficulties of differentiating low occlusive coronary flow velocity signals from vascular wall motion artefacts (Fig. 2.80), respectively, to time-consuming efforts of wire repositioning in order to obtain true flow velocity signals. Also in the presence of low-velocity signals, artefacts almost mirroring the true signals are visible with the baseline as reflector rendering it difficult to define the flow direction. This is not a limitation for

Fig. 2.80 Instantaneous coronary Doppler flow velocity spectrum (*upper part*) and flow velocity trend (*lower part*) obtained distal to a coronary occlusion (*left side*) and during vessel patency (*right side*) at identical location. Instantaneous flow velocity during occlusion (V_{occl}; *vertical axis*) is low and the signal quality difficult to discern from noise

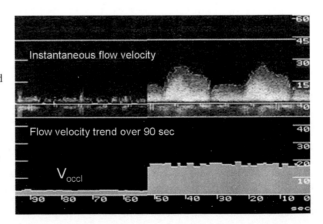

the calculation of occlusive flow velocity, since the sum of flow velocity time integral averaged over several cardiac cycles irrespective of its direction towards or away from the Doppler sensor is taken as V_{occl}.[124,128] However, it highlights the difficulty of distinguishing between true and artificial signals. Such technical problems influence low-flow velocity measurements much more than high-velocity measurements. Non-occlusive, high-flow velocity signals may be overestimated by the fact that not enough time has been allowed to elapse following ischaemic hyperaemia due to vascular occlusion. Since coronary flow velocity is taken as a surrogate for flow, a constant vascular calibre has to be ascertained during the course of the study protocol by the systematic and regular application of nitroglycerin. Even if the epicardial arterial cross-sectional area (A) remains constant, the A-times-V relationship reflecting coronary flow (Q) may not be constant depending on varying flow velocity profiles during different states of Q and on different measurement sites of V within the coronary tree.[132] Despite these shortcomings of Doppler-derived collateral assessment, they are helpful instead of or, ideally, in addition to CFI_p measurements. However, combined coronary pressure and flow velocity measurements were limited in the past by the necessary and time-consuming placement of two sensor guidewires, and are still negatively influenced by the prolonging signal optimization procedure using the current combined pressure-/Doppler-sensor wires (Volcano). In case of collateral assessment as opposed to coronary haemodynamic measurements during vessel patency (coronary and FFR), the limitations just mentioned manifest themselves much more often.

   In comparison to currently used non-sensor angioplasty guidewires, the technical performance of sensor guidewires of any type or brand is still clearly inferior, although it has improved substantially over the past years.

2.5.4.3 Influence of Pharmacologically Induced Hyperaemia on CFI Measurements

In approximately two-third of the patients with chronic CAD, coronary occlusion causes myocardial ischaemia (Fig. 2.76),[54] which is regarded as a very strong hyperaemic stimulus. An additional pharmacological hyperaemic stimulus (e.g. by intravenous adenosine) does probably not induce further reduction in microvascular resistance in this population, i.e. does not alter CFI. However, among individuals not revealing signs of ischaemia during occlusion (Fig. 2.77), pharmacological vasodilation may further decrease collateral and peripheral vascular resistance and increase CFI, and thus, CFI may be underestimated in the absence of pharmacological hyperaemia. Alternatively, microvascular resistance in the collateral supplying region may predominantly decline, and collateral flow may be re-directed away from the collateral-receiving area (i.e. collateral steal; see also under Chapter 4).[133] A study by Perera et al. confirmed the above hypothesis in 18 of 33 CAD patients with CFI<0.25, in whom the average CFI was 0.16 without and with intravenous adenosine at an infusion rate of 140 µg/min/kg.[134] Among the 15 of

33 patients with CFI≥0.25, CFI was 0.37 without adenosine and 0.33 with adenosine (p = 0.001); seven of those 15 patients revealed no change under adenosine and eight showed collateral steal. The CFI distribution in that study with almost half the patients manifesting well-developed collaterals indicates that the small study population was not representative for patients with chronic CAD as a whole. This impression is corroborated by the fact that among patients with non-occlusive chronic CAD, collateral steal occurs only in about 10% and not in 25% of the cases.[133] Nevertheless, it can be argued that CFI measurements with and without pharmacological hyperaemia provide more information than without vasodilation and that induction of maximal vasodilation is theoretically sound.[120] The simplicity of a measurement protocol without, e.g. intravenous adenosine, and thus, possibly also safety aspects have to be weighed against additional gain of information.

2.5.4.4 Safety of CFI Measurements in Normal Coronary Arteries

Theoretically, angioplasty balloon occlusion of a normal coronary artery for the purpose of CFI measurement may pose a risk for endothelial injury and development of a stenotic lesion at the occlusion site. This ethical issue was considered early-on before our group initiated a study in which the hypothesis was tested that there are preformed, functional coronary collaterals in normal human coronary arteries.[27] At that time, data on the risk of a very soft vascular balloon occlusion using an inflation pressure of ~1 atmosphere, as we specifically performed it in our protocol, were absent. The only experimental investigation, which employed balloon inflation pressures comparable to ours, performed *30 times longer* inflation durations.[135] Using such long-lasting inflation periods, it is not unexpected that after 3 months, neointima formation could be observed in 60% of the vessel segments. Aside from the shortness of a 1-minute vessel occlusion, the principal feature of our protocol with regard to preventing vessel injury was and still is the use of a balloon inflation pressure just sufficient to occlude the artery. This minimal occlusion pressure is reached very slowly, and imminent occlusion is sensed using the start of decline of the pressure obtained distal to the balloon and not primarily of angiographic detection of occlusion which only follows later. Using this protocol and a rather oversized, compliant angioplasty balloon, abrading the endothelium of an artery appears unlikely to happen. In the context of these considerations, the senior author of the mentioned study on collateral flow in normal coronary arteries (CS[27]) served as a study subject for invasive CFI measurements on four occasions.[136,137] Mid-LAD occlusions according to the described protocol did not reveal a de novo stenotic lesion at the occlusion site during angiographic follow-up between August 2000 and October 2007, and adenosine-induced coronary flow velocity reserve ranged between 4.4 at baseline and 5.5 during follow-up. While these are the only *functional* follow-up measurements, 176 of a total of 488 CFI measurements in angiographically normal vessels have been performed during repeat coronary angiography at our institution so far (average follow-up duration 36 weeks). In 2 of 176 patients with repeat coronary angiography following CFI measurement in a non-stenotic vessel, coronary de-novo stenosis at the site of CFI measurement was alleged.

2.6 Quantitative Collateral Perfusion Measurements

Simultaneous assessment of pressure-derived CFI (CFI_p) and absolute myocardial blood flow has been lacking until recently. Direct comparison of CFI_p and absolute myocardial perfusion to a briefly and artificially occluded vascular region requires a bedside quantitative method for blood flow measurements, the condition of which is fulfilled by MCE. Significant and direct correlations have been documented between collateral myocardial blood flow and the simultaneously obtained haemodynamic parameters of coronary occlusive pressure, coronary occlusive pressure normalized for aortic pressure and the difference between coronary occlusive pressure and CVP. Collateral-to-normal myocardial perfusion as obtained by MCE has been shown to be tightly associated with the mentioned haemodynamic parameters, whereby the relevance of directly obtaining CVP for computing CFI_p has become evident. The distinction between patients revealing ECG signs or no signs of myocardial ischaemia during a brief coronary occlusion appears to be most accurate using absolute collateral myocardial blood flow at a threshold of $0.374 \, \mathrm{ml \cdot min^{-1} \cdot g^{-1}}$. Side-by-side comparison of the two different quantitative methods for collateral assessment verifies that chronic CAD pressure-derived CFI measurements accurately reflect collateral relative to normal antegrade flow in humans even in the low range. In terms of collateral relative to normal antegrade flow, the overestimation of myocardial contrast-derived collateral perfusion index (CPI) by CFI_p is approximately 5%.

2.6.1 *Myocardial Contrast Echocardiography for Collateral Perfusion Measurement*

As outlined above, the current reference method for quantitative collateral assessment measures collateral flow invasively as a fraction of normal flow using CFI that is derived from simultaneous measurements of mean aortic pressure, coronary wedge pressure and CVP during angioplasty. Pressure-derived CFI is theoretically defined and its validity has been confirmed by several invasive studies.[86,112,124,128] Moreover, Matsuo et al. validated the index against perfusion defects using ^{99m}Tc-Sestamibi during angioplasty.[138] However, the direct verification of pressure-derived CFI versus the reference of myocardial blood supply assessment, i.e. absolute myocardial blood flow (ml/min/g), has been lacking until recently. Myocardial blood flow, defined as blood flow (ml/min) into a region relative to its mass (g), can be obtained by

PET and lately by MCE.[21] In Section 2.3 on the coronary occlusion model, a few existing studies using PET in a total of 59 patients with chronic coronary occlusion but viable downstream myocardium are described, in which the average collateral perfusion was 0.79 ml/min/g (see Table 2.1).[79-82] For technical reasons, it is not feasible to employ quantitative PET using oxygen-labelled water or ^{13}N-ammonia for collateral perfusion measurement in CAD without chronic total occlusions. To obtain simultaneous values of pressure-derived CFI and absolute myocardial perfusion to a briefly and artificially occluded vascular region, a bedside quantitative method for blood flow measurements has to be used, the conditions of which are fulfilled by MCE.

MCE has been proposed for the assessment of collateral-derived myocardial perfusion by several authors.[139-143] Two human studies fulfilling the mandatory requirements, i.e. documented chronic total occlusion to avoid concomitant contrast flow via the native vessel, compared MCE and invasive collateral assessment. In patients with recent acute myocardial infarction,[140] angiographically visible collaterals correlated poorly with the size of the collateralized area as well as normalized ultrasound contrast agent transit rates. In patients with stable CAD undergoing PCI,[142] CFI_p has been shown to modestly correlate with peak signal intensity of ultrasound contrast agent transit curves but not with contrast transit rates. Based on the MCE technique of ultrasound contrast agent destruction by high mechanical index with subsequent observation of contrast refill (expressed by the volume exchange rate β; Fig. 2.83) within a vascularized myocardial region of interest (providing the parameter of relative myocardial blood volume, rBV), absolute collateral myocardial perfusion or collateral myocardial blood flow was obtained during coronary angioplasty balloon occlusion in 30 patients who underwent PCI.[127] MBF was calculated according to the continuity equation as the product of β and rBV divided by myocardial tissue density (Fig. 2.81). The precision of this MCE method has been previously documented in comparison to a perfusion phantom model, to PET and to invasive coronary flow velocity measurements.[21] To be directly comparable with simultaneously obtained CFI, MCE-derived CPI was calculated in our study as the ratio between collateral myocardial blood flow and coronary blood flow as obtained in the identical myocardial region after PCI and after cessation of reactive hyperaemia (Fig. 2.82). Collateral myocardial blood flow ranged between 0.060 and 0.876 ml/min/g.[127] There were direct correlations between collateral myocardial blood flow and the simultaneously obtained haemodynamic parameters (Fig. 2.83). CPI also correlated significantly with the haemodynamic parameters (Fig. 2.84), whereby the relevance of directly obtaining CVP became evident by the marked decrease of the y intercept when it was accounted for.[127] The distinction between patients revealing ECG signs or no signs of myocardial ischaemia during 1 minute of coronary occlusion appears to be most accurate using absolute MCE-derived collateral myocardial blood flow at a threshold of 0.374 ml/min/g (Fig. 2.85).[144]

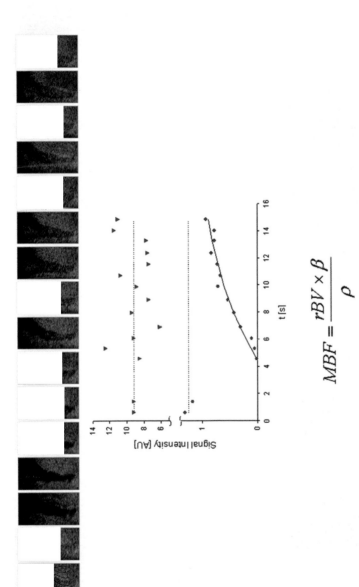

$$MBF = \frac{rBV \times \beta}{\rho}$$

Fig. 2.81 Measurement of myocardial perfusion or blood flow (MBF; ml/min/g) using contrast echocardiography. Sequence of contrast-echocardiographic images of the inter-ventricular septum and the adjacent right and left ventricular (LV) cavity (*upper part*). The red and blue regions of interest are positioned in the septum and the adjacent LV. The video signal intensity (arbitrary units, AU; *vertical axis of the middle panel*) within the LV is plotted against time (*horizontal axis*), and it represents the reference level for the calculation of relative myocardial blood volume (rBV, ml/ml; calculated as the ratio of signal intensity in the septum divided by LV signal intensity). β, the blood volume exchange rate following contrast microbubble destruction (occurring between the second and third image of the *top row*) is obtained on the basis of the exponential refill curve (*red symbols*). MBF is the product of rBV and b divided by the density of blood (*lower row*).[21]

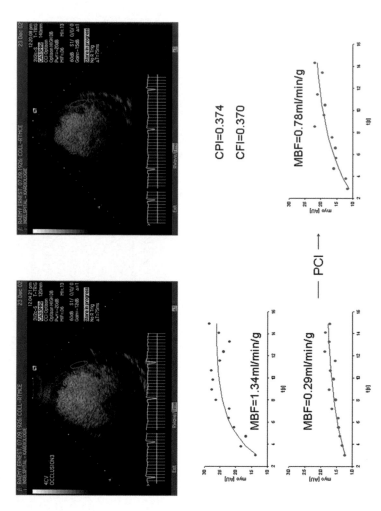

Fig. 2.82 Measurement of myocardial blood flow (MBF) using contrast echocardiography in collateralized (*upper left panel*; blue region of interest) and a normally perfused (*upper left panel*; red region of interest) area during coronary occlusion and after percutaneous intervention (PCI; *right upper panel*) of the respective vessel. The video signal intensity/time plots (*lower rows*) show the different dynamics of myocardial contrast refill following microbubble destruction by an increased ultrasonic mechanical index (yielding β). Collateral perfusion index (CPI) is calculated as MBF ratio between the collateralized and the normally perfused region. Abbreviation: CFI = collateral flow index

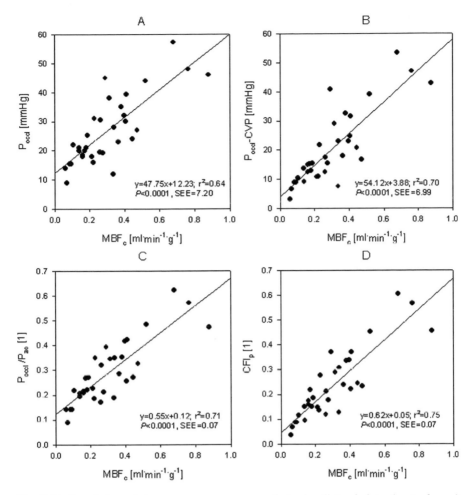

Fig. 2.83 Correlations between coronary pressure-derived collateral data (*vertical axes*) and absolute collateral-derived myocardial blood flow as obtained by quantitative contrast echocardiography (*horizontal axis*)[127]

2.6.2 Relevance of Direct Coronary Pressure-Flow Measurements

In the context of our study with side-by-side comparison of two different quantitative methods for collateral assessment,[127] it is reasonable to state that in chronic CAD pressure-derived CFI measurements accurately reflect collateral relative to normal antegrade flow in humans even in the low range and despite the above-outlined theoretical constraints. Actually, the above-discussed problem of a curvilinear coronary pressure-flow relationship in the lower range of pressures appears to be confirmed by our study

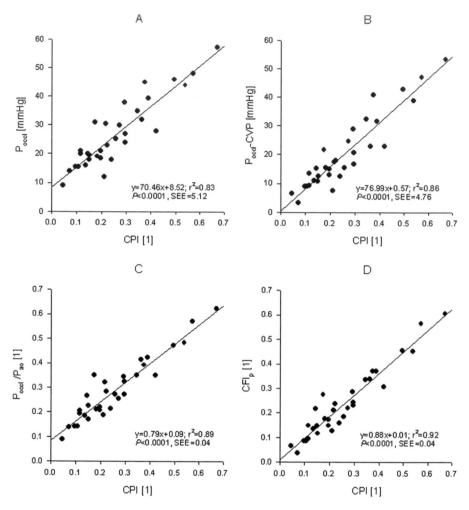

Fig. 2.84 Correlations between coronary pressure-derived collateral data (*vertical axes*) and relative collateral-derived myocardial blood flow (collateral perfusion index, CPI) as obtained by quantitative contrast echocardiography (*horizontal axis*)[127]

(Fig. 2.83A), but after accounting for CVP, the pressure intercept at zero-collateral-flow amounts only to <5 mmHg (Fig. 2.83B), i.e. the extravascular myocardial pressure determinants of P_{occl} related to LV diastolic pressure and cardiac contraction are not of high relevance in patients with chronic CAD (Table 2.2). This finding certainly challenges the recently expressed notion that a P_{occl}<25 mmHg is not likely a measure of collateral flow.[119] In terms of collateral relative to normal antegrade flow, the overestimation of

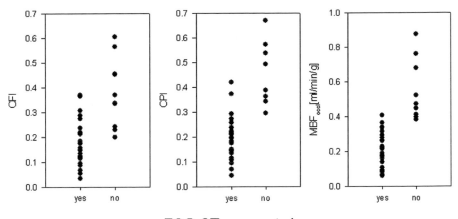

ECG ST segment changes

Fig. 2.85 Plots of different quantitative parameters of collateral flow (*vertical axes*) in relation to simultaneously obtained intracoronary ECG ST segment changes indicative for or against myocardial ischaemia during a 1-minute coronary occlusion (*horizontal axis*). Abbreviations: CFI = coronary pressure-derived collateral flow index; CPI = collateral perfusion index as obtained by myocardial contrast echocardiography; MBF_{coll} = collateral myocardial blood flow as obtained by myocardial contrast echocardiography. All three parameters are taken simultaneously[144]

CPI by pressure-derived CFI is much less than the abovementioned of Doppler-derived CFI,[124] and it amounts to approximately 2–7% depending on whether the CFI-intercept or the standard error of estimate of the CFI_p–CPI relation is considered (Fig. 2.84D).

Abbreviations

AR	area at risk for myocardial infarction
C	vascular conductance (ml/min/mmHg)
C_{coll}	collateral conductance
C_{myo}	myocardial conductance
C_s	stenosis conductance
CAD	coronary artery disease
CPI	collateral perfusion index
IS	infarct size
L	regional coronary artery branchlength (cm)
LAD	left anterior descending coronary artery
LCA	left coronary artery
LCX	left circumflex coronary artery
L_{tot}	total summed coronary artery branchlength (cm)
LV	left ventricle
M	regional myocardial mass (g)

MCE   myocardial contrast echocardiography
MR   magnetic resonance imaging
M_{tot} total myocardial mass (g)
Q   coronary blood flow rate (ml/min)
P_{ao} aortic pressure (mmHg)
P_d distal coronary pressure (mmHg)
PET   positron emission tomography
P_{occl} distal coronary occlusive or wedge pressure (mmHg)
PCI   percutaneous coronary intervention
R   vascular resistance (mmHg/ml/min)
R_m microvascular resistance (mmHg/ml/min)
RCA   right coronary artery
SPECT   single photon emission computer tomography

References

1. Helfant RH, Vokonas PS, Gorlin R. Functional importance of the human coronary collateral circulation. *N Engl J Med.* 1971;284:1277–1281.
2. Seiler C. The human coronary collateral circulation. *Heart.* 2003;89:1352–1357.
3. Fujita M, Tambara K. Recent insights into human coronary collateral development. *Heart.* 2004;90:246–250.
4. Prinzen F, Bassingthwaighte J. Blood flow distributions by microsphere deposition methods. *Cardiovasc Res.* 2000;45:13–21.
5. Utley J, Carlson E, Hoffman J, Martinez H, Buckberg G. Total and regional myocardial blood flow measurements with 25 micron, 15 micron, 9 micron, and filtered 1–10 micron diameter microspheres and antipyrine in dogs and sheep. *Circ Res.* 1974;33:391–405.
6. Rudolph A, Heymann M. The circulation of the fetus in utero. Methods for studying distribution of blood flow, cardiac output and organ blood flow. *Circ Res.* 1967;21: 163–184.
7. Hale S, Vivaldi M, Kloner R. Fluorescent microspheres: a new tool for visualization of ischemic myocardium in rats. *Am J Physiol.* 1986;251:H863–H868.
8. Glenny R, Bernard S, Brinkley M. Validation of fluorescent-labeled microspheres for measurement of regional organ perfusion. *J Appl Physiol.* 1993;74:2585–2597.
9. Bassingthwaighte J, King R, Roger S. Fractal nature of regional myocardial blood flow heterogeneity. *Circ Res.* 1989;65:578–590.
10. Kleiber M. Body size and metabolism. *Hilgardia.* 1932;6:315–353.
11. Weibel E. Early stages in the development of collateral circulation to the lung in the rat. *Circ Res.* 1960;8:353–376.
12. West GB, Brown JH, Enquist BJ. A general model for the origin of allometric scaling laws in biology. *Science.* 1997;276:122–126.
13. West G, Brown J. The origin of allometric scaling laws in biology from genomes to ecosystems: towards a quantitative unifying theory of biological structure and organization. *J Exp Biol.* 2005;208:1575–1592.
14. Glenny R, Bernard S, Neradilek B, Polissar N. Quantifying the genetic influence on mammalian vascular tree structure. *Proc Natl Acad Sci USA.* 2007;104:6858–6863.
15. Seiler C, Kirkeeide RL, Gould KL. Basic structure-function relations of the epicardial coronary vascular tree. Basis of quantitative coronary arteriography for diffuse coronary artery disease. *Circulation.* 1992;85:1987–2003.

16. Maroko P, Kjekshus J, Sobel B, et al. Factors influencing infarct size following experimental coronary artery occlusions. *Circulation.* 1971;43:67–82.

17. Murray C. The physiological principle of minimum work: I. The vascular system and the cost of blood volume. *Proc Natl Acad Sci USA.* 1926;12:207–214.

18. Murray C. The physiological principle of minimum work: II. Oxygen exchange in capillaries. *Proc Natl Acad Sci USA.* 1926;12:299–304.

19. Bergmann S, Herrero P, Markham J, Weinheimer C, Walsh M. Noninvasive quantitation of myocardial blood flow in human subjects with oxygen-15-labeled water and positron emission tomography. *J Am Coll Cardiol.* 1989;14:639–652.

20. Chareonthaitawee P, Kaufmann P, Rimoldi O, Camici P. Heterogeneity of resting and hyperemic myocardial blood flow in healthy humans. *Cardiovasc Res.* 2001;50:151–161.

21. Vogel R, Indermuhle A, Reinhardt J, et al. The quantification of absolute myocardial perfusion in humans by contrast echocardiography: algorithm and validation. *J Am Coll Cardiol.* 2005;45:754–762.

22. Kucher N, Lipp E, Schwerzmann M, Zimmerli M, Allemann Y, Seiler C. Gender differences in coronary artery size per 100 g of left ventricular mass in a population without cardiac disease. *Swiss Med Wkly.* 2001;131:610–615.

23. Windecker S, Allemann Y, Billinger M, et al. Effect of endurance training on coronary artery size and function in healthy men: an invasive followup study. *Am J Physiol Heart Circ Physiol.* 2002;282:H2216–H2223.

24. Seiler C, Kirkeeide R, Gould K. Measurement from arteriograms of regional myocardial bed size distal to any point in the coronary vascular tree for assessing anatomic area at risk. *J Am Coll Cardiol.* 1993;21:783–797.

25. Cohnheim J, von Schulthess-Rechberg A. Ueber die Folgen der Kranzarterienverschliessung für das Herz. *Virchows Arch.* 1881;85:503–537.

26. Pitt B. Interarterial coronary anastomoses. Occurence in normal hearts and in certain pathologic conditions. *Circulation.* 1959;20:816–822.

27. Wustmann K, Zbinden S, Windecker S, Meier B, Seiler C. Is there functional collateral flow during vascular occlusion in angiographically normal coronary arteries? *Circulation.* 2003;107:2213–2220.

28. Dole W. Autoregulation of the coronary circulation. *Prog Cardiovasc Dis.* 1987;29:293–323.

29. Olsson R. Myocardial reactive hyperemia. *Circ Res.* 1975;37:263–270.

30. Laxson D, Homans D, Bache R. Inhibition of adenosine-mediated coronary vasodilatation exacerbates myocardial ischemia during exercise. *Am J Physiol.* 1993;265: H1471–H1477.

31. Heberden W. Commentaries on the history and cure of diseases. In: Wilius F, Kays T, eds. *Classics of Cardiology.* New York: Dover; 1961:220–224.

32. Birnbaum Y, Kloner R. Percutaneous transluminal coronary angioplasty as a model of ischemic preconditioning and preconditioning-mimetic drugs. *J Am Coll Cardiol.* 1999;33:1036–1039.

33. Hillis L, Askenazi J, Braunwald E, et al. Use of changes in the epicardial QRS complex to assess interventions which modify the extent of myocardial necrosis following coronary artery occlusion. *Circulation.* 1976;54:591–598.

34. Guo X, Yap Y, Chen L, Huang J, Camm A. Correlation of coronary angiography with "tombstoning" electrocardiographic pattern in patients after acute myocardial infarction. *Clin Cardiol.* 2000;23:347–352.

35. Sobel B, Bresnahan G, Shell W, Yoder R. Estimation of infarct size in man and its relation to prognosis. *Circulation.* 1972;46:640–647.

36. Reimer K, Jennings R. The "wavefront phenomenon" of myocardial ischemic cell death. II. Transmural progression of necrosis within the framework of ischemic bed size (myocardium at risk) and collateral flow. *Lab Invest.* 1979;40:633–644.

37. Schaper W, Frenzel H, Hort W. Experimental coronary artery occlusion. I. Measurement of infarct size. *Basic Res Cardiol.* 1979;74:46–53.

38. Ortiz-Perez J, Meyers S, Lee D, et al. Angiographic estimates of myocardium at risk during acute myocardial infarction: validation study using cardiac magnetic resonance imaging. *Eur Heart J*. 2007;28:1750–1758.
39. Rentrop K, Cohen M, Blanke H, Phillips R. Changes in collateral channel filling immediately after controlled coronary artery occlusion by an angioplasty balloon in human subjects. *J Am Coll Cardiol*. 1985;5:587–592.
40. Bourassa M, Roubin G, Detre K, et al. Bypass Angioplasty Revascularization Investigation: patient screening, selection, and recruitment. *Am J Cardiol*. 1995;75:3C–8C.
41. Pohl T, Hochstrasser P, Billinger M, Fleisch M, Meier B, Seiler C. Influence on collateral flow of recanalising chronic total coronary occlusions: a case-control study. *Heart*. 2001;86:438–443.
42. Lee CW, Park SW, Cho GY, Hong MK, Kim JJ, Kang DH, Song JK, Lee HJ, Park SJ. Pressure-derived fractional collateral blood flow: a primary determinant of left ventricular recovery after reperfused acute myocardial infarction. *J Am Coll Cardiol*. 2000;35:949–955.
43. Billinger M, Fleisch M, Eberli FR, Garachemani AR, Meier B, Seiler C. Is the development of myocardial tolerance to repeated ischemia in humans due to preconditioning or to collateral recruitment? *J Am Coll Cardiol*. 1999;33:1027–1035.
44. Murry C, Jennings R, Reimer K. Preconditioning with ischemia: a delay of lethal cell injury in ischemic myocardium. *Circulation*. 1986;74:1124–1136.
45. Lambiase PD, Edwards RJ, Cusack MR, Bucknall CA, Redwood SR, Marber MS. Exercise-induced ischemia initiates the second window of protection in humans independent of collateral recruitment. *J Am Coll Cardiol*. 2003;41:1174–1182.
46. Hausenloy D, Yellon D. The evolving story of "conditioning" to protect against acute myocardial ischaemia-reperfusion injury. *Heart*. 2007;93:649–651.
47. Lim S, Davidson S, Hausenloy D, Yellon D. Preconditioning and postconditioning: the essential role of the mitochondrial permeability transition pore. *Cardiovasc Res*. 2007;75:530–535.
48. MacAlpin R, Weidner W, Kattus AJ, Hanafee W. Electrocardiographic changes during selective coronary cineangiography. *Circulation*. 1966;34:627–637.
49. Dupouy P, Geschwind H, Pelle G, et al. Repeated coronary artery occlusions during routine balloon angioplasty do not induce myocardial preconditioning in humans. *J Am Coll Cardiol*. 1996;27:1374–1380.
50. Tomai F. Warm up phenomenon and preconditioning in clinical practice. *Heart*. 2002;87:99–100.
51. Leesar M, Jneid H, Tang X, Bolli R. Pretreatment with intracoronary enalaprilat protects human myocardium during percutaneous coronary angioplasty. *J Am Coll Cardiol*. 2007;49:1607–1610.
52. Leesar M, Stoddard M, Ahmed M, Broadbent J, Bolli R. Preconditioning of human myocardium with adenosine during coronary angioplasty. *Circulation*. 1997;95:2500–2507.
53. Piek JJ, Koolen JJ, Hoedemaker G, David GK, Visser CA, Dunning AJ. Severity of single-vessel coronary arterial stenosis and duration of angina as determinants of recruitable collateral vessels during balloon occlusion. *Am J Cardiol*. 1991;67:13–17.
54. Pohl T, Seiler C, Billinger M, et al. Frequency distribution of collateral flow and factors influencing collateral channel development. Functional collateral channel measurement in 450 patients with coronary artery disease. *J Am Coll Cardiol*. 2001;38:1872–1878.
55. Piek J, van Liebergen R, Koch K, Peters R, David G. Comparison of collateral vascular responses in the donor and recipient coronary artery during transient coronary occlusion assessed by intracoronary blood flow velocity analysis in patients. *J Am Coll Cardiol*. 1997;29:1528–1535.
56. Iwata S, Hozumi T, Matsumura Y, et al. Cut-off value of coronary flow velocity reserve by transthoracic Doppler echocardiography for the assessment of significant donor left anterior descending artery stenosis in patients with spontaneously visible collaterals. *Am J Cardiol*. 2006;98:298–302.
57. Garza D, White F, Hall R, Bloor C. Effect of coronary collateral development on ventricular fibrillation threshold. *Basic Res Cardiol*. 1974;69:371–378.

58. Wright A, Hudlicka O. Capillary growth and changes in heart performance induced by chronic bradycardial pacing in the rabbit. *Circ Res.* 1981;49:469–478.
59. Brown M, Davies M, Hudlicka O. Angiogenesis in ischaemic and hypertrophic hearts induced by long-term bradycardia. *Angiogenesis.* 2005;8:253–262.
60. Zheng W, Brown M, Brock T, Bjercke R, Tomanek R. Bradycardia-induced coronary angiogenesis is dependent on vascular endothelial growth factor. *Circ Res.* 1999;85:192–198.
61. Hudlicka O. Mechanical factors involved in the growth of the heart and its blood vessels. *Cell Mol Biol Res.* 1994;40:143–152.
62. Patel S, Breall J, Diver D, Gersh B, Levy A. Bradycardia is associated with development of coronary collateral vessels in humans. *Coron Artery Dis.* 2000;11:467–472.
63. Turakhia M, Tseng Z. Sudden cardiac death: epidemiology, mechanisms, and therapy. *Curr Probl Cardiol.* 2007;32:501–546.
64. Airaksinen K, Ikaheimo M, Huikuri HV. Stenosis severity and the occurrence of ventricular ectopic activity during acute coronary occlusion during balloon angioplasty. *Am J Cardiol.* 1995;76:346–349.
65. Gheeraert P, Henriques J, De Buyzere M, et al. Out-of-hospital ventricular fibrillation in patients with acute myocardial infarction: coronary angiographic determinants. *J Am Coll Cardiol.* 2000;35:144–150.
66. Gheeraert P, De Buyzere M, Taeymans Y, et al. Risk factors for primary ventricular fibrillation during acute myocardial infarction: a systematic review and meta-analysis. *Eur Heart J.* 2006;27:2499–2510.
67. Gerson M, Phillips J, Morris S, McHenry P. Exercise-induced U-wave inversion as a marker of stenosis of the left anterior descending coronary artery. *Circulation.* 1976;60:1014–1020.
68. Miwa K, Nakagawa K, Hirai T, Inoue H. Exercise-induced U-wave alterations as a marker of well-developed and well-functioning collateral vessels in patients with effort angina. *JACCM.* 2000 March 1;35(3):757–763.
69. Suzuki M, Nishizaki M, Arita M, et al. Increased QT dispersion in patients with vasospastic angina. *Circulation.* 1998;98:435–440.
70. Tandogan I, Aslan H, Aksoy Y, et al. Impact of coronary collateral circulation on QT dispersion in patients with coronary artery disease. *Coron Artery Dis.* 2006;17:623–628.
71. Christian T, Gibbons R, Clements I, Berger P, Selvester R, Wagner G. Estimates of myocardium at risk and collateral flow in acute myocardial infarction using electrocardiographic indexes with comparison to radionuclide and angiographic measures. *J Am Coll Cardiol.* 1995;26:388–393.
72. Aldrich H, Wagner N, Boswick J, et al. Use of initial ST-segment deviation for prediction of final electrocardiographic size of acute myocardial infarcts. *Am J Cardiol.* 1988;61:749–753.
73. Palmeri S, Harrison D, Cobb F, et al. A QRS scoring system for assessing left ventricular function after myocardial infarction. *N Engl J Med.* 1982;306:4–9.
74. Suero J, Marso S, Jones P, et al. Procedural outcomes and long-term survival among patients undergoing percutaneous coronary intervention of a chronic total occlusion in native coronary arteries: a 20-year experience. *J Am Coll Cardiol.* 2001;38:409–414.
75. Aziz S, Stables R, Grayson A, Perry R, Ramsdale D. Percutaneous coronary intervention for chronic total occlusions: improved survival for patients with successful revascularization compared to a failed procedure. *Catheter Cardiovasc Interv.* 2007;70:15–20.
76. Heil M, Eitenmuller I, Schmitz-Rixen T, Schaper W. Arteriogenesis versus angiogenesis: similarities and differences. *J Cell Mol Med.* 2006;10:45–55.
77. Colombo A, Chieffo A. Drug-eluting stent update 2007: part III: technique and unapproved/unsettled indications (left main, bifurcations, chronic total occlusions, small vessels and long lesions, saphenous vein grafts, acute myocardial infarctions, and multivessel disease). *Circulation.* 2007;116:1424–1432.

78. Wahl A, Billinger M, Fleisch M, Meier B, Seiler C. Quantitatively assessed coronary collateral circulation and restenosis following percutaneous revascularization. *Eur Heart J*. 2000;21:1776–1784.

79. Vanoverschelde JLJ, Wijns W, Depré C, et al. Mechansims of chronic regional postischemic dysfunction in humans. New insights from the study of non-infarcted collateral-dependent myocardium. *Circulation*. 1993;87:1513–1523.

80. Uren N, Crake T, Tousoulis D, Seydoux C, Davies G, Maseri A. Impairment of the myocardial vasomotor response to cold pressor stress in collateral dependent myocardium. *Heart*. 1997;78:61–67.

81. Sambuceti G, Parodi O, Giorgetti A, et al. Microvascular dysfunction in collateral-dependent myocardium. *J Am Coll Cardiol*. 1995;26:615–623.

82. McFalls E, Araujo L, Lammertsma A, et al. Vasodilator reserve in collateral-dependent myocardium as measured by positron emission tomography. *Eur Heart J*. 1993;14:336–343.

83. Muehling O, Huber A, Cyran C, et al. The delay of contrast arrival in magnetic resonance first-pass perfusion imaging: a novel non-invasive parameter detecting collateral-dependent myocardium. *Heart*. 2007;93:842–847.

84. Demer LL, Gould KL, Goldstein RA, Kirkeeide RL. Noninvasive assessment of coronary collaterals in man by PET perfusion imaging. *J Nucl Med*. 1990;31:259–270.

85. Meier P, Gloekler S, Zbinden R, et al. Beneficial effect of recruitable collaterals: a 10-year follow-up study in patients with stable coronary artery disease undergoing quantitative collateral measurements. *Circulation*. 2007;116:975–983.

86. Werner G, Ferrari M, Heinke S, et al. Angiographic assessment of collateral connections in comparison with invasively determined collateral function in chronic coronary occlusions. *Circulation*. 2003;107:1972–1977.

87. Matsubara T, Minatoguchi S, Matsuo H, et al. Three minute, but not one minute, ischemia and nicorandil have a preconditioning effect in patients with coronary artery disease. *J Am Coll Cardiol*. 2000;35:345–351.

88. Faircloth M, Redwood S, Marber M. Ischaemic preconditioning and myocardial adaptation to serial intracoronary balloon inflation: cut from the same cloth? *Heart*. 2004;90:358–360.

89. Ambepityia G, Kopelman P, Ingram D, Swash M, Mills P, Timmis A. Exertional myocardial ischemia in diabetes: a quantitative analysis of anginal perceptual threshold and the influence of autonomic function. *J Am Coll Cardiol*. 1990;15:72–77.

90. Chiariello M, Indolfi C, Cotecchia M, Sifola C, Romano M, Condorelli M. Asymptomatic transient ST changes during ambulatory ECG monitoring in diabetic patients. *Am Heart J*. 1985;110:529–534.

91. Friedman P, Shook T, Kirshenbaum J, Selwyn A, Ganz P. Value of the intracoronary electrocardiogram to monitor myocardial ischemia during percutaneous transluminal coronary angioplasty. *Circulation*. 1986;74:330–339.

92. Cohen M, Yang X, Downey J. Attenuation of S-T segment elevation during repetitive coronary occlusions truly reflects the protection of ischemic preconditioning and is not an epiphenomenon. *Basic Res Cardiol*. 1997;92:426–434.

93. de Marchi S, Meier P, Oswald P, Seiler C. Variable ECG signs of ischemia during controlled occlusion of the left and right coronary artery in humans. *Am J Physiol*. 2006;291:H351–H356.

94. Surber R, Schwarz G, Figulla H, Werner G. Resting 12-lead electrocardiogram as a reliable predictor of functional recovery after recanalization of chronic total coronary occlusions. *Clin Cardiol*. 2005;28:293–297.

95. Engelstein E, Terres W, Hofmann D, Hansen L, Hamm C. Improved global and regional left ventricular function after angioplasty for chronic coronary occlusion. *Clin Invest*. 1994;72:442–447.

96. Elhendy A, Cornel J, Roelandt J, et al. Impact of severity of coronary artery stenosis and the collateral circulation on the functional outcome of dyssynergic myocardium after

revascularization in patients with healed myocardial infarction and chronic left ventricular dysfunction. *Am J Cardiol.* 1997;79:883–888.

97. Werner G, Surber R, Kuethe F, et al. Collaterals and the recovery of left ventricular function after recanalization of a chronic total coronary occlusion. *Am Heart J.* 2005;149:129–317.

98. Blanke H, Cohen M, Karsch K, Fagerstrom R, Rentrop K. Prevalence and significance of residual flow to the infarct zone during the acute phase of myocardial infarction. *J Am Coll Cardiol.* 1985;5:827–831.

99. Hirai T, Fujita M, Nakajima H, et al. Importance of collateral circulation for prevention of left ventricular aneurysm formation in acute myocardial infarction. *Circulation.* 1989;79:791–796.

100. Habib GB, Heibig J, Forman SA, et al. Influence of coronary collateral vessels on myocardial infarct size in humans. Results of phase I thrombolysis in myocardial infarction (TIMI) trial. The TIMI Investigators. *Circulation.* 1991;83:739–746.

101. Perez-Castellano N, Garcia E, Abeytua M, et al. Influence of collateral circulation on in-hospital death from anterior acute myocardial infarction. *J Am Coll Cardiol.* 1998;31:512–518.

102. Rentrop K, Thornton J, Feit F, Van Buskirk M. Determinants and protective potential of coronary arterial collaterals as assessed by an angioplasty model. *Am J Cardiol.* 1988;61:677–684.

103. Seiler C, Pohl T, Lipp E, Hutter D, Meier B. Regional left ventricular function during transient coronary occlusion: relation with coronary collateral flow. *Heart.* 2002;88:35–42.

104. Fulton WFM. Arterial anastomoses in the coronary circulation. I. Anatomical features in normal and diseased hearts demonstrated by stereoarteriography. *Scottish Med J.* 1963;8:420–434.

105. Fulton WFM. Arterial anastomoses in the coronary circulation. II. Distribution, enumeration and measurement of coronary arterial anastomoses in health and disease. *Scott Med J.* 1963;8:466–474.

106. Rockstroh J, Brown B. Coronary collateral size, flow capacity, and growth. Estimates from the angiogram in patients with obstructive coronary disease. *Circulation.* 2002;105:168–173.

107. Gibson C, Ryan K, Sparano A, et al. Angiographic methods to assess human coronary angiogenesis. *Am Heart J.* 1999;137:169–179.

108. Levin D. Pathways and functional significance of the coronary collateral circulation. *Circulation.* 1974;50:831–837.

109. Gensini GG, Bruto da Costa BC. The coronary collateral circulation in living man. *Am J Cardiol.* 1969;24:393–400.

110. Carroll R, Verani M, Falsetti H. The effect of collateral circulation on segmental left ventricular contraction. *Circulation.* 1974;50:709–713.

111. Zierler K. Circulation times and theory of indicator dilution mehtods for detemining blood flow and volume. In: Society AP, ed. *Handbook of Physiology.* Washington DC: American Phyiological Society; 1962:585–615.

112. Seiler C, Billinger M, Fleisch M, Meier B. Washout collaterometry: a new method of assessing collaterals using angiographic contrast clearance during coronary occlusion. *Heart.* 2001;86:540–546.

113. Feldman R, Pepine C. Evaluation of coronary collateral circulation in conscious humans. *Am J Cardiol.* 1984;53:1233–1238.

114. Cohen M, Sherman W, Rentrop K, Gorlin R. Determinants of collateral filling observed during sudden controlled coronary artery occlusion in human subjects. *J Am Coll Cardiol.* 1989;13:297–303.

115. Probst P, Zangl W, Pachinger O. Relation of coronary arterial occlusion pressure during percutaneous transluminal coronary angioplasty to presence of collaterals. *Am J Cardiol.* 1985;55:1264–1269.

116. Macdonald R, Hill J, Feldman R. ST segment response to acute coronary occlusion: coronary hemodynamic and angiographic determinants of direction of ST segment shift. *Circulation.* 1986;74:973–979.
117. Meier B, Luethy P, Finci L, Steffenino G, Rutishauser W. Coronary wedge pressure in relation to spontaneously visible and recruitable collaterals. *Circulation.* 1987;75:906–913.
118. de Marchi S, Oswald P, Windecker S, Meier B, Seiler C. Reciprocal relationship between left ventricular filling pressure and the recruitable human coronary collateral circulation. *Eur Heart J.* 2005;26:558–566.
119. Spaan J, Piek J, Hoffman J, Siebes M. Physiological basis of clinically used coronary hemodynamic indices. *Circulation.* 2006;113:446–455.
120. Pijls NHJ, van Son JAM, Kirkeeide RL, de Bruyne B, Gould KL. Experimental basis of determining maximum coronary, myocardial, and collateral blood flow by pressure measurements for assessing functional stenosis severity before and after percutaneous coronary angioplasty. *Circulation.* 1993;86:1354–1367.
121. Spaan J, Kolyva C, van den Wijngaard J, et al.Coronary structure and perfusion in health and disease. *Philos Transact A Math Phys Eng Sci.* 2008;366:3137–3153.
122. Hoefer I, van Royen N, Buschmann I, Piek J, Schaper W. Time course of arteriogenesis following femoral artery occlusion in the rabbit. *Cardiovasc Res.* 2001;49:609–617.
123. Pijls NH, Bech GJ, el Gamal MI, et al. Quantification of recruitable coronary collateral blood flow in conscious humans and its potential to predict future ischemic events. *J Am Coll Cardiol.* 1995;25:1522–1528.
124. Seiler C, Fleisch M, Garachemani A, Meier B. Coronary collateral quantitation in patients with coronary artery disease using intravascular flow velocity or pressure measurements. *J Am Coll Cardiol.* 1998;32:1272–1279.
125. Christian T, Berger P, O'Connor M, Hodge D, Gibbons R. Threshold values for preserved viability with a noninvasive measurement of collateral blood flow during acute myocardial infarction treated by direct coronary angioplasty. *Circulation.* 1999;100:2392–2395.
126. Cornelissen A, Dankelman J, VanBavel E, Stassen H, Spaan J. Myogenic reactivity and resistance distribution in the coronary arterial tree: a model study. *Am J Physiol.* 2000;278:H1490–H1499.
127. Vogel R, Zbinden R, Indermuhle A, Windecker S, Meier B, Seiler C. Collateral-flow measurements in humans by myocardial contrast echocardiography: validation of coronary pressure-derived collateral-flow assessment. *Eur Heart J.* 2006;27:157–165.
128. van Liebergen RA, Piek JJ, Koch KT, de Winter RJ, Schotborgh CE, Lie KI. Quantification of collateral flow in humans: a comparison of angiographic, electrocardiographic and hemodynamic variables. *J Am Coll Cardiol.* 1999;33:670–677.
129. Kattus A, Gregg D. Some determinants of coronary collateral blood flow in the open-chest dog. *Circ Res.* 1959;7:628–642.
130. Conway R, Kirk E, Eng C. Ventricular preload alters intravascular and extravascular resistances of coronary collaterals. *Am J Physiol.* 1988;254:H532–H541.
131. Perera D, Biggart S, Postema P, et al. Right atrial pressure: can it be ignored when calculating fractional flow reserve and collateral flow index? *J Am Coll Cardiol.* 2004;44:2089–2091.
132. Jenni R, Büchi M, Zweifel H, Ritter M. Impact of Doppler guidewire size and flow rates on intravascular velocity profiles. *Catheter Cardiovasc Diagn.* 1998;45:96–100.
133. Seiler C, Fleisch M, Meier B. Direct intracoronary evidence of collateral steal in humans. *Circulation.* 1997;96:4261–7.
134. Perera D, Patel S, Blows L, Tomsett E, Marber M, Redwood SR. Pharmacological vasodilatation in the assessment of pressure-derived collateral flow index. *Heart.* 2006;92:1149–1150.
135. Strotmann J, Bauersachs J, Fraccarollo D, et al. Trauma induced by nontraumatic coronary devices and its impact on vascular reactivity and morphology. *Am J Physiol.* 2002;283:H2356–2362.

136. Zbinden R, Zbinden S, Windecker S, Meier B, Seiler C. Direct demonstration of coronary collateral growth by physical endurance exercise in a healthy marathon runner. *Heart*. 2004;90:1350–1351.

137. Zbinden R, Meier P, Hutter D, et al. Coronary collateral flow in response to endurance exercise training. *Eur J Cardiovasc Prev and Rehab*. 2007;14:250–257.

138. Matsuo H, Watanabe S, Kadosaki T, et al. Validation of collateral fractional flow reserve by myocardial perfusion imaging. *Circulation*. 2002;105:1060–1065.

139. Grill H, Brinker J, Taube J, et al. Contrast echocardiographic mapping of collateralized myocardium in humans before and after coronary angioplasty. *J Am Coll Cardiol*. 1990;16:1594–1600.

140. Sabia PJ, Powers ER, Jayaweera AR, Ragosta M, Kaul S. Functional significance of collateral blood flow in patients with recent acute myocardial infarction: a study using myocardial contrast echocardiography. *Circulation*. 1992;85:2080–2089.

141. Mills J, Fischer D, Villanueva F. Coronary collateral development during chronic ischemia: serial assessment using harmonic myocardial contrast echocardiography. *J Am Coll Cardiol*. 2000;36:618–624.

142. de Marchi S, Schwerzmann M, Fleisch M, Billinger M, Meier B, Seiler C. Quantitative contrast echocardiographic assessment of collateral derived myocardial perfusion during elective coronary angioplasty. *Heart*. 2001;86:324–329.

143. Coggins M, Sklenar J, Le D, Wei K, Lindner J, Kaul S. Noninvasive prediction of ultimate infarct size at the time of acute coronary occlusion based on the extent and magnitude of collateral-derived myocardial blood flow. *Circulation*. 2001;104:2471–2477.

144. Vogel R, Indermühle A, Seiler C. Determination of the absolute perfusion threshold preventing myocardial ischemia in humans. *Heart*. 2007;93:115–116.

145. Murray C. A relationship between circumference and weight in trees and its bearing on branching angles. *J Gen Physiol*. 1927;10:725–729.

Chapter 3
Pathogenesis of the Human Coronary Collateral Circulation

3.1 Introduction

The term pathogenesis relates to the Greek, πάθος, *pathos* and γένεσις, *genesis*, i.e. the origin and development of a disease with all its associated factors. Additionally, the expressions *causal* and *formal* pathogenesis are distinguished, whereby the former concentrates on the predisposition of the individual to become sick, and the latter describes the functional and structural disease processes. The disease in the centre of collateral development is atherosclerosis. In this context, the development of collateral vessels is a reaction to the disease atherosclerosis, i.e. an adaptive process of divergent body function(s) in response to the disease atherosclerosis. By strict definition, this procedure is covered by the term pathophysiology. However, in this book, *pathophysiology* of the collateral circulation (see Chapter 4) is reserved for its patho-*biophysical* behaviour resulting from the specific collateral feature of connecting adjacent vascular areas with their individual resistances to blood flow. Thus, 'pathogenesis of the (human) coronary collateral circulation' relates to the genesis and growth of collateral vessels in coronary artery disease (CAD) with its determinant factors. The term genesis specifically includes vasculogenesis, angiogenesis and arteriogenesis (Fig. 3.1).[1,2]

Vasculogenesis describes the process of vessel development in the embryo, whereby they arise from endothelial precursors, which share an origin with haematopoietic progenitor cells (Figs. 3.1, 3.2, and 3.3).[1] These progenitors assemble into a primitive vascular labyrinth of small capillaries.

Angiogenesis is defined as sprouting of new capillaries from pre-existing vessels resulting in new capillary networks[2,3] (Fig. 3.1). Alternatively, intussusception is described as a mechanism of angiogenesis. The capillary networks consist of endothelial cell tubes without additional wall structures such as smooth muscle cells or adventitial stabilizing structures. The driving force for angiogenesis is hypoxia in the adjacent tissue. Sprouting of capillaries leads to an increase in their density, which is equivalent to a decrease in interspaces between neighbouring vessels. Since diffusion distances are, thus, reduced, angiogenic growth augments oxygen supply to hypoxic tissue, provided that the upstream epicardial arteries are not obstructed.

C. Seiler, *Collateral Circulation of the Heart*, DOI 10.1007/978-1-84882-342-6_3,

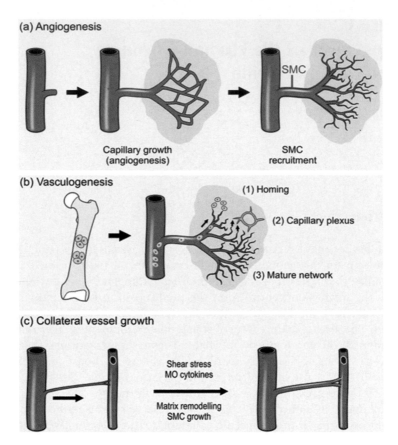

Fig. 3.1 Schematic illustration of the development of vascular systems. See text for details

Arteriogenesis (Fig. 3.1), in contrast, describes the growth of functional collateral arteries from pre-existing arterio-arteriolar anastomoses.[2,4] According to the law of Hagen-Poiseuille, the volume flow rate in a vessel changes with the product of the perfusion pressure and the vessel radius raised to the fourth power. Thus physically, the focus of this section will be on arteriogenesis and not on angiogenesis, since large-sized natural bypasses or anastomoses are clinically more relevant than small ones, because they are able to provide the bulk flow of blood relevant for the salvage of myocardium. Development of collateral arteries is initially triggered by augmented tangential shear force manifesting within the preformed collateral arteriole after a blood flow rise, which itself is caused by a perfusion pressure gradient along the collateral vessel connecting branches upstream (i.e. the collateral supplying artery) and down-stream of the occluded or obstructed coronary artery. Arteriogenesis comprises not just passive vasodilatation, but induction of vascular wall cell proliferation and migration and includes remodelling processes.

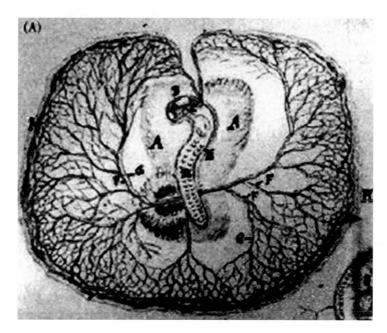

Fig. 3.2 Drawing by Marcello Malpighi (1661) showing the vascular network of arteries, capillaries and veins in a developing chicken embryo

In this context, the subsequent sections focus on the prevalence of functional collaterals in humans in the absence and presence of CAD, the dynamics of developing existence following coronary occlusion and the clinical, cellular and molecular determinants of the coronary collateral circulation.

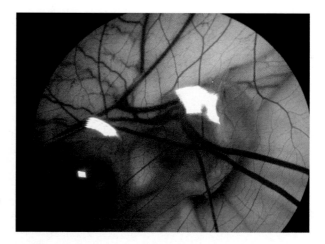

Fig. 3.3 Chicken embryo showing numerous vascular anastomoses between different branches

3.2 Frequency Distribution of Collateral Flow in Humans

In post-mortem studies, coronary collateral vessels sized > 40 μm and up to 500 μm have been documented to occur not only in human hearts with CAD, cor pulmonale cardiac hypertrophy and valvular lesions but also in normal hearts from patients with and without anaemia.

The prevalence of individuals with well-developed *preformed* collaterals is probably closer to one-fifth as indicated by intracoronary electrocardiogram (ECG) than to one-third as suggested by the absence of angina pectoris during a 1-minute coronary occlusion. Irrespective of the method employed for collateral assessment in patients without CAD, bradycardia appears to be consistently related to more prevalent, sufficient preformed collaterals.

In the presence of CAD, the occurrence of spontaneously visible collaterals during coronary angiography varies widely between 25 and 60%. The prevalence of angiographically *recruitable* collaterals is consistently higher. Coronary collaterals sufficient to prevent ECG signs of myocardial ischaemia during a 1-minute occlusion occur in 20–30%. Every third patient with chronic stable CAD has a collateral relative to normal antegrade flow (collateral flow index, CFI) of ≥0.21. CFI≥0.21 distinguishes best between patients without and with intracoronary ECG signs of ischaemia during a 1-minute coronary occlusion. Aside from coronary stenosis severity and irrespective of the method employed for collateral assessment in patients with CAD, the following factors appear to be related to better functioning collaterals: right coronary artery (RCA) as the collateral receiving artery, smoking and absence of prior myocardial infarction.

In the presence of permanent coronary occlusion, angiographic coronary collaterals are visible in 50–100% of patients after acute myocardial infarction; the prevalence increases with the age of the infarct. In chronic total occlusion, well-developed collaterals are present in 80–90% when assessed quantitatively by CFI measurements.

3.2.1 Introduction

The methodology in pathogenetic research on determinants of the human (coronary) collateral circulation differs principally from the experimental animal model in that the former is based to a high degree on epidemiological observation, while the latter can rely much more on techniques such as exposure of the animal to artificial inhibition or promotion of previously found potential factors. The collection of epidemiologically relevant data requires exact knowledge of the 'naturally' occurring prevalence of human coronary collateral flow in order to prevent misinterpretation of biologically unrepresentative data. Therefore, the subsequent chapter provides insight into different aspects of the frequency with which coronary collaterals occur in humans.

3.2.2 Prevalence of Collaterals in the Absence of CAD

In 1951, Zoll et al. published the results of the largest pathoanatomic study on the occurrence of interarterial coronary anastomoses ever performed in human hearts.[5] In an unselected series of 1,050 human hearts, the coronary arteries were uniformly injected at necropsy with a radiopaque mass, the heart was then 'unrolled' and the occurrence of interarterial anastomoses studied with respect to their frequency and pathogenesis (Fig. 3.4). Zoll et al. concluded that coronary collateral vessels sized >40 μm were increased in hearts with coronary artery occlusion or marked narrowing, cor pulmonale, cardiac hypertrophy and valvular lesions, and also in normal hearts from patients with anaemia.[5] Using a refined technique of post-mortem coronary arteriography, Fulton found inter-coronary anastomoses between 10 and 40 μm and up to 500 μm in diameter much more frequently (Fig. 3.5), namely 144 times in nine normal hearts.[6]

Thus, the prevalence and frequency distribution of differently sized collaterals appear to depend substantially on the technique used for their detection, but as the following study illustrates,[7] they also change under the influence of

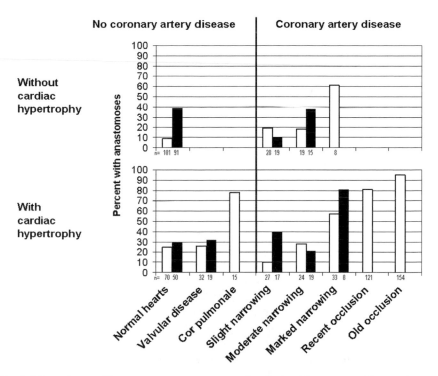

Fig. 3.4 Prevalence of intercoronary anastomoses (vertical axis) as assessed in a pathoanatomic study among 1,050 patients according to different cardiac conditions (*horizontal axis*). Black bars: patients with anaemia; white bars: patients without anaemia or total number (cor pulmonale, old occlusions) of patients

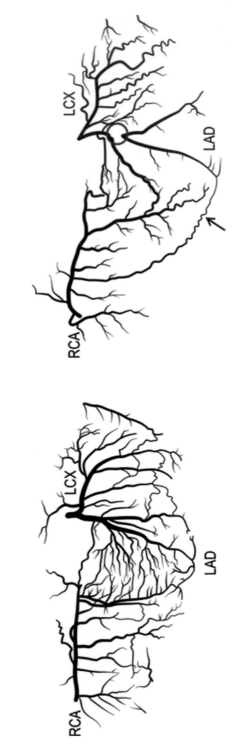

Fig. 3.5 Drawings of post-mortem coronary arteriograms in 'unrolled' hearts from an individual without cardiac disease (*left*) and a patient with coronary artery disease (CAD) and an occlusion of the left anterior descending coronary artery (LAD, *red circle*; *right panel*). In the case with normal heart, numerous anastomoses between the LAD and the right coronary (RCA) territory via the interventricular septum are visible. In the presence of occlusive CAD, a few enlarged collateral arteries between the LAD and the RCA are discernible; one of them distal to the occlusion is a branch collateral artery between the RCA with proximal origin and distal orifice in the LAD (→). LCX=left circumflex coronary artery[118]

various physical conditions. It is known that the restoration of maximal blood flow conductance in animals after arterial occlusion is equal to approximately 35% of the value in the non-occluded condition of the canine coronary circulation and 40% in the rabbit hindlimb, despite the fact that normal blood flow at rest is reached early.[4,8] Eitenmüller et al. tested the hypothesis whether this deficit of adenosine-induced hyperaemic collateral flow is diminished by artificial increase in vascular fluid shear stress.[7] Fluid shear stress was chronically increased by creating an arterio-venous shunt between the distal stump of the occluded femoral artery and the adjacent vein in the rabbit model, thus inducing and maintaining a steep pressure gradient. Figure 3.6 provides an example of how wide the range of adaptation can be in collateral arteries following femoral artery occlusion. After temporary reclosure of the shunt, collateral flow was measured at maximum vasodilatation, and maximum conductance reached the value of the non-ligated vessel at day 7 and had, after 4 weeks, surpassed the value before occlusion by a factor of 2 (Fig. 3.7).[7] With regard to the pressure value in the peripheral, i.e. collateralized artery, it fell to values *at rest* of $31 \pm 4\%$ of the aortic pressure immediately following femoral artery occlusion and rose to $50 \pm 8\%$ after 7 days.[7] In animals with arterial occlusion plus arterio-venous shunt, peripheral artery pressure dropped to $6 \pm 1\%$ of the arterial pressure immediately after the shunt operation, and it increased to values during shunt re-occlusion of $60 \pm 3\%$, respectively $73 \pm 1\%$ following 1, respectively 4 weeks of arterial occlusion.[7] This model of permanently increased vascular fluid shear stress can certainly not be regarded as a therapeutic model for the promotion of collateral growth, because the pathophysiological prize to be paid is that of chronic cardiac volume overload with development of chronic

Femoral artery ligature   **Ligature plus A-V shunt**

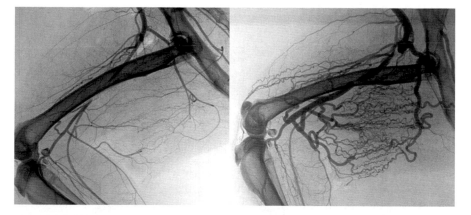

Fig. 3.6 Post-mortem angiographies of rabbit hindlimbs, 4 weeks after femoral artery ligature (*left panel*) and 4 weeks after ligature with arteriovenous (A-V) shunt treatment of the distal stump. In the shunt-treated animal, there is a multitude of large collateral arteries (corkscrew appearance) in comparison to fewer and much smaller anastomoses in the control animal without shunt treatment

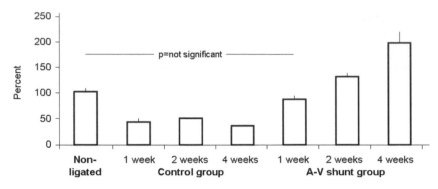

Fig. 3.7 Maximum collateral conductances (C_{max}) after control-ligature (control) and after ligature in combination with shunt-treatment (shunt) in percent of C_{max} without ligation (non-ligated). C_{max} after ligature is not able to reach C_{max} of non-ligated femoral arteries. One week after ligature in combination with arteriovenous shunt treatment C_{max} is similar to that of non-ligated arteries, and after 4 weeks, it is twice as high ($p<0.01$)[7]

heart failure. However, it represents a valuable pathogenetic model elucidating not only the full range of possible haemodynamic adaptation, but also the molecular factors involved in the process (see below).

In humans, a situation comparable to the mentioned study can be, for obvious reasons, encountered just accidentally. Figure 3.8 illustrates the case of a 22-year-old woman who underwent heart transplantation 2 years earlier (April 2005) and who suffered an iatrogenic fistula between the left anterior descending coronary artery (LAD) and the right ventricle in the course of myocardial biopsy. The maximum diastolic flow velocity of >1.20 m/s indicates a high LAD-to-right-ventricular shunt volume. An extensive, spontaneously visible collateral artery developed between the RCA and the middle part of the LAD in the absence of obstructive CAD.

In humans without CAD, there are obviously no systematic investigations using coronary angiography for the detection of spontaneously visible inter-arterial anastomoses. As in CAD, a pressure gradient between the collateral supplying and receiving vessels is required in order for the collateral artery to become visible during angiography (Fig. 3.9). In the absence of an artificial coronary occlusion, this is possible in congenital coronary artery agenesis (Fig. 3.9) or when the origin of the collateral vessel is located much more proximal than the insertion site at the recipient vessel (i.e. creating a pressure gradient of 5–10 mmHg).

Wustmann et al. analysed ECG signs indicative of myocardial ischaemia (Fig. 3.10; example of absence of signs of ischaemia) and angina pectoris during a 1-minute angioplasty balloon occlusion in a normal coronary artery of 100 patients with either atherosclerotic lesions in the other vessels (n = 49) or with entirely normal coronary arteries (n = 51).[9] Using an intracoronary ECG lead, signs indicative of myocardial ischaemia were defined as ≥ 0.1 mV or 1 mm ST segment elevation. Among 10 of 51 (20%) patients without coronary stenoses, there were no ECG signs of ischaemia indicating sufficient collaterals to prevent

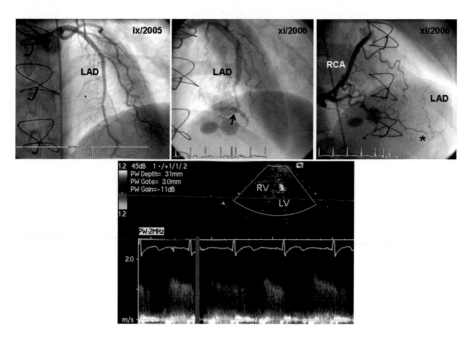

Fig. 3.8 Left (*left and middle upper panel*) and right coronary angiogram (*right upper panel*) of a heart transplant recipient with iatrogenic fistula between the left anterior descending coronary artery (LAD) and the right ventricle in the course of myocardial biopsy (2005: normal left coronary angiogram; anteroposterior cranial view; 2006: fistula →). In 2006, the LAD distal to the fistula is occluded with regard to antegrade flow (*middle upper panel*, anteroposterior cranial view). Contrast injection into the right coronary artery (RCA) reveals a branch collateral artery (*) to the LAD filling it retrogradely up to the site of the fistula. *Lower panel*: transthoracic Doppler echocardiography (apical view) of the same patient showing a diastolic flow velocity signal at a speed of >1.2 m/s (normal mid LAD coronary flow velocity ~20–40 cm/s) between the antero-septal region of the left ventricle (LV) and the right ventricle (RV). This arteriovenous shunt constitutes also a permanent pressure gradient across preformed collaterals between the RCA and LAD, which in turn triggers arteriogenesis

them (Table 3.1 and Fig. 3.10). This value corresponded to that of 13 patients (25%) who did not suffer angina pectoris during artificial coronary occlusion (Table 3.1). In a larger series of our laboratory comprising 110 individuals without coronary atherosclerotic lesions, 18 (16%) did not reveal ECG ST segment elevation and 36 (33%) did not suffer angina pectoris during the 1-minute balloon occlusion (Fig. 3.11). Among 7 of the 18 patients without ECG signs of ischaemia (39%), there was a discrepancy to the presence of angina pectoris, and in 25 of the 36 patients without angina pectoris (69%), ECG signs of ischaemia were present, i.e. they had silent ischaemia. Since ECG ST elevation ≥0.1 mV is much easier to detect than the presence or absence of angina pectoris, the absence of ECG signs for ischaemia is likely more reliable for the characterization of sufficient collaterals (see also Chapter 2). Thus, the frequency of individuals with well-developed *preformed* collaterals is probably

Fig. 3.9 Right coronary artery (RCA) angiogram (anteroposterior view) in an individual with agenesis of the left main coronary artery. The left coronary artery system is filled with contrast medium via collateral arteries (→) originating from the RCA. Abbreviation: LAD = left anterior descending artery

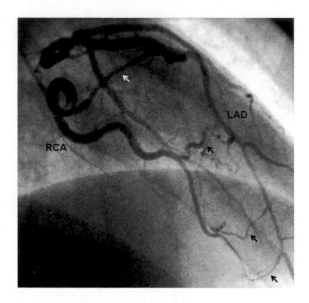

closer to one-fifth as indicated by intracoronary ECG than to one-third as suggested by the absence of angina pectoris. This figure seems to depend on the subgroup of patients focused on. According to dichotomous qualification of either well- or poorly developed collaterals (ECG or angina pectoris during vessel occlusion), men have consistently more often sufficient collaterals than women, and there appear to be more sufficient collaterals supplying the RCA than the left coronary artery (LCA) (Fig. 3.12; $p < 0.02$). These results are based on just a univariate factorial analysis, but they were obtainable irrespective of the qualitative method used for collateral assessment. The following may illustrate the point: the higher prevalence of absence of ECG signs for ischaemia in case of the RCA as the collateral receiving artery could be alternatively related not only to better collateral function, but also to a smaller myocardial mass at risk for ischaemia in the RCA than the LCA territory (→smaller ECG amplitude). That patients with the RCA as the collateral recipient artery also suffered less often from angina during occlusion than those with the LCA as the ipsilateral vessel is a strong argument for the presence of good collaterals. However, the appropriate way to analyse such problems consists of multivariate regression analysis, which requires greater patient populations (see below).

The just-described nominal data on collateral supply during a brief coronary occlusion in patients without CAD were obtained by Wustmann et al. and by Meier et al. in the course of *quantitative* collateral assessment (see also Fig. 3.10). Quantitative collateral assessment consisted of simultaneous measurement of mean aortic pressure, mean coronary occlusive pressure obtained distal to the balloon occlusion site and central venous pressure (CVP) yielding relative collateral flow in comparison to normal antegrade flow (CFI; Fig. 3.10; see also Chapter 2). Among 110 individuals without CAD, the median CFI

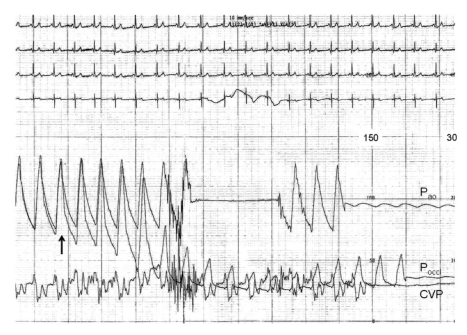

Fig. 3.10 Coronary collateral assessment in a patient with normal coronary arteries and absence of ECG signs indicative of ischaemia (*upper part*; the lowest lead is that of an intracoronary ECG obtained via the sensor guidewire) during a 1-minute coronary occlusion. Collateral flow index (CFI) expressing collateral flow to the balloon-occluded coronary artery relative to normal antegrade flow during vessel patency is determined using simultaneous aortic pressure, coronary pressure and central venous pressure (CVP) measurements (phasic recordings of these pressures obtained during coronary patency are shown on the left middle and lower side of the figure). After vascular occlusion ($\rightarrow$), phasic and mean coronary artery occlusive or wedge pressure (P_{occl}) starts to decrease and plateaus at a level of 36 mmHg (*right lower side*). Note the different scale for mean aortic pressure (P_{ao}), mean occlusive pressure and CVP. CFI is calculated as $(P_{occl}-CVP)/(P_{ao}-CVP)$

value was equal to 0.174 (Fig. 3.13). Twenty-four of the 110 patients had a CFI value of ≥ 0.25 (22%; Table 3.1).[10] The mean value was 0.178 ± 0.092, which was not significantly lower than the mean CFI value of 0.193 ± 0.133 among CAD patients (p = 0.25; Fig. 3.13). However, the skew of the distribution towards higher CFI values observed in the presence of CAD was absent in individuals without CAD. The pattern of CFI frequency distribution did not differ from the entire group with regard to gender or the vessel undergoing collateral assessment. Thus, the results obtained using dichotomous, ECG-based collateral assessment could not be reproduced by CFI measurements (see Fig. 3.12). However, irrespective of the method employed for collateral assessment in patients without CAD (CFI, ECG ST segment or angina pectoris during coronary occlusion), bradycardia (n = 12) as opposed to normo- or tachycardia (n = 98) was consistently related to more prevalent, sufficient pre-formed collaterals (Fig. 3.14).

Table 3.1 Prevalence of coronary collateral vessels

No CAD / CAD	Coronary occlusion duration	Prevalence of (sufficient*) collaterals (%)	Method for collateral assessment	Number of patients	Reference
No CAD	1 minute	20*	Intracoronary ECG	51	{Wustmann, 2003 94}[9]
No CAD	1 minute	25*	Angina pectoris during occlusion	51	{Wustmann, 2003 94}[9]
No CAD	1 minute	22*	Collateral flow index ≥0.25	110	{Meier, 2007 436}[10]
CAD	No occlusion	32	Angiography, spontaneously visible collaterals	19	{Feldman, 1984 434}[11]
CAD	No occlusion	44	Angiography, spontaneously visible collaterals	16	{Rentrop, 1985 433}[12]
CAD	90 seconds	94	Angiography, recruitable collaterals	16	{Rentrop, 1985 433}[12]
CAD	No occlusion	61	Angiography, spontaneously visible collaterals	49	{Meier, 1987 435}[13]
CAD	>30 seconds	75	Angiography, recruitable collaterals	49	{Meier, 1987 435}[13]
CAD	30 seconds	68	Angiography recruitable collaterals	57	{Piek, 1997 438}[14]
CAD	No occlusion	25	Angiography, spontaneously visible collaterals	51	{Seiler, 1998 74}[15]
CAD	2 minutes	25*	Surface lead ECG	120	{Pijls, 1995 440}[16]
CAD	1 minute	22*	Intracoronary ECG	51	{Seiler, 1998 74}[15]
CAD	1 minute	57*	Surface lead ECG	63	{van Liebergen, 1999 439}[17]
CAD	1 minute	34*	Intracoronary ECG	450	{Pohl, 2001 152}[18]
CAD	1 minute	20*	Intracoronary ECG	925	{Meier, 2007 436}[55]
CAD	1 minute	32*	Angina pectoris during occlusion	925	{Meier, 2007 436}[55]
CAD	2 minutes	32	Collateral flow index >0.24	120	{Pijls, 1995 440}[16]
CAD	1 minute	33	Collateral flow index ≥0.25	450	{Pohl, 2001 152}[18]
CAD	1 minute	24	Collateral flow index ≥0.25	925	Own data
CAD	1 minute	36	Collateral flow index ≥0.21	925	Own data
CTO	6 hours	48	Coronary angiography	116	{Schwartz, 1984 423}[19]
CTO	1–14 days	92	Coronary angiography	116	{Schwartz, 1984 423}[19]

Table 3.1 (continued)

No CAD / CAD	Coronary occlusion duration	Prevalence of (sufficient*) collaterals (%)	Method for collateral assessment	Number of patients	Reference
CTO	14–45 days	100	Coronary angiography	116	{Schwartz, 1984 423}[19]
CTO	<3 hours	66	Coronary angiography	700	{Waldecker, 2002 424}[20]
CTO	>6 hours	75	Coronary angiography	700	{Waldecker, 2002 424}[20]
CTO	Permanent	85	Collateral perfusion >0.5 ml/min/g	26	{Vanoverschelde, 1993 442}[21]
CTO	>14 days	93	Collateral flow index ≥0.25	100	{Werner, 2003 444}[23]
CTO	Permanent	60*	Intracoronary ECG	61	Own data
CTO	Permanent	60*	Angina pectoris during occlusion	61	Own data
CTO	Permanent	79	Collateral flow index ≥0.21	61	Own data
CTO	Permanent	66	Collateral flow index ≥0.25	61	Own data

*Sufficient to prevent signs of myocardial ischaemia during coronary occlusion.
CAD = coronary artery disease; CTO = chronic total coronary occlusion.

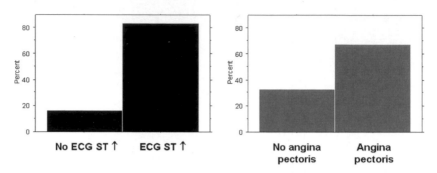

Fig. 3.11 Prevalence in individuals with normal coronary arteries (vertical axis) of absence or presence of ECG signs of ischaemia (intracoronary ECG ST segment elevations, ECG ST↑ ≥0.1 mv; *left panel*; black bars) and absence or presence of angina pectoris (*right panel*; *grey bars*) during a 1-minute coronary balloon occlusion

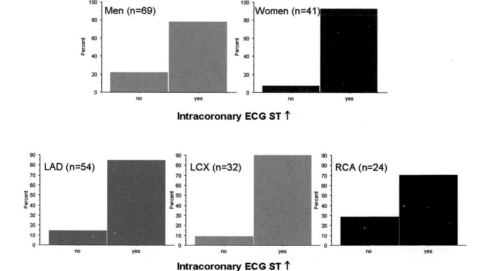

Fig. 3.12 Prevalence in individuals with normal coronary arteries (*vertical axis*) of absence or presence of ECG signs of ischaemia (intracoronary ECG ST segment elevations, ECG ST↑ ≥0.1 mv) according to gender (*upper panels*) and according to the vessel (*lower panels*) undergoing a 1-minute coronary balloon occlusion

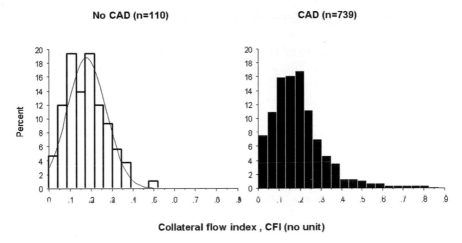

Fig. 3.13 Frequency distribution (*vertical axis*) in individuals without (*left panel*) and with (*right panel*) coronary artery disease (CAD) of invasively obtained coronary collateral flow index (CFI; horizontal axis; see also Fig. 3.10) showing a rightward shift in the prevalence of CFI in the presence of CAD

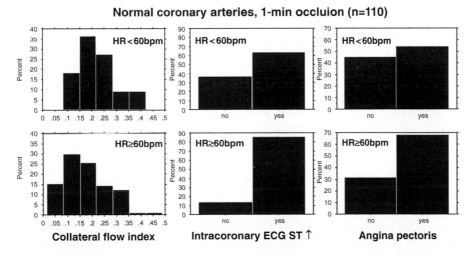

Fig. 3.14 Prevalence in individuals with normal coronary arteries (*vertical axis*) of seven different degrees of quantitatively obtained collateral flow index (*left panels*), of absence or presence of ECG signs of ischaemia (intracoronary ECG ST segment elevations, ECG ST↑ $\geq$0.1 mv; *middle panels*) and absence or presence of angina pectoris (*right panels*) during a 1-minute coronary balloon occlusion according to the presence of resting bradycardia (*blue bars*) or normo-/tachycardia (*red bars*). Bradycardia is related to a consistently better collateral function than normo-/tachycardia

3.2.3 Prevalence of Collaterals in Non-occlusive CAD

The above-cited post-mortem coronary arteriographic study by Zoll et al. reported an incidence of interarterial anastomoses >40 μm in 10–80% of patients with non-occlusive CAD.[5] The wide range of frequency was directly influenced by left ventricular (LV) hypertrophy by the presence of anaemia and by the degree of atherosclerotic narrowing (see Fig. 3.4), i.e. >80% patients with LV hypertrophy and anaemia presented with coronary collaterals if, in addition, they had a severe coronary artery stenosis. In comparison, Fulton detected coronary collaterals sized 300–800 μm (22 hearts with CAD) in high numbers and anastomotic vessels between 1000 and 1200 μm less frequently.[6]

The first small in vivo coronary angiographic studies on the prevalence of collateral vessels in patients with CAD were performed by Feldman et al.[11], and Rentrop et al.[12] Feldman et al. investigated 19 men with an LAD stenosis and observed angiographic filling via collaterals of the non-occluded LAD in six patients and no filling by collaterals in 13 patients (Table 3.1).[11] Rentrop et al. were the first to demonstrate that angiographic appearance of collaterals substantially depends on the fact whether the artery of interest is occluded or not.[12] In their study among 16 patients with isolated LAD stenosis, nine had no collaterals and seven had grade 1 (of 3) collaterals during LAD patency (Table 3.1). All patients except for one showed an increase in collateral grade during LAD balloon occlusion and with radiographic contrast injection from the contralateral vessel (RCA), and thus, collateral recruitment occurred in the vast majority of the study population (Fig. 3.15).[12] Since angiographic grade 1 collaterals (filling of side branches of the collateral recipient vessel) are not considered clinically relevant, the frequency of (probably) sufficient recruitable collaterals according to Rentrop et al. seems to be less (13/16, 81%).[12] The frequency of spontaneously visible collaterals is quite variable depending on factors such as interobserver differences, the threshold of collateral grade for the definition of visibility (>0 or >1) and the inclusion of patients with complete coronary obstructions. To illustrate the latter, the study by Meier et al. found in patients with coronary stenosis or complete obstruction that spontaneously visible collaterals occurred in 61% of the 49 individuals.[13] The respective number in 57 patients with one-vessel CAD was 68% (39 patients), whereby visibility in the study by Piek et al. was defined as the presence of angiographic score ≥2.[14] In a population of 51 CAD patients without chronic total occlusion, angiographic collaterals were spontaneously visible at our laboratory only in 13 cases (=25%; visibility: grade ≥2; Table 3.1).[15] The assessment of spontaneously visible collaterals on coronary angiography appears to be subjected to higher variability than that of recruitable collaterals, which is mainly due to the various degrees of stenotic obstructions using the former technique. For scientific purposes, spontaneously visible collaterals on coronary angiography ought to be employed only in the context of other endpoints characterizing collaterals.

Strictly speaking, coronary angiography is unable to provide information on the ability of visible collaterals to prevent myocardial ischaemia (possibility of

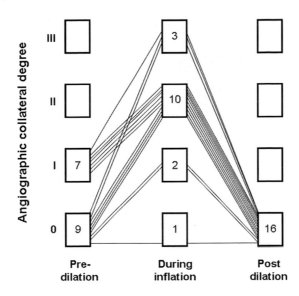

Fig. 3.15 Angiographic collateral degree (0–III) before and during occlusion of the collateral receiving artery and following percutaneous coronary intervention of the stenotic lesion in the collateral receiving artery (spontaneously visible versus recruitable collaterals and collaterals without stenosis). Grade 0 = no collaterals; grade I = side branch filling of the recipient artery without filling of the main epicardial artery; grade II = partial filling of the main epicardial recipient artery; grade III = complete filling of the main epicardial recipient artery

post-infarction development of collaterals), because it cannot characterize collaterals as sufficient or insufficient for ischaemia prevention. Therefore, other methods of assessing recruitable collaterals during a systematically applied, brief coronary occlusion should be employed for determining the prevalence of collaterals. As presented above, the occurrence of ECG ST segment elevation of ≥0.1 mV and of angina pectoris during occlusion, as well as CFI measurements fulfil these requirements. The frequency of absence of ST elevation during a ≥1-minute occlusion in patients with non-occlusive CAD and without previous myocardial infarction in the vascular area of interest has been described to range between 20 and 57% (Table 3.1).[15–17] Thus and with one exception,[17] coronary collaterals sufficient to prevent myocardial ischaemia during a 1-minute occlusion in patients with chronic stable CAD occur in 20–30%. In comparison and consistent with the situation in individuals without CAD, absence of angina pectoris during brief coronary occlusion could be observed at our institution more frequently, i.e. in 32% (Fig. 3.16). The general prevalence of 1/5 sufficient collaterals as defined by absence of ECG ST elevation varied depending on the presence of smoking, prior myocardial infarction and the vessel undergoing brief occlusion (Fig. 3.17).

Similarly as with angiographic collateral assessment, the quantitative CFI does not 'automatically' provide a value beyond which sufficient collaterals to prevent ischaemia are present. Conversely and per definition, absence of ECG

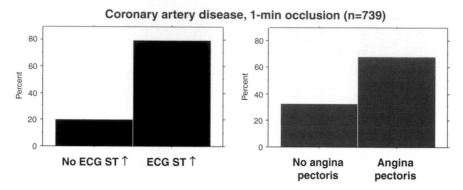

Fig. 3.16 Prevalence in individuals with coronary artery disease (*vertical axis*) of absence or presence of ECG signs of ischaemia (intracoronary ECG ST segment elevations, ECG ST↑ ≥0.1 mv; *left panel; black bars*) and absence or presence of angina pectoris (*right panel; grey bars*) during a 1-minute coronary balloon occlusion

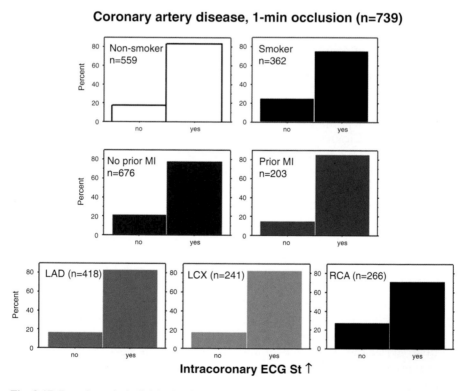

Fig. 3.17 Prevalence in individuals with coronary artery disease (*vertical axis*) of absence or presence of ECG signs of ischaemia (intracoronary ECG ST segment elevations, ECG ST↑ ≥0.1 mv) according to the history of smoking (*upper panels*) of previous myocardial infarction (MI in an area remote from the collateralized region; *middle row panels*) and according to the vessel (*lower panels*) undergoing a 1-minute coronary balloon occlusion

signs of ischaemia do indicate sufficient collaterals. The theoretically estimated
CFI threshold suggesting sufficient collaterals is related to the inverse of the
coronary flow reserve, which is equal to 4–5, thus a sufficient CFI $\geq$0.20–0.25.
Empirically, the best CFI cutoff indicating functional collaterals for the prevention
of intracoronary ECG signs of myocardial ischaemia (ST elevation $\geq$0.1 mV)
during a 1-minute balloon occlusion is $\geq$0.210 (n = 1025, sensitivity = 76%,
specificity = 76%, area under the curve = 0.826; see also Chapter 2). In small
studies, the respective value has been reported to range between 0.25 and 0.30.[15–17]
Using a 2-minute coronary occlusion protocol, Pijls et al. described the prevalence
of CFI>0.24 to be 32% (Table 3.1).[16] Pohl et al. found that in 450 patients with
CAD, sufficient collaterals according to a CFI$\geq$0.25 occurred in 1/3 (Fig. 3.18).[18]
However, in relatively small studies, the question may be raised whether the study
population obtainable is representative for the entire population with chronic stable
CAD. Among over 900 patients with CAD, the rate of those with a CFI at rest
$\geq$0.25 is approximately one-fourth (Table 3.1) and the prevalence of those with a
CFI$\geq$0.21 is about one-third. The above-described observation, using the ECG or
angina pectoris for collateral assessment of more prevalent sufficient collaterals in
the RCA, smokers and patients without prior myocardial infarction, is reproducible

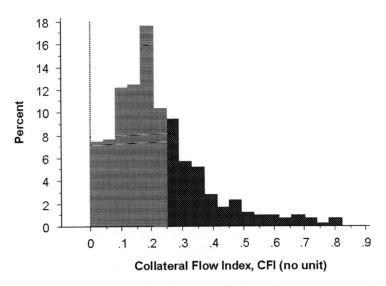

Fig. 3.18 Frequency distribution (*vertical axis*) in individuals with coronary artery disease of
invasively obtained coronary collateral flow index (CFI; *horizontal axis*; see also Fig. 3.10).
The border between the light and dark areas marks CFI = 0.25; in that study, this threshold
defined insufficient (*light grey area*) and sufficient (*dark area*) collaterals to prevent myocardial ischaemia during a 1-minute coronary occlusion

Coronary artery disease, 1-min occlusion (n=739)

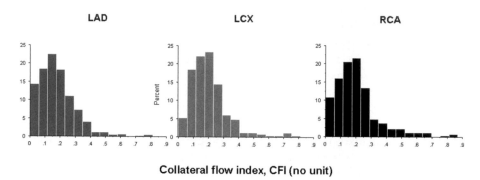

Fig. 3.19 Frequency distribution (*vertical axis*) in individuals with coronary artery disease of invasively obtained coronary collateral flow index (CFI; *horizontal axis*; see also Fig. 3.10) according to the vessel in which the 1-minute balloon occlusion was performed for collateral assessment. Left anterior descending coronary artery (LAD; *left panel*); left circumflex coronary artery (LCX; *middle panel*); right coronary artery (RCA; *right panel*)

by quantitative collateral measurement (Figs. 3.19 and 3.20). The prevalence of sufficient collaterals according to any measurement technique varies substantially with the fraction of patients with chronic total coronary occlusion (CTO) included in the study population. All of the above-cited investigations examined also individuals with total occlusion as part of the entire population. The number of patients with CTO in the study by Meier et al. was 20 of the 49 patients (41%), the fact of which may explain the high frequency of coronary wedge pressures above 20 mmHg (37/49).[13]

3.2.4 Prevalence of Collaterals in Occlusive CAD

The high prevalence of well-developed coronary collaterals in the presence of a CTO has been undisputed already in the era of pathoanatomic studies with respective figures ranging between 80 and 95% (see Fig. 3.4).[5] Part of the variability of collateral occurrence in CTO appears to be due to a certain dynamic of collateral growth depending on whether the occlusion has taken place recently or is old. In that context, Schwartz et al. studied the temporal evolution of the human coronary collateral circulation in 116 patients after myocardial infarction and with persistence of 100% occlusion of the infarct artery.[19] Patients were classified into four groups according to the interval between acute infarction and angiography. Of the 42 patients studied within 6 hours of infarction, 48% had evidence of any coronary collateral development

Coronary artery disease, 1-min occlusion (n=739)

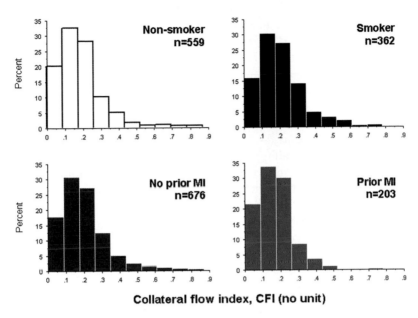

Collateral flow index, CFI (no unit)

Fig. 3.20 Frequency distribution (*vertical axis*) in individuals with coronary artery disease of invasively obtained coronary collateral flow index (CFI; *horizontal axis*; see also Fig. 3.10) according to the history of smoking (*upper panels*) and of previous myocardial infarction (MI in an area remote from the collateralized region; *lower panels*). The sum of the numbers in the panels exceeds the number of patients (given in the title) because of multiple measurements in some patients

as compared with 92% studied from 1 day to 2 weeks after infarction (Table 3.1). Virtually all patients studied beyond 2 weeks after myocardial infarction and later than 45 day had visible collateral flow. Waldecker et al. obtained coronary angiograms from 700 consecutive and unselected patients with an acute transmural infarction within 3.7 ± 3 hours (range 0.5–12 hours) of symptom onset.[20] Patients who had undergone angiography within 3 hours of symptom onset had collaterals detected less frequently than patients who had angiography beyond 6 hours (66% vs. 75%, p < 0.05).

In an attempt to elucidate the mechanism of chronic regional wall motion abnormalities in entirely collateralized vascular regions, Vanoverschelde et al. performed an elegant study using ^{14}N-ammonia positron emission tomography in 26 anginal patients with CTO of a major coronary artery but without previous infarction.[21] Positron emission tomography was performed to measure absolute regional myocardial blood flow at rest. Regional LV function was evaluated by contrast ventriculography at baseline. In nine patients, there was normal regional wall motion, and in 17 there was regional systolic dysfunction. Myocardial blood flow in the collateralized regions without wall motion abnormalities was similar as that in remote, non-collateralized regions (Fig. 3.21).[21] Interestingly, it even exceeded that of the adjacent regions: on average 0.85 ml/min/g in the collater-alized area and 0.83 ml/min/g in the normally supplied area. In other words, there was a calculated collateral myocardial perfusion index comparable to the mentioned CFI >1, the fact of which can be explained by a highly heterogeneous regional myocardial perfusion. In the 17 patients with regional LV dysfunc-tion, collateral-dependent segments had lower myocardial blood flow (Fig. 3.21). Since this study was one with a highly selected population, no conclusion could be drawn on the frequency distribution of collateral flow in the presence of CTO. However, Fig. 3.22 as adapted from that publication illustrates that 24 of 26 collateral flow values were distributed between 0.5 and 1.3 ml/min/g, whereby 1.0 ml/min/g is considered normal myocardial blood flow, and 0.374 ml/min/g has been found to be the absolute threshold beyond which no ECG changes indicative of ischaemia become visible during a 1-minute coronary balloon occlusion.[22]

In a larger series of 100 patients with CTO of >2 weeks duration, Werner et al. assessed the angiographic collateral connections in comparison with

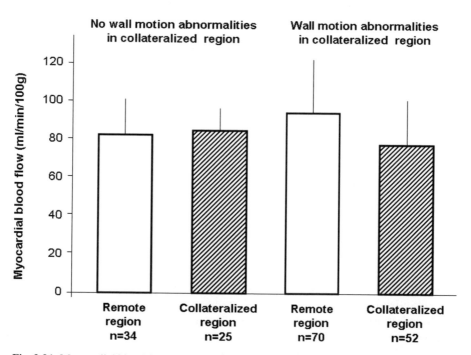

Fig. 3.21 Myocardial blood flow (*vertical axis*) in remote myocardial areas (*white bars*) and in permanently collateralized regions (*hatched bars*) as obtained by ^{14}N-ammonia positron emission tomography in 26 patients with chronic total coronary occlusion and normal or dysfunctional left ventricular wall motion at rest[21]

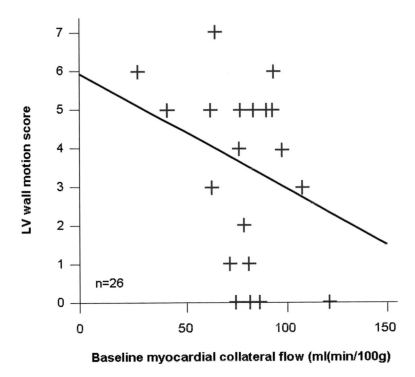

Fig. 3.22 Same study as in Fig. 3.21. Relationship between left ventricular (LV) systolic wall motion score in the entirely collateralized region (*vertical axis*) and the respective (collateral) myocardial blood flow (*horizontal axis*). The wall motion score directly indicates the severity of wall motion abnormality (0: no wall motion abnormality)

invasively determined collateral function.[23] It is evident from Fig. 3.23 as adapted from the cited work that only 7 of 100 patients had a coronary pressure derived CFI < 0.25 (Table 3.1). In addition, Fig. 3.23 illustrates the relatively high number of 11 of 100 patients showing no angiographic collateral connections, despite a CFI value which was mostly >0.25.[23]

Among 960 CAD patients examined at our institution for quantitative collateral measurement, 61 had a CTO. The majority of the patients with CTO did not reveal ECG signs of ischaemia during reocclusion of the recanalized vessel and 60% of them did not experience chest pain (Fig. 3.24 and Table 3.1). Since only patients without myocardial infarction in the vascular territory who underwent collateral assessment were included in the database, absence of ischaemia signs can be really interpreted as indicative of sufficient collateralization. In the presence of previous myocardial infarction in the region of interest, absence of ECG signs of ischaemia and/or absence of angina pectoris would not provide information on the adequacy of collateral supply. Conversely, presence of ischaemia would indicate myocardial viability within the occluded vascular area. The frequency distribution of CFI in comparison to

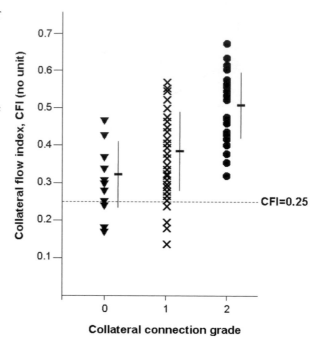

Fig. 3.23 Individual data of pressure-derived collateral flow index (CFI; *vertical axis*) in relation to different angiographic collateral connection grades (*horizontal axis*). Irrespective of angiographic appearance, the majority of CFI values in the patients with chronic total coronary occlusion is above a threshold of 0.25 indicating collaterals sufficient to prevent myocardial signs of ischaemia[23]

patients with non-occlusive CAD is depicted in Fig. 3.25. The prevalence of CFI≥0.21 and CFI≥0.25 was 48/61 and 40/61, respectively (Table 3.1).

3.3 Clinical Determinants of Collateral Flow

Pathoanatomic studies have suggested the following to be the predictors for coronary collaterals in the absence of CAD: gestational age, maternal age at birth, congenital heart disease, anaemia, ventricular hypertrophy and cor pulmonale. As opposed to the situation in CAD with a multitude of candidate determinants, in vivo studies on factors related to preformed human coronary collaterals are lacking.

Every candidate for 'clinical predictor of collateral function' should be scrutinized for an a priori relation to the endpoint collateral function before accepting it as a statistically determined 'independent predictor'. The factor most consistently reported as the determinant of coronary collaterals in the presence of CAD has been its severity. A history of angina pectoris is rather a marker for the severity of CAD than an independent predictor of well-developed collaterals. Inconsistently described cardiovascular risk factors related to impaired collateral development in patients with CAD are old age, female gender, diabetes mellitus, arterial hypertension, hyperlipidaemia, smoking and alcohol intake. Smoking in the clinical setting of patients with

Non-occlusive CAD (n=899)   **Chronic total occlusion (n=61)**

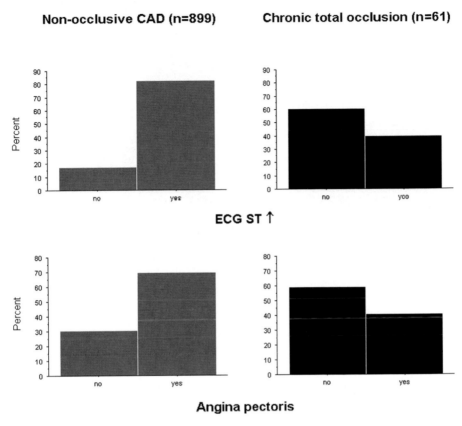

Fig. 3.24 Prevalence in individuals with coronary artery disease (CAD; vertical axis) of absence or presence of ECG signs of ischaemia (intracoronary ECG ST segment elevations, ECG ST↑ ≥0.1 mv; *upper panels*) and absence or presence of angina pectoris (*lower panels*) during a 1-minute coronary balloon of a stenotic, non-occlusive coronary artery (*grey bars*) or of a recanalized chronic total occlusion (*black bars*). The majority of patients with non-occlusive CAD has insufficient collaterals, whereas the majority of patients with chronic total occlusions has sufficient collaterals

chronic CAD is likely a co-variable of CAD severity rather than an independent predictor of collateral growth. The use of nitrates and of statins have been inconsistently described to influence the human coronary collateral circulation.

3.3.1 Introduction

The content of the present and the subsequent chapters on the pathogenesis of the coronary collateral circulation is dedicated to the question, as to which factors contribute to the entirely divergent outcome of a permanent coronary occlusion in a similarly sized myocardial area at risk for infarction. Considering

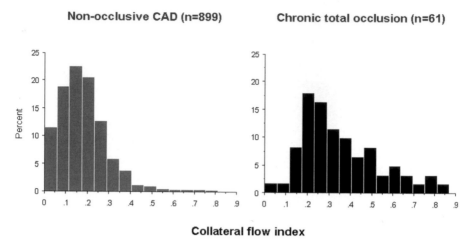

Non-occlusive CAD (n=899)   **Chronic total occlusion (n=61)**

Collateral flow index

Fig. 3.25 Frequency distribution of invasively obtained coronary collateral flow index (CFI; see also Fig. 3.10) in patients with non-occlusive coronary artery disease (CAD; *left panel*) and with chronic total occlusion (*right panel*) showing a rightward shift in the prevalence of CFI in the latter

the main contributors to infarct size, i.e. coronary occlusion duration, area at risk, collateral supply, myocardial preconditioning and oxygen demand, the presence or absence of collateral supply to an occluded artery (Fig. 3.26) may be responsible for a normal post-occlusive systolic LV function in one case and an extensive dyskinesis in the second patient. The knowledge of determinants or

Fig. 3.26 Right coronary angiogram (left anterior oblique cranial view) in a patient with multiple chronic occlusions of the right coronary artery (RCA) and contrast filling of the posterolateral and interventricular posterior branch of the RCA by a branch collateral artery originating from the proximal RCA (→; so called Kugel's collateral artery)

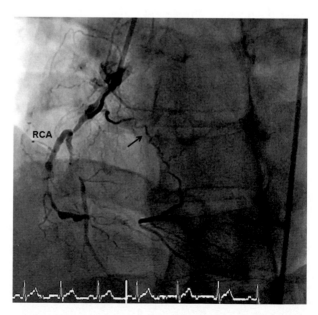

predictors of collateral development may be a key to finding potentially efficient therapeutic means for collateral promotion. The access to potential determinants with regard to the *human* coronary collateral circulation may occur
most easily via clinically determinable factors, and less simple, via the examination of potential cellular or molecular predictors. Directly associated with the
simplicity of access to clinical candidates for collateral growth is probably the
high number of 'suspects' under discussion. From a statistical standpoint of
view, the majority of declared clinical predictors for collaterals in CAD are very
likely artefacts related to insufficient power of the study, repetitive testing
without appropriate correction and inadequate use of multivariate regression
analysis. With regard to the latter statistical procedure, the final result of the
'independent predictors' of collateral growth is substantially influenced by
each of the following: regression model used, completeness of data set,
number of variables entered into the analysis, adherence to the rule of
inserting only variables significant in univariate analysis and exclusion of
variables with a priori biological interdependence (e.g. heart rate and cardiac
output or CFI and CVP). The risk of falsely detecting an 'independent
predictor' appears to rise with the degree of reliance on purely statistical
methods of analysis instead of the use of several methods of assessing the
endpoint. The knowledge about a biological foundation of the link between
a candidate factor and the collateral circulation does not prevent, but often
even advance the mentioned dependence on statistical methods. As opposed
to the situation in CAD with a multitude of associated candidate determinants, in vivo studies on factors related to preformed human coronary
collaterals are lacking.

3.3.2 Determinants of Preformed Coronary Collaterals

Table 3.2 provides a synopsis of the numerous candidate clinical determinants
of the human coronary collateral circulation. A minority is unrelated to the
presence of CAD. In this context of incongruence between some predictors
(e.g. gestational age) and CAD, Fulton stated that it would be teleological and
unscientific to assume that coronary collaterals are there for the benefit of
salvaging myocardium in the course of CAD, but that they are remnants of
the early stages of arterial development in foetal life, and the advantages they
provide are fortunate but fortuitous.[24] Nevertheless, it would be interesting to
be able of stratifying healthy people according to their innate natural escape
mechanism of preformed collaterals in case of developing CAD. The only
information available so far in this respect comes from pathoanatomic studies,
which have suggested, on the basis of partly few individuals with the respective
condition, that the following are predictors for coronary collaterals in the
absence of CAD: gestational age, maternal age at birth, congenital heart disease, anaemia, ventricular hypertrophy and cor pulmonale (Table 3.2).[5,25–27]

Table 3.2 Candidate clinical determinants of collateral flow

Potential determinant	Association	Method for collateral assessment	N	Reference
No coronary artery disease (CAD)				
Gestational age	Direct	Post-mortem arteriography	55	{Reiner, 1961 #449}[25]
Maternal age at birth	Inverse	Post-mortem arteriography	55	{Reiner, 1961 #449}[25]
Congenital heart disease	Direct	Coronary wax sphere injection; 20 controls	55	{Bloor, 1966 #448}[26]
Racial background	Related to anaemia	Post-mortem arteriography	188	{Pepler, 1960 #447}[27]
Anaemia	Direct	Post-mortem arteriography	188	{Pepler, 1960 #447}[27]
Anaemia	Direct	Post-mortem arteriography	165	{Zoll, 1951 #429}[5]
LV hypertrophy (LVH)	Direct	Post-mortem arteriography	215	{Zoll, 1951 #429}[5]
Valvular heart disease	Related to LVH	Post-mortem arteriography	75	{Zoll, 1951 #429}[5]
Cor pulmonale	Direct	Post-mortem arteriography	15	{Zoll, 1951 #429}[5]
Heart rate	Inverse	Collateral flow index	110	Own data
CAD				
Narrowing of the coronary artery	Direct	Coronary angiography (contralateral artery)	67	{Cohen, 1989 #452}[29]
Narrowing of the coronary artery	Direct	Coronary angiography (contralateral artery)	58	{Piek, 1991 #455}[30]
Duration of angina pectoris	Related to CAD severity	Coronary angiography (contralateral artery)	58	{Piek, 1991 #455}[30]
Narrowing of the coronary artery	Direct	Coronary angiography (contralateral artery)	105	{Piek, 1997 #456}[33]
Proximal location of the stenotic lesion	Related to angina	Coronary angiography (contralateral artery)	105	{Piek, 1997 #456}[33]
Ischemic area at risk	Related to angina	Collateral flow index	450	{Pohl, 2001 #152}[18]
Duration of angina pectoris	Related to CAD severity	Coronary angiography (contralateral artery)	105	{Piek, 1997 #456}[33]
Duration of angina pectoris	Related to preconditioning	Coronary angiography in CTO	58	{Juillière, 1990 #454}[35]
Cardiac ischemic score	Related to CAD severity	Coronary angiography	244	{Koerselman, 2005 #419}[37]

Table 3.2 (continued)

Potential determinant	Association	Method for collateral assessment	N	Reference
Age	Inverse	Coronary angiography	102	{Nakae, 2000 #457}[32]
Age	Inverse	Coronary angiography	1934	{Kurotobi, 2004 #459}[38]
Age	Trend to inverse relation	Collateral flow index	1068	Own data
Male gender	Direct	Coronary angiography	410	{Abaci, 1999 #460}[39]
Cardiovascular risk factors				
Diabetes mellitus	Inverse	Coronary angiography	410	{Abaci, 1999 #460}[39]
Diabetes mellitus	No relation	Collateral flow index	200	{Zbinden, 2005 #461}[44]
Arterial hypertension	Direct	Coronary angiography	313	{Kyriakides, 1991 #462}[41]
Arterial hypertension	Inverse	Coronary angiography	237	{Koerselman, 2005 #418}[37]
Hypercholesterolemia	No relation	Collateral flow index	500	{Zbinden, 2004 #463}[46]
Smoking	Direct	Coronary angiography	242	{Koerselman, 2007 #465}[43]
Alcohol	Bivariate	Coronary angiography	242	{Koerselman, 2007 #465}[43]
Heart rate	Inverse	Coronary angiography	61	{Patel, 2000 #468}[51]
Cardiovascular medication				
Nitrates	Inverse	Coronary angiography (contralateral artery)	105	{Piek, 1997 #456}[14]
Nitrates	Direct	Collateral flow index	500	{Zbinden, 2004 #463}[48]
Statins	Direct	Coronary angiography	94	{Pourati, 2004 #470}[53]
Statins	No relation	Collateral flow index	500	{Zbinden, 2004 #463}[48]

CTO = chronic total coronary occlusion.

3.3.2.1 Gestational Age and Maternal Age at Birth

Reiner et al. stated that in full-term neonates, coronary anastomoses >40 μm in calibre were present in 78%, and they further indicated an involution of these channels during childhood in the absence of stimuli known to promote their growth, such as cardiac hypertrophy, anoxia or anaemia.[25] The incidence of collaterals was not dependent on gender in pre- or full-term neonates, but interarterial coronary anastomoses were encountered more frequently in newborns of women younger than 23 years of age than in those born of women above that age. Congenital cardiac anomalies (n = 6: subpulmonic stenosis, endocardial fibroelastosis, aortic atresia) and pre-eclampsia were associated with a more developed collateral circulation. The authors suspected intrauterine hypoxia to be related to collateral growth.

3.3.2.2 Congenital Heart Disease

In the pathoanatomic investigation of Bloor et al. that included 35 children aged 3.4 ± 0.9 years (range 0–19 years) with congenital heart disease (21 with cyanosis, 14 acyanotic) and 20 children aged 4.2 ± 0.9 years (range 0–14 years) with normal hearts, the majority of those with congenital heart disease (19 of 35) had shown collaterals sized up to 120 μm, whereas all of the control group had had smaller collaterals of up to 74 μm[26] (Table 3.2). Within the group of congenital heart disease, those operated on had developed larger collaterals than those treated medically (the former had also been older than the latter). No difference in collateral size could be found between the groups of cyanotic and acyanotic congenital heart defects.

3.3.2.3 Racial Differences

In an attempt to test the hypothesis that there are racial differences in preformed coronary collaterals, Pepler et al. investigated 90 hearts from Europeans and 98 from Bantus (Table 3.2).[27] A significantly better-developed coronary collateral circulation was found in Bantu hearts, which was present from early age on, and not related to cardiac hypertrophy, gross anatomical differences in coronary tree structure (third primary division of the LCA, i.e. intermediary branch) or CAD. However, there was an association of well-developed collaterals to the presence of chronic megaloblastic or iron-deficiency anaemia in Bantu children.[27] Thus, based on that study, the conclusion of racial differences influencing collateral preformation cannot be drawn.

3.3.2.4 Anaemia

The above cited, large pathoanatomic study by Zoll et al.[5] particularly focused on the influence of absolute or relative cardiac anoxia and its association to collateral development. Among the 1,050 hearts examined by post-mortem coronary arteriography, 647 had not been affected by CAD. Figure 3.26 illustrates that in the presence of normal heart weight, the existence of anaemia had a direct influence on the incidence of coronary anastomoses.[5]

3.3.2.5 Non-atherosclerotic Heart Diseases

In the presence of cardiac hypertrophy, the occurrence of collaterals increased irrespective of a co-existing anaemia (Fig. 3.26; Table 3.2).[5] In 62 of 75 cases with valvular heart disease, there was simultaneous cardiac hypertrophy, so that the direct association between valvular heart disease and coronary collaterals appears questionable. Although the absolute number of patients with cor pulmonale was low in the study by Zoll et al. (Fig. 3.27, Table 3.2),[5] 11 of 15 were documented to have coronary anastomoses.

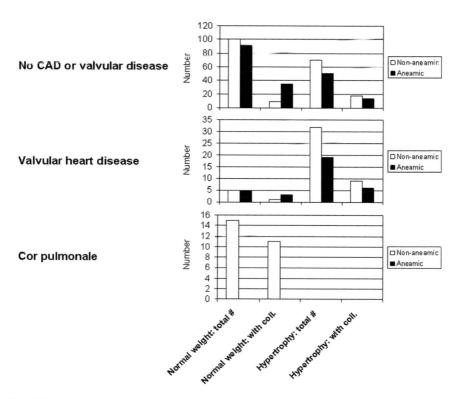

Fig. 3.27 Number of hearts with intercoronary anastomoses (*vertical axis*) as assessed in a pathoanatomic study among 1,050 patients according to the absence of cardiovascular disease, the presence of valvular heart disease or cor pulmonale with normal heart weight or cardiac hypertrophy (*horizontal axis*). Black bars: patients with anaemia; white bars: patients without anaemia[5]

3.3.2.6   In Vivo Obtained Determinants of Preformed Coronary Collaterals

Except for the studies by Goldstein et al. in 1975 (n = 7, aortic valve disease),[28] Wustmann et al. in 2003 and Meier et al. in 2007[10], no investigations on the function of human coronary collaterals in the absence of CAD have been performed so far. Until now, there have been no in vivo studies on predicting factors of preformed collaterals. Analysis of our own data indicates that bradycardia not induced by β-blocking agents as the only clinical parameter may be related to well-functioning preformed collateral vessels.

3.3.3   Determinants of Collateral Function in CAD

Aside from listing the determinants for preformed collaterals in humans, Table 3.2 provides an overview of the much larger 'catalogue' of more than a dozen clinical candidates having been declared or accepted relevant in collateral pathogenesis.

3.3.3.1   Severity of CAD, Duration of Angina Pectoris and Ischaemic Area at Risk

The factor most consistently reported as the determinant of coronary collaterals in the presence of CAD has been its severity.[29–33] As Fig. 3.28 shows, severity of CAD can be defined on the basis of atherosclerotic luminal narrowing in percent of an adjacent reference diameter. Cohen et al. obviously rather qualified than quantified the stenosis severity as evidenced by the discrete 5%-point steps between lesion severities (Fig. 3.28). Notwithstanding, lesion severity was the only independent variable associated with angiographic filling during

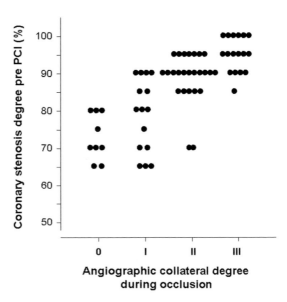

Fig. 3.28 Direct relationship between the degree of visually estimated percent diameter coronary stenosis before percutaneous coronary intervention (PCI; *vertical axis*) and angiographic collateral degree as obtained during stenosis occlusion (*horizontal axis*). See legend of Fig. 3.15 for definition of angiographic collateral degree

balloon occlusion of the collateral recipient vessel.[29] More appropriately, CAD severity is *quantitatively* obtained as percent diameter reduction of the stenotic lesion in the collateral receiving vessel of interest. Alternatively, CAD severity could also be defined as the number of main coronary arteries affected by stenotic lesions >50% in diameter narrowing, or by the total number of such stenoses, or by the number of also less severe atherosclerotic lesions, or by the presence, severity and duration of angina pectoris, or by a history of previous myocardial infarction. From a purely pathogenetic standpoint of view of collateral growth in CAD, the measurement of percent-diameter luminal narrowing is most reasonable because of the primary importance of a coronary pressure gradient between collateral supplying and receiving arteries as *the* trigger for arteriogenesis.[34] Among the above-listed possible indicators for CAD severity, percent-diameter luminal reduction is most closely related to the pressure drop across the stenosis during hyperaemia, and at the same time, it is most universally obtainable. A more elaborated structural measurement of the stenosis including its length, shape, curvature would more accurately reflect the haemodynamic relevance, i.e. the resulting pressure drop, but such a degree of quantification would not be universally available. Likewise, directly obtaining the hyperaemic lesion pressure gradient also lacks common case of use. Furthermore, hyperaemic coronary pressure obtained distal to a stenosis relative to aortic pressure (myocardial fractional flow reserve) is influenced by both the structural stenosis severity and collateral perfusion pressure (see also Section 3.3), and thus, such a value is a priori dependent on the variable being tested for the influence of independent factors. In analogy, every candidate for 'predictor of collateral function' should be scrutinized for a possible a priori relationship to the endpoint collateral function before entering it into a multivariate regression analysis or before accepting it as a declared 'independent predictor' following such an analysis. Figure 3.29 supports the notion that

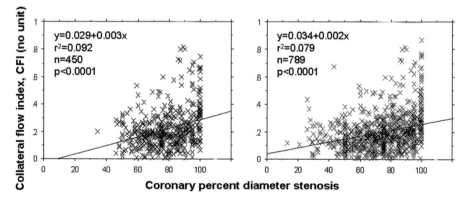

Fig. 3.29 Correlation between invasively obtained coronary collateral flow index (*vertical axes*) and percent diameter stenosis as measured by quantitative coronary angiography (*horizontal axis*) in the first 450 patients with collateral function assessment at our laboratory (*left panel, black symbols*), and after more than 1,000 measurements (*right panel*)

percent-diameter stenosis is a highly consistent factor associated with collateral function. Plotting 450 and close to 800, respectively, data pairs of percent-diameter stenosis and CFI as the dependent variable hardly alters the slope of the regression equation and the data variability increases most in measurement areas with primarily missing data. The respective data are taken from our CFI-database. The y intercept of the regression equation alters during acquisition of new data from –0.029 to +0.034, indicating that relative collateral flow in the absence of a coronary stenosis is equal to –0.03 (i.e. on average coronary steal via collaterals in the vessel of interest) and +0.03, respectively. The variable y intercept instantaneously reveals one major limitation of the statistical association between percent-diameter stenosis and CFI, namely the effects of missing data points in the low range of percent-diameter stenosis. Considering the above-mentioned average CFI in the absence of CAD of 0.178 ± 0.092, it is obvious that the size of the gap of missing data points between 0 and 50% stenosis is directly related to the dimension of the erroneous information given by the y intercept.

Similarly as the above-cited work of Cohen et al.,[29] Piek et al. aimed to determine the factors that influence the presence of collateral vessels during coronary occlusion.[30] In 58 patients with one-vessel CAD and without previous myocardial infarction, a standardized contrast injection of the contralateral coronary artery was performed. The angiographic appearance of collateral vessels during a 1-minute balloon inflation showed a statistically significant correlation to the percent-diameter stenosis before angioplasty (r = 0.28; p = 0.03) and to the duration of angina pectoris (r = 0.37; p = 0.004).[30] In a subsequent study among 105 patients with single-vessel CAD and normal systolic LV function, Piek et al. performed angiography of the contralateral artery during balloon coronary occlusion and angiographic grading of collateral vessels.[33] A multivariate logistic analysis of clinical and angiographic variables revealed duration of angina ($\geq$3 months, p < 0.0001), severity of the lesion ($\geq$75% diameter stenosis, p < 0.0001) and location of proximal lesion (p = 0.02) as independent factors positively associated with recruitability of collateral vessels.[33] The statistical independence of the determinants for collateral angiographic degree may be questioned on biological grounds, since the history of angina pectoris is a marker of the severity of CAD. Likewise, the extent of myocardial ischaemia being directly related to the proximity of a culprit stenotic lesion can be doubted, because a larger ischaemic region causes more severe angina pectoris. In fact, the quantitatively obtained size of the ischaemic risk area was related to CFI by univariate statistical analysis in a study by Pohl et al., but it did not become an independent predictor of collateral function during further analysis (Fig. 3.30). Further biological support along this line is provided by accumulating experimental evidence that it is not primarily ischaemia, but perfusion pressure gradient between different vascular areas, that drives collateral development (i.e. arteriogenesis rather than angiogenesis).[34] Alternatively to a *direct* association between area at risk for infarction and collateral function, an inverse one can be easily assumed based on the

Fig. 3.30 Correlation between coronary collateral flow index (CFI; *vertical axes*) and angiographically obtained myocardial area at risk for infarction at the site of CFI measurement (*horizontal axis*)

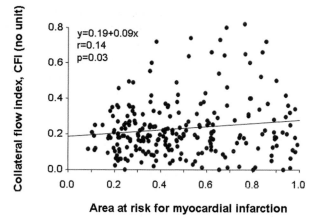

imaged temporal sequence of angiographic filling of an occluded collateral recipient artery (Fig. 3.31): the ischaemic area at risk of the LAD in the present example becomes smaller with progressive retrograde LAD filling from the contralateral side (RCA).

The aim of a study by Juillière et al. was to determine whether previous angina pectoris and collateral circulation influenced myocardial function after isolated coronary occlusion. In 58 consecutive patients, coronary angiography showed a complete isolated occlusion of the LAD; 43 patients (74%) had suffered a previous myocardial infarction.[35] In contrast to the above-cited studies on CAD severity and collateral function, the present study elegantly resolved the problem of an association between chest pain and CAD severity by

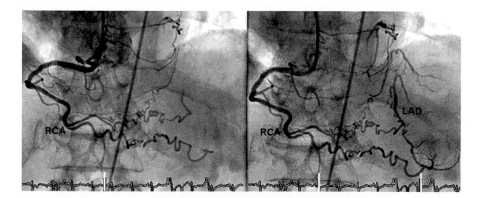

Fig. 3.31 Right coronary angiogram (right anterior oblique cranial view) in a patient with chronic total occlusions of the proximal and mid left anterior descending coronary artery (LAD). The dynamics of the gradual retrograde contrast filling of the LAD via numerous collaterals from the RCA illustrates the concept of an inverse relationship between collateral flow and (in this case LAD-) area at risk for infarction

rendering the latter constant, i.e. at 100%. Duration of previous angina pectoris was defined as the time from the first ischaemic symptom to the date of myocardial infarction or of coronary angiography in the absence of myocardial infarction. Forty patients with angiographic collaterals had higher LV ejection fraction (57 vs. 38%; p < 0.0001) and longer duration of previous angina pectoris (11 vs. 0.1 months; p < 0.002) than 18 patients without collaterals.[35] The results of this study may tamper the above remarks on the dependence between angina and CAD severities in case the role of ischaemic preconditioning (dependent on the severity of CAD) in the development of myocardial tolerance to ischaemia is not considered.[36] In a study by Fujita et al. (n = 248), the prevalence of well-developed collaterals was 57% in patients with a history of angina pectoris prior to acute myocardial infarction at study onset, which was significantly (p < 0.0001) higher than the 26% in those without a history of angina.[31] Despite the finding of angina pectoris being an independent determinant of collateral function, the interpretation of Fujita et al., that a history of angina pectoris prior to acute myocardial infarction is a clinical marker for coronary stenoses, is very likely correct.[31] Thus, it is unlikely that 'Cardiac ischemic score *determines* the presence of coronary collateral circulation' as the title of a recent publication on that subject has stated,[37] but that the ischaemic burden of CAD is rather a diagnostic indicator of collateral function (see also Table 3.2).

3.3.3.2 Age

Based on the above-presented evidence of angina pectoris duration as a factor associated with the collateral circulation, it could be hypothesized that old age of the patient would be related to well-developed collaterals. There has been evidence in the literature that the contrary might be the case, i.e. advanced age is an anti-arteriogenic factor. In a relatively small study, Nakae et al. evaluated the extent of collateral development using coronary angiography in 102 patients with an acutely occluded infarct-related artery within 12 hours after the onset of the first acute myocardial infarction, and who had a history of long-standing effort angina.[32] A well-developed collateral circulation was observed in 54 (53%) of the patients. The prevalence of good collaterals in the younger group (≤64 years, n = 48) was 69% (33/48), being significantly (p = 0.003) higher than 39% (21/54) in the older group (>64 years, n = 54).[32] In comparison, Piek et al., in the above study on predictors of recruitable collateral flow among 105 patients,[33] did not confirm age as a factor inversely related to collateral function. The sizeable study by Kurotobi et al. in 1,934 patients with acute myocardial infarction and angiographic collateral grading may explain the elusive nature of the correlation, since they found only small, though significant differences in the prevalence of collaterals among the four age groups (Fig. 3.32).[38] Univariate analysis of our database on quantitatively assessed collateral function revealed an insignificant trend towards decreasing CFI with increasing age (Fig. 3.33; p = 0.0981).

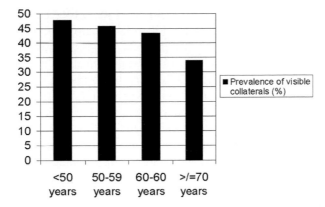

Fig. 3.32 Prevalence of angiographically visible coronary collaterals (*vertical axis*) in patients with acute myocardial infarction and total coronary occlusion according to age (*horizontal axis*). Angiographically visible coronary collaterals were defined according to the presence of first- to third-degree collaterals. The prevalence was significantly lower in the age group ≥70 years as compared to the younger age categories

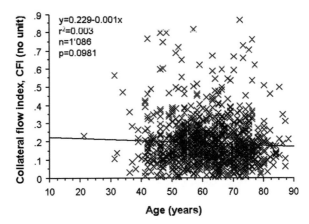

Fig. 3.33 Correlation between collateral flow index (CFI; *vertical axis*) and age (*horizontal axis*) in 739 patients with coronary artery disease

3.3.3.3 Gender

The study by Abaci et al., in 205 diabetic patients with CAD matched with 205 control individuals without diabetes mellitus, found the male gender to be a covariate (aside from diabetes) of angiographic collateral score.[39] This finding cannot be confirmed by our database, i.e. both men and women have an average CFI of 0.193 with a similar standard deviation of 0.132 and 0.120, respectively.

3.3.3.4 Cardiovascular Risk Factors

Inconsistently described pathogenetic factors related to impaired collateral development in patients with CAD are diabetes mellitus,[39,40] arterial hypertension,[41] hyperlipidemia,[42] smoking,[43] and, in part, alcohol.[43]

The principal finding of the above-mentioned study by Abaci et al. was that the patients with diabetes mellitus developed less angiographically visible collateral vessel than non-diabetic control patients.[39] This was the case despite the existence of a more severe CAD in the diabetic patients. The main limitation of that sizeable investigation is its use of a very blunt instrument for collateral assessment, i.e. detection of spontaneously visible collaterals in non-occlusive CAD. A study by Zbinden et al. using quantitative CFI measurements in 100 diabetic and 100 non-diabetic patients matched for clinical, haemodynamic and angiographic parameters revealed no difference in collateral function between the groups (Fig. 3.34).[44] Likewise, CFI did not differ when only angiographically normal vessels (0.20 ± 0.09 vs. 0.15 ± 0.08, not significant; Fig. 3.35) or

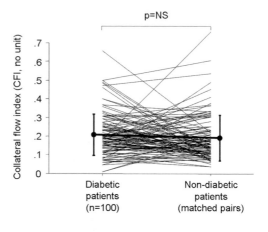

Fig. 3.34 Collateral flow index (CFI; *vertical axis*) in diabetic and non-diabetic patients (*horizontal axis*) matched 1:1 for clinical, haemodynamic and angiographic parameters

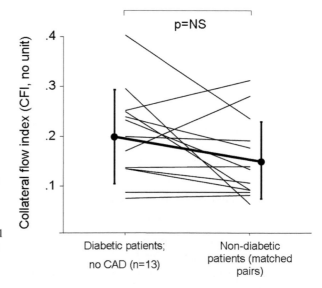

Fig. 3.35 Collateral flow index (CFI; *vertical axis*) in diabetic and non-diabetic patients without coronary angiographic stenoses (*horizontal axis*) matched 1:1 for clinical, haemodynamic and angiographic parameters

Fig. 3.36 Collateral flow index (CFI; *vertical axis*) in diabetic and non-diabetic patients with (recanalized) chronic total coronary occlusion (*horizontal axis*) matched 1:1 for clinical, haemodynamic and angiographic parameters

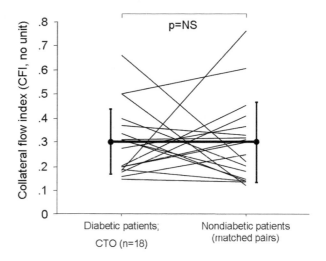

CTO (0.30 ± 0.14 vs. 0.30 ± 0.17, not significant; Fig. 3.36) were compared.[44] Akin to the topic of diabetes mellitus, Olijhoek et al. did not find an association between the presence of metabolic syndrome (impaired glucose metabolism, high blood pressure, dyslipidaemia and central obesity) in 103 of 227 patients with CAD and the angiographic formation of collateral vessels.[45]

Kyriakides et al. studied 313 patients with CAD to evaluate the coronary collateral circulation in relation to the presence of systemic hypertension and LV hypertrophy.[41] The patients had greater than or equal to 95% diameter luminal obstruction of either the left anterior descending artery or the RCA. The hypertensive group (n = 61) had more extensive angiographic coronary collaterals than the normotensive group (n = 252; p < 0.01). There was a positive relationship between coronary collateral circulation and LV wall thickness (p < 0.001) (Table 3.2).[41] Koerselman et al. found the opposite in a cross-sectional study among 237 patients admitted for elective coronary angioplasty[46] (Table 3.2). Systolic blood pressure, diastolic blood pressure, mean arterial pressure, systolic hypertension (systolic blood pressure > 140 mmHg) and antihypertensive treatment each were inversely associated with the presence of angiographically visible collaterals.[46]

An effect of hypercholesterolemia or statin treatment on collateral development has been described only in the experimental animal model,[47] and could not be confirmed in a clinical study using quantitative collateral assessment (Table 3.2).[48]

The extent to which smoking and alcohol use affect the presence of coronary collateral circulation was investigated by Koerselman et al. using coronary angiography for collateral characterization in 242 patients.[43] Current smoking was positively associated, while pack years of smoking was not related.[43] Current alcohol intake showed a J-shaped tendency with coronary collateral presence, while past moderate alcohol consumption was inversely associated (Table 3.2).[43] By univariate analysis of our database, current smoking (n = 401) was related to an increased CFI of 0.203 ± 0.134 as compared to 0.185 ± 0.127 in non-smokers (n = 664; p = 0.0333), but concurrently, smokers had a more extended CAD than non-smokers. Similarly, a study by Kornowski in 112 patients with a CTO did not find a relationship between smoking and the development of collaterals.[49] The methodological advantage of the investigation just mentioned consists of the identical degree of CAD (chronic total occlusion), thus excluding this important determinant of the collateral circulation as a co-variable of smoking. In comparison, the prevalence of two- and three-vessel CAD in the study by Koerselman et al. was significantly higher among patients with angiographic collaterals than in those without, and the same pattern could be observed for the prevalence of smoking.[43] However, the number of vessels affected by CAD as a potential confounding variable of the relationship between smoking and collaterals was not entered into the multivariate logistic regression model in that study.[43] Thus, despite fitting well into the picture of a pro-arteriogenic effect of nicotine in rabbits,[50] smoking in the clinical setting of patients with chronic CAD is likely rather a co-variable of CAD severity than an independent predictor of collateral growth.

3.3.3.5 Heart Rate

Low heart rate as a determinant for well-developed coronary collaterals was described only in the retrospective investigation by Patel et al. [51]. In that study, angiograms of patients with heart rates ≤ 50 beats/min (n = 30) were reviewed. An equivalent number of patients with heart rates ≥ 60 beats/min served as controls. Patients with acute myocardial infarction, with rhythms other than sinus, and without high-grade obstructive CAD were excluded from the study. A significantly greater proportion of patients in the group with bradycardia than of matched controls was demonstrated to have developed collaterals (97 vs. 55% in the group with normocardia, $p < 0.005$).[51]

3.3.3.6 Cardiovascular Medication

The use of nitrates has been described both to impair,[33] and to promote, respectively, the coronary collateral circulation (Table 3.2).[48] In both studies, a dichotomous analysis did not reveal a relevant influence of the use of nitrates, and their effect was unveiled only after multivariate analysis. Piek et al. speculated that the use of nitrates reduces the ischaemic burden and, hence, the stimulus of collateral development.[33] Such an interpretation does not take into account that the major trigger of collateral development, i.e. arteriogenesis, is the biophysical pressure gradient along preformed coronary anastomoses and not the degree of ischaemia.

The use of statins has been inconsistently described to influence the human coronary collateral circulation.[48,52,53] In the study by Pourati et al., 51 patients were taking statins before hospital admission and 43 were not. Their angiograms were reviewed and coronary collaterals graded from 0 to 3. The statin-treated group had significantly more angiographic collaterals than the group not taking statins (Table 3.2).[53] As indicated above, Zbinden et al. did not find an association between statin use and quantitatively assessed coronary collateral function.[48] The reason for the apparently controversial results probably is related to the small sample size of the study by Pourati et al. in combination with their use of coronary angiography for collateral assessment.

Drug-eluting stents have an inhibitory effect on the production of cytokines, chemotactic proteins and growth factors, and may therefore negatively affect coronary collateral growth.[54] In this context, the study by Meier et al. was designed to compare coronary collateral function in patients after bare-metal stent or drug-eluting stent implantation.[55] A total of 120 patients with long-term stable CAD after stent implantation were included. Both the bare-metal stent group and the drug-eluting stent group comprised 60 patients matched for in-stent stenosis severity of the vessel who underwent CFI measurement at follow-up and for the duration of follow-up. Despite equal in-stent stenosis severity and equal follow-up duration (6.2 ± 10 months and 6.5 ± 5.4 months), CFI was diminished in the drug-eluting stent versus bare-metal stent group (0.154 ± 0.097 vs. 0.224 ± 0.142; $p = 0.0049$), (Fig. 3.37).[55]

Other cardiovascular substances such as acetylsalicylic acid and spironolactone have been described to negatively influence collateral development only in the experimental animal model.[56,57]

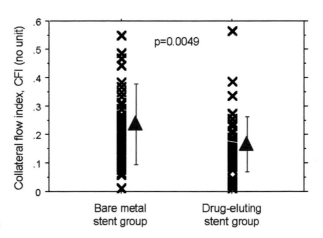

Fig. 3.37 Individual values of collateral flow index (CFI; vertical axis) in patients with similar restenosis long after bare metal or drug-eluting stent implantation (*horizontal axis*). Red symbols with error bars indicate mean values ± standard deviation

3.4   Cellular Determinants of Collateral Flow

The trigger of arterial remodelling in native as well as collateral vessels is increased tangential fluid shear stress at the endothelial surface. Early after fluid shear stress increase, the number of endothelial cells increases and longitudinal bulges appear in growing collaterals as opposed to the flat inner surface of small normal coronary arteries (endothelial activation). Mechanotransducers for altering fluid shear stress may be aAdhesion molecules on the endothelial cell surface, tyrosine kinase receptors and stretch-sensitive sodium and chloride channels. The actin cytoskeleton of the endothelial cell may have an intermediate function by transmitting the mechanical signal to the nucleus. Endothelial activation in response to augmented fluid shear stress reflected by initial cell swelling coincides with a number of processes conditioning for the attraction of circulating mononuclear cells. Transfer of monocyte chemoattractant protein-1 (MCP-1) to the cell surface with immobilization by proteoglycans generates a chemotactic gradient for monocyte adhesion at the endothelium. Following adhesion, trans-migration of monocytes into deeper parts of the collateral wall and surrounding tissue can be observed. Monocytes with their function as 'power plants' of chemokines, proteases and growth factors appear to play a pivotal role in the induction and proliferation of vascular wall cells as well as in arterial remodelling, an essential step in arteriogenesis. Additionally, lymphocytes, tissue-resident mononuclear progenitor cells and bone marrow-derived stem cells may play a role in arteriogenesis.

3.4.1 Introduction

Although mechanisms of collateral growth, i.e. arteriogenesis have been well elucidated in experimental animal models, knowledge of cellular, growth factor and molecular factors that mediate the process in humans is still limited.[2,34] Therefore, this and the subsequent section will be based on experimental evidence relating to determinants of arteriogenesis with particular focus on available clinicopathogenetic studies in support of the basic concept(s).

In the animal model of an occluded femoral artery, arteriogenesis is induced independently of tissue hypoxia,[2] i.e. the occlusion of an artery, and thus, the region in which collateral vessels grow is much more proximal than the hypoxic zone of the foot. In this context, Deindl et al. could detect neither an increased expression level of hypoxia-inducible factor-1alpha (HIF-1) mRNA nor an up-regulation of the HIF-1-controlled vascular endothelial growth factor (VEGF) gene expression in a rabbit ischaemic hindlimb model.[58] The transcription factor HIF-1 is a strong mediator of reactions to tissue hypoxia. However, the mentioned investigation was performed in the hindlimb model, and it cannot be ruled out, in case of other organs and tissues including the myocardium, that collateral growth does take place under hypoxic conditions. To which degree the presence of hypoxia would contribute to collateral development, i.e. to which extent angiogenesis in addition to arteriogenesis plays a role particularly in human collateral development, remains unknown.

3.4.2 Trigger of Arteriogenesis

It has been known for years that the structure of blood vessels can adapt to altered flow conditions.[59] The cross-sectional area of an artery changes with its volume flow rate according to a 2/3-power law,[60] i.e. it enlarges in response to chronically increased flow or it regresses when not constantly perfused. Very recently, it has been elegantly demonstrated in rabbits that underwent femoral artery occlusion with drainage of the arterial stump into the adjacent vein that tangential wall fluid shear stress is the major trigger of arterial remodelling, and thus, of collateral growth (see also Fig. 3.6).[7] The augmented fluid shear stress was induced by the arterio-venous pressure gradient and the related chronic left-to-right shunt flow.

In humans, a similar situation of chronically augmented fluid shear stress within a coronary artery can be present following an iatrogenic right-ventricular-coronary-artery fistula in the context of myocardial biopsy (see Fig. 3.8), or it occurs in congenital coronary malformation with, e.g. coronary-to-right atrial fistula (Fig. 3.38). Obviously, such circumstances occur accidentally and cannot be created systematically. Methodical augmentation of arterial fluid shear stress takes place during repetitive increases of cardiac output, such as during physical exercise. Windecker et al. found that in eight healthy volunteers who underwent a physical endurance exercise programme of >5 months duration with coronary angiography before and after the training programme, the nitro-glycerin-induced left coronary calibres increased significantly (Fig. 3.39).[61] They remodelled to bigger luminal size in direct relation to the exercise-induced increase in LV myoacardial mass, which in physiological terms has to be perfused at a higher coronary volume flow rate ($\sim$1 ml/min/g of LV mass). Similarly, Zbinden et al. demonstrated that in 40 patients with CAD who underwent a 3-month endurance exercise training programme with baseline and follow-up assessments of coronary CFI, the respective changes in normal coronary arteries were from 0.176 ± 0.075 to 0.227 ± 0.070 in the exercise group (n = 24; p = 0.0002) and from 0.219 ± 0.103 to 0.238 ± 0.086 in the sedentary group (n = 16; Fig. 3.40).[62] Clinical studies focusing also on normal coronary arteries

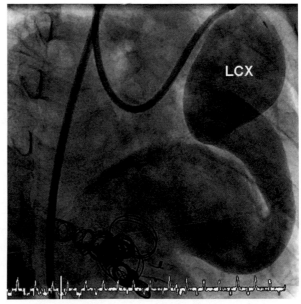

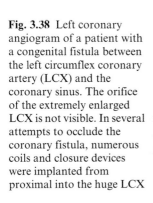

Fig. 3.38 Left coronary angiogram of a patient with a congenital fistula between the left circumflex coronary artery (LCX) and the coronary sinus. The orifice of the extremely enlarged LCX is not visible. In several attempts to occlude the coronary fistula, numerous coils and closure devices were implanted from proximal into the huge LCX

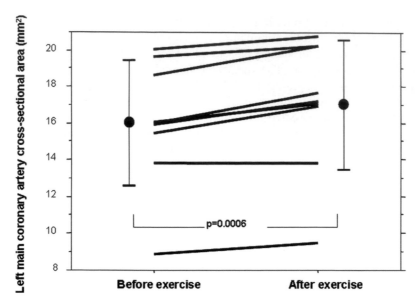

Fig. 3.39 Individual changes of coronary artery cross-sectional area before (*before exercise*) and at the end (*after exercise*) of a physical endurance exercise programme. Circular symbols with error bars denote mean values ± standard deviation

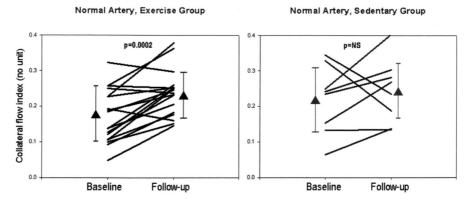

Fig. 3.40 Individual changes of collateral flow index (CFI; *vertical axes*) obtained in angiographically normal coronary arteries before and after treatment (*horizontal axes*) among patients who underwent exercise training (*black lines*) or belonging to the sedentary group (*blue lines*). The triangles with error bars indicate mean values ± standard deviation

are selected here for better comparison with experimental studies, in which the vessels are generally free of atherosclerotic obstructions. Passive augmentation of organ perfusion especially during diastole can be induced by ECG-triggered, lower limb external counterpulsation. Figure 3.41 illustrates that sequential lower limb cuff inflation of 300 mmHg from distal to proximal leads to a large increase

Diastolic augmentation of radial artery flow velocity

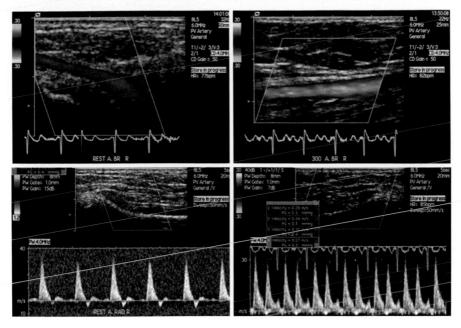

Fig. 3.41 Duplex sonographic images of the radial artery in a patient who underwent diastolic lower leg external counterpulsation at 300 mmHg (*right panels*) in comparison to the situation without counterpulsation (*left panels*). The *upper panels* show the colour Doppler flow images of the right radial artery. The *lower panels* show the radial artery pulsed Doppler flow spectra with a very low diastolic flow velocity signal at rest, and with diastolic and systolic flow velocity signals at identical speeds during high-pressure counterpulsation (*lower right panel*)

in diastolic radial artery flow velocity, the fact of which most likely mirrors the situation in the coronary circulation. A protocol of 30 hours of external counter-pulsation (90 minutes per session, 20 sessions over the course of 4 weeks) leads to a consistent increase in coronary collateral flow in stenotic as well as normal vessels (Fig. 3.42).

3.4.3 Endothelial Activation

How is augmented vascular fluid shear stress as initial trigger for arteriogenesis transmitted to the cellular and molecular level? The primary physiological response to fluid shear stress is an activation of endothelial cells.[2] Early after coronary occlusion, the number of endothelial cells per unit inner vascular surface increases and longitudinal bulges appear in growing collaterals as opposed to the completely flat inner surface of small normal coronary arteries

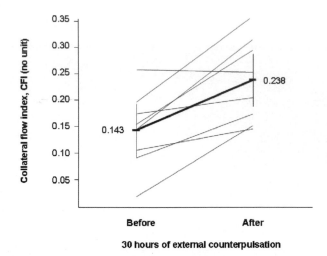

Fig. 3.42 Coronary collateral flow index (CFI; *vertical axis*) before and after a total of 30 hours of lower leg external counterpulsation (*horizontal axis*) as obtained in 8 vessels of four patients with coronary artery disease. Figures 3.41 and 3.42 illustrate the concept of shear rate (change of flow velocity per change vessel radius)-triggered collateral arterial remodelling (i.e. arteriogenesis) by direct demonstration of doubled flow velocity signals during counterpulsation and augmented collateral function in response to it

(Fig. 3.43).[63] The surface of many endothelial cells appears rough, and large numbers of monocytes adhere to the inner vascular surface (Fig. 3.43). Mechanotransducers or mechanosensing elements for altering fluid shear stress may be integrins (adhesion molecules) on the endothelial cell surface.[64] They serve as anchors of the endothelium to the extracellular compartment of the vascular wall. In addition, tyrosine kinase receptors (transcription factor early growth response-1 switching on MCP-1 gene expression) and stretch sensitive sodium and chloride channels may act as mechanotransducers of fluid shear stress [65] (Fig. 3.44). The actin cytoskeleton of the endothelial cell may have an intermediate function by transmitting the mechanical signal to the nucleus.[66] Furthermore, expression of endothelial nitric oxide synthase is modulated by shear stress.[67] Its product nitric oxide permeabilizes the endothelium. However, recent evidence from a murine model of distal femoral artery ligation has demonstrated that endothelial nitric oxide synthase activity is crucial for nitric oxide-mediated vasodilation but not for collateral artery growth.[68] Numerous genes have been reported to be controlled by shear stress responsive elements in their promoter region, and an influence of fluid shear stress on the expression of these genes has been documented (see also below).[69] In this context, Eitenmüller et al. performed gene expression profiling in their rabbit hindlimb model with arterio-venous shunt and found an upregulation of the Rho-pathway (RhoA, cofilin, focal adhesion kinase, vimentin).[7] Endothelial cell activation in response to

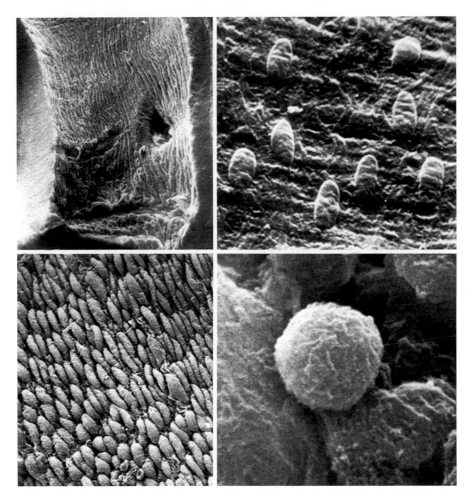

Fig. 3.43 Images of normal and collateral vessel in the scanning electron microscope. *Upper left panel*: The endothelium is continuous and oriented in the direction of blood flow. The endothelial cells are oriented towards the side branch. *Upper right panel*: Larger magnification showing the regular direction of the endothelial nuclei. *Lower left panel*: The endothelium in growing collaterals is more prominent but still regularly arranged. Lower right panel: Adhesion of a monocyte to an endothelial cell

augmented fluid shear stress is reflected by initial cell swelling (Fig. 3.43),[70] which coincides with a number of processes conditioning for the attraction of circulating cells. Upregulated genes encode for chemoattractant or activating cytokines or for adhesion molecules,[71] whereby MCP-1 plays a pivotal role in monocyte recruitment. Transfer of MCP-1 to the cell surface with immobilization by proteoglycans generates a chemotactic gradient for endothelial monocyte adhesion (Fig. 3.44).

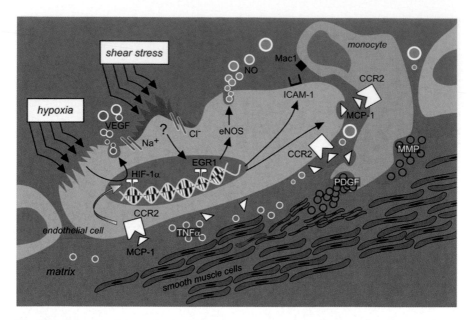

Fig. 3.44 Scheme of hypothesized molecular pathways in human coronary collateral growth. At the onset of arteriogenesis, fluid shear stress activates endothelial mechanotransducers such as stretch sensitive sodium (Na+) and chloride (Cl–) channels, and in turn the transcription factor early growth response-1 (EGR-1) leading to a cascade of permeability increase of the endothelium (through nitric oxide, NO, via endothelial nitric oxide synthase, eNOS), upregulated intercellular adhesion molecule (ICAM-1) promoting docking of monocyte chemoattractant protein (MCP-1) through its CC-motif chemokine receptor (CCR-2). This is related to transmigration of peripheral blood mononuclear cells. Matrix metalloproteinases (MMP) degrade intercellular matrix and platelet-derived growth factor (PDGF) stimulates smooth muscle cell proliferation. Tumour necrosis factor-alpha may act by yet unidentified mechanisms, playing a dual role depending on local concentrations. The role of the angiogenesis pathway is disputed in collateral formation. Angiogenesis is promoted by hypoxia which upregulates the transcription-factor hypoxia-inducible factor-1-alpha, (HIF-1α) which leads to upregulation of vascular endothelial growth factor (VEGF)

Within the same framework, Werner et al. performed a study on growth factors in the collateral circulation of 104 patients with CTO.[72] Collateral function was assessed invasively during recanalization by intracoronary Doppler and pressure recordings (CFI). Blood samples were drawn from the distal coronary bed supplied by the collaterals and from the aortic root to measure MCP-1, basic fibroblast growth factor (bFGF), transforming growth factor-β (TGFβ), placenta growth factor (PlGF) and tumour necrosis factor-α (TNFα).[72] Not only MCP-1 but also PlGF and TGFβ were significantly increased in patients with small or no angiographic collaterals and in those with recent coronary occlusion (Fig. 3.45).

Fig. 3.45 Monocyte chemoattractant protein-1 (MCP-1) concentration (*vertical axis*) as obtained in the distal coronary artery (*grey bars*) and aorta (*white bars*) of patients with chronic total coronary occlusions according to angiographically determined collateral connection grades (*horizontal axis*). The distal coronary MCP-1 concentration in the absence of collaterals is significantly elevated (p<0.05)[74]

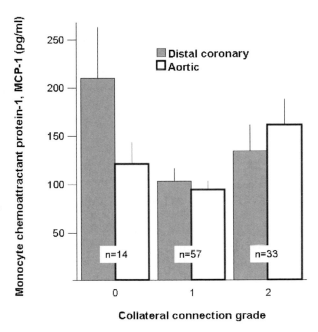

3.4.4 The Role of Monocytes

Ito et al. demonstrated, in a rabbit femoral artery occlusion model, that an increase in the above-mentioned chemotactic gradient by chronic local infusion of MCP-1 enhanced arteriogenesis substantially to magnitudes above all tested growth factor treatments.[4] Additionally, alterations in the expression and conformation of adhesion molecules convert the collateral endothelium from a quiescent vessel layer into an adhesive surface supporting invasion of leucocytes (Fig. 3.44).[2] Expression of selectins, intercellular adhesion molecules (ICAM-1 and –2; Fig. 3.44) and vascular cell adhesion molecules (VCAM-1) has been observed to be not only increased, but also clustered in focal adhesion complexes.[73] The cellular elements being attracted to the 'primed' endothelial surface and having been studied most extensively in relation to arteriogenesis are circulating blood monocytes. Beginning in the mid-1970s, where electron microscopic images of canine cardiac collaterals showed extensive adhesion of monocytes at the activated endothelium (see also Fig. 3.43),[63] relevant parts of the mechanism of arteriogenesis have been unravelled. Being attracted by MCP-1 and likely by other chemoattractants, monocyte binding to the collateral surface is mediated by integrin receptors such as Mac-1 (Fig. 3.44). The heterodimeric molecule is the counterpart of endothelial ICAM and VCAM, and their expression on monocytes has been described to be upregulated by growth factors such as VEGF, PlGF and TGFβ and chemokines such as MCP-1.[74,75] Following adhesion, transmigration of monocytes into deeper parts of the collateral wall and surrounding tissue can be observed (Fig. 3.44). Monocytes and macrophages with their function as 'power plants' of chemokines, proteases and growth factors appear to play a pivotal role in the induction and proliferation of vascular wall cells as well as in arterial remodelling, an essential step in arteriogenesis.[2] For example, monocytes potently produce proteases such as matrix metalloproteinases and uPA.[76,77] The proteolytic degradation of extracellular structures during monocyte migration through the collateral wall may generate the proliferation signal for smooth muscle cells by elastin fragments derived from proteolytic cleavage of the elastic lamina.[2] Also, it has been shown that the release of growth factors by macrophages such as bFGF and TNFα directly enhances proliferation within the collateral wall.[78] In the study by Arras et al.,[78] the effects of an increase in monocyte recruitment by lipopolysaccharide on capillary density as well as on collateral and peripheral conductance after 7 days of femoral artery occlusion in the rabbit were investigated. Monocytes accumulated around day 3 in collateral arteries when maximal proliferation was observed (Fig. 3.46) and stained strongly for bFGF and TNFα. In a study where blood monocyte concentrations were pharmacologically manipulated, it could be demonstrated that even peripheral blood monocyte concentration is crucial for the course of arteriogenesis (Fig. 3.47).[79]

Akin to the above- mentioned study, a small investigation in humans with extensive CAD who underwent a pro-arteriogenic treatment with granulocyte-macrophage colony stimulating factor (GM-CSF, n = 10) versus placebo (n = 11) during 2 weeks observed a direct relationship between the peripheral blood concentration of monocytes at follow-up and the degree of change in collateral function (Fig. 3.48).[80] Translational research in the field of cellular and also humoral mechanisms underlying the development of well-conductive collateral vessels (i.e. arteriogenesis) is limited.

3.4.4.1 Acute Coronary Syndrome

There has been clinical evidence that certain, partly monocyte-derived cytokines play a pathophysiological role in acute coronary syndromes and myocardial infarction.[81–83] Recently, Heeschen et al. observed in 547 patients with acute coronary syndrome that elevated PlGF levels (>27.0 ng/L; 41% of patients) indicated an increased risk of major adverse cardiac events at 30 days (15% vs. 5%; unadjusted hazard ratio, 3.34; 95% confidence interval [CI], 1.79–6.24; p < 0.001).[83] In a similar study, de Lemos et al. found in 4,244 patients with acute coronary syndrome that rates of major adverse cardiovascular events increased across baseline quartiles of MCP-1 and among patients with MCP-1 > vs. ≤ 238 pg/ml (Fig. 3.49).[84] That elevated levels of MCP-1 but also increased PlGF indicate a poor prognosis in patients following acute myocardial infarction appears to contradict the above-described experimental evidence of a pro-arteriogenic effect of these substances, which would rather salvage than spend myocardium. Since monocytes are intimately involved in both atherogenesis and

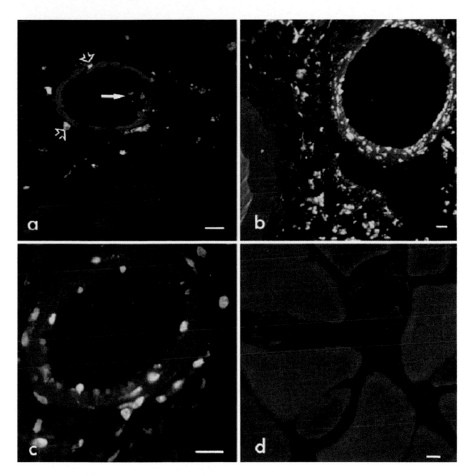

Fig. 3.46 Monocyte accumulation and proliferation in excised collateral arteries after 3 days of femoral artery ligation in the rabbit. *Upper left panel*: Several macrophages are distributed in the adventitia and the connective tissue surrounding the vessels. Macrophages adhere to the endothelium (→) and penetrate the vascular wall (*open arrow*). *Upper right panel*: BrdU staining reveals extensive proliferation of endothelial and smooth muscle cells. *Lower left panel*: K1 67 staining shows proliferation of endothelial and smooth muscle cells at day 3. *Lower right panel*: Similarly sized vessel adjacent to the excised collateral artery stained with an antibody against rabbit monocytes/macrophages. The absence of macrophages in neighbouring control vessels indicates that monocyte migration is specific for growing collateral vessels. Bars: 20 μm[78]

arteriogenesis, the apparent contradiction is none and indicates the involvement of monocytes in the acute event of an atherosclerotic plaque rupture with more or less extensive endothelial injury on one hand, and conversely, activation by augmented fluid shear forces of the uninjured endothelium in the course of arteriogenesis. With the use of an enzyme-linked immunosorbent assay, Fujita et al. measured the concentrations of bFGF and VEGF in pericardial fluids of

Fig. 3.47 Blood flow ratio (*vertical axis*) in hindlimbs from mice without treatment (control, *black line*; only femoral artery ligation), with rebound monocytosis following treatment with 5-fluorouracil (*red line*), or monocyte depletion during treatment with 5-fluorouracil (*blue line*) assessed postoperatively and 3, 7, 14 and 21 days after femoral artery ligation [79]

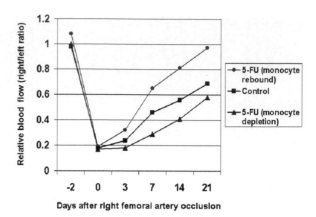

Fig. 3.48 Change in collateral flow index during a 2-week treatment protocol (CFI2 minus CFI1; *vertical axis*) with placebo or granulocyte macrophage colony-stimulating factor (GM-CSF) in relation to the blood monocyte concentration at follow-up (*horizontal axis*)

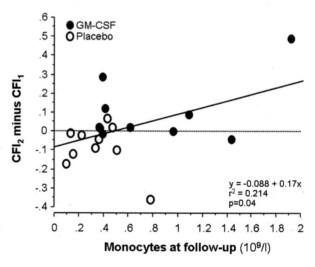

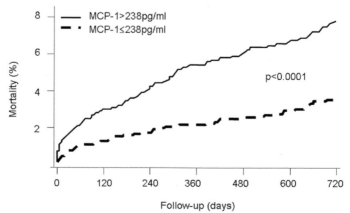

Fig. 3.49 Cumulative mortality (*vertical axis*) in 4,244 patients after acute myocardial infarction (*horizontal axis*) according to baseline monocyte chemoattractant protein-1 concentration above (*solid line*) or below (*dashed line*) 238 pg/ml

12 patients with unstable angina and of 8 patients with non-ischaemic heart diseases.[85] The concentration of bFGF in pericardial fluids among patients with CAD was 2036 ± 357 pg/mL, significantly ($p < 0.001$) higher than the concentration of 289 ± 72 pg/mL in patients without CAD. Without directly obtaining collateral function, Fujita et al. concluded that 'bFGF plays an important role in mediating collateral growth in humans'.[85] Knowledge of the frequency distribution of different levels of collateral function among patients with and without CAD (see also Fig. 3.13) supports this untested notion.

3.4.4.2   Chronic Stable CAD

In comparison, Fleisch et al. directly measured collateral function in the presence of chronic stable CAD and simultaneously, serum concentrations of bFGF and VEGF, sampled from the ostium of the collateralized coronary artery and from the distal position of the occluded coronary artery.[86] Focusing on the proximal sampling site, there was a direct correlation between CFI and both bFGF ($r = 0.29$, $p = 0.01$) and VEGF concentrations ($r = 0.44$, $p < 0.0001$). The sum of the concentrations of both growth factors was directly associated with CFI irrespective of the proximal ($r = 0.51$, $p < 0.0001$) or distal sampling site ($r = 0.34$, $p = 0.048$; Fig. 3.50).[86] The above-cited investigation by Werner et al. in 104 patients with CTO revealed also a consistent inverse

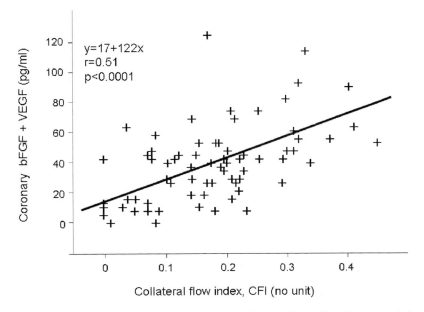

Fig. 3.50 Combined coronary concentration (*vertical axis*) of basic fibroblast growth factor (bFGF) and vascular endothelial growth factor (VEGF) in relationship to collateral flow index (CFI, *horizontal axis*)

association between distal coronary bed bFGF concentration and angiographic collateral degree as well as duration of arterial occlusion (Fig. 3.51).[72] In 18 CAD patients with inadequate (CFI < 0.25) compared with those with adequate (CFI ± 0.25, n = 12) collateral support, Lambiase et al. observed lower concentrations of coronary sinus growth factors (VEGF and PlGF).[87] The results of the humoral factor concentrations (bFGF, VEGF and PlGF) in both the studies by Fleisch et al.[86] and Lambiase et al.[87] apparently contradict those of Werner et al.,[72] in that there is a direct relationship between growth factors and collateral function in the former, but an inverse in the latter investigation. Possibly, the divergent experimental setting between the mentioned studies of a 1-minute acute coronary balloon occlusion as opposed to the chronic total occlusion renders a comparison difficult. In a study among 100 patients with chronic stable CAD, our group found a significant, inverse correlation between plasma TNFα concentrations and invasively obtained collateral function (CFI).[88] In a study that included 14 patients randomized to treatment with GM-CSF (n = 7) or to placebo (n = 7), the treatment-induced change in collateral function (CFI) was predicted by the respective change in TNFα concentration.[89]

Sources alternative to peripheral blood monocytes have been suggested such as proliferation of tissue-resident monocyte progenitors.[90] However, considering the fast recovery of blood flow deficits within days, it can be

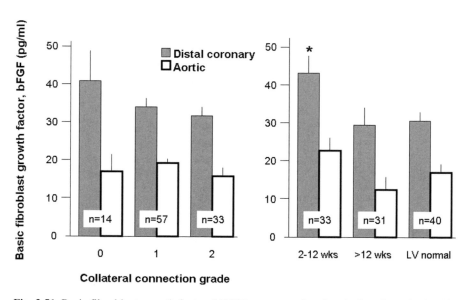

Fig. 3.51 Basic fibroblast growth factor (bFGF) concentration (*vertical axis*) as obtained in the distal coronary artery (*grey bars*) and aorta (*white bars*) of patients with chronic total coronary occlusions according to angiographically determined collateral connection grades (*horizontal axis; right panel*) and according to the time of coronary occlusion respectively to the presence of normal left ventricular (LV) systolic function. *p<0.01 versus aortic value

extrapolated that recruitment of tissue resident cells with the subsequent proliferation may not represent a relevant pathway for monocyte recruitment.

3.4.5 The Role of Lymphocytes

A previous investigation by Stabile et al. observed lymphocytes as a second blood-derived cell population in the vicinity of growing collaterals.[91] They found that in mice with a genetic deficiency of the T-cell marker CD4, arteriogenesis was markedly diminished in the experimental hindlimb ischaemia model, which could be rescued by injecting purified CD4[+] cells. Also, the lack of CD4[+] T lymphocytes led to a reduced inflammatory response in this model including a reduction in the number of monocytes, which were detected in growing collaterals of CD4 knock-out mice. Stabile et al. concluded that T lymphocytes contribute to arteriogenesis by releasing chemoattracting cytokines, thus supporting monocyte recruitment. Similarly, van Weel documented in a murine model of hindlimb ischaemia that lymphocytes, detected with markers for natural killer cells (NK) 1.1, CD3 and CD4, invaded the collateral vessel wall and that arteriogenesis was impaired in C57BL/6 mice depleted for NK cells and in NK-cell-deficient transgenic mice.[92] Furthermore, arteriogenesis was impaired in C57BL/6 mice depleted for CD4[+] T-lymphocytes by anti-CD4 antibodies and in major histocompatibility complex-class-II-deficient mice that more selectively lack mature peripheral CD4[+] T lymphocytes.[92]

3.4.6 The Role of Stem and Progenitor Cells

Two studies by Asahara et al., which suggested the existence of circulating endothelial progenitor cells within the blood and later their contribution to compensatory vessel growth,[93,94] were later followed by a multitude of investigations, demonstrating the contribution of adult stem or progenitor cells to different kinds of vessel growth.[95] Experiments were performed in different animal species such as mice, rabbits and rats, and different cell populations such as bone marrow-derived mononuclear cells, defined stem cell populations and progenitor cells isolated from peripheral blood were tested in pre-clinical studies. Initially, findings predominated suggesting that bone marrow-derived stem cells are incorporated into the wall of growing blood vessels, predominantly as elements of the endothelium or vascular smooth muscle layer.[2] Ziegelhoeffer et al. investigated whether bone marrow-derived progenitor cells incorporate into vessels using mouse models of hindlimb ischaemia (arteriogenesis and angiogenesis) and tumour growth.[96] C57BL/6 wild-type mice were lethally irradiated and transplanted with bone marrow cells from littermates expressing enhanced green fluorescent protein. Six weeks after bone marrow transplantation, the animals underwent unilateral femoral artery occlusions or were subcutaneously implanted with methylcholanthrene-induced fibrosarcoma cells. After 7 and 21 days of surgery, proximal hindlimb muscles with growing collateral arteries and ischaemic gastrocnemius muscles as well as grown tumours and various organs were excised for histological analysis. The authors failed to co-localize green fluorescent protein signals with endothelial or smooth muscle cell markers.[96] Green fluorescent protein positive cells adjacent to growing collateral were identified as fibroblasts, pericytes and primarily leucocytes that stained positive for several growth factors and chemokines, thus indicating a possible paracrine role of adult stem cells for vessel growth.

Clinical studies investigating the relevance of progenitor cells with regard to directly obtained coronary collateral function have been scarce. In the above-mentioned small study by Lambiase et al.,[87] there was a strong positive correlation between numbers of CD34/CD133-positive circulating haemopoietic precursor cells and CFI (r = 0.75, p < 0.001). Preliminary data from our laboratory in 52 patients with chronic CAD randomized to a 2-week treatment protocol with granulocyte colony-stimulating factor (G-CSF) (n = 26) or to placebo (n = 26) showed an increase in CD34-postive cells after 14 days, the change of which was associated with collateral function during follow-up (Fig. 3.52). It is worth emphasizing that the absolute majority of clinical studies in the field of cardiac applications of progenitor or stem cell therapy has not directly obtained coronary collateral function, but only claimed their effect on angiogenesis or arteriogenesis. For example, Hill et al. administered 10 μg/kg/day of G-CSF for 5 days to 16 chronic CAD patients. Progenitor cells were measured by flow cytometry; ischaemia was assessed by exercise stress testing and by dobutamine stress cardiac magnetic resonance imaging.[97] G-CSF increased $CD34^+/CD133^+$ cells in the circulation from 1.5 ± 0.2 to 52.4 ± 10.4 μl (p < 0.001). At 1 month after treatment, there was no improvement from baseline values in wall motion score or segments with abnormal perfusion and a trend towards a greater number of ischaemic segments.[97] In the setting of acute myocardial infarction, the direct effect of progenitor cells on

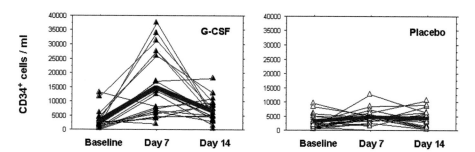

Fig. 3.52 Individual $CD34^+$ progenitor cell counts (*vertical axis; red line*: mean value) before, during and immediately after the course of a 2-week treatment with granulocyte colony-stimulating factor (G-CSF) or placebo. The value obtained after 14 days was related to collateral function

the collateral circulation was not tested either. Schächinger et al. randomly assigned 204 patients with acute myocardial infarction to receive an intracoronary infusion of progenitor cells derived from bone marrow or placebo medium into the infarct artery 3–7 days after successful reperfusion therapy.[98] At 1 year, intracoronary infusion of bone marrow cells was associated with a reduction in the pre-specified combined clinical end point of death, recurrence of myocardial infarction and any revascularization procedure (p = 0.01; entirely driven by the lower number of revascularization procedures in the bone marrow cells group), which appeared to be related to improved LV ejection fraction (primary endpoint).[98] Intracoronary bone marrow cell infusion in 75 patients with stable CAD following myocardial infarction (≥3 months previously) resulted in an absolute change in LV ejection fraction of +2.9% points among patients receiving bone marrow cells (vs. –0.4% points in patients receiving circulating blood infusion, p = 0.003) or no infusion (–1.2% points, p < 0.001).[99]

3.5 Genetic Determinants of Collateral Flow

Genes influence the presence and extent of coronary collateral vessels principally in two ways, namely by determining the innate collateral network, from which functioning collaterals arise. Experimental studies have, so far, investigated exclusively the first aspect, and not the second, i.e. collateral growth in the presence of coronary atherosclerosis as it is the case in humans. Thus, evidence from experimental animal models for the existence of a genetic programme during collateral growth is likely not representative of the situation in human CAD. In mice, femoral artery ligation has caused a ≥2-fold differential expression of 783 genes at one or multiple time points as determined by microarray analysis: 518 were induced and 265 were repressed. Cluster analysis generated four temporal patterns: early upregulated genes (early transcriptional factors, angiogenesis, inflammation and stress-related genes); mid-phase upregulated genes (cell cycle and cytoskeletal and inflammatory genes); late upregulated genes (angiostatic, anti-inflammatory, and extracellular matrix-associated genes) and downregulated genes involved in energy metabolism, water channel and muscle contraction.

In humans with and without CAD, respectively, and direct collateral function assessment (n = 160), microarray gene expression analysis has found 203 and 56 genes, respectively, to be significantly correlated with collateral function. Biological pathway analysis has revealed 76 of those genes belonging to four different pathways: angiogenesis, integrin signalling, platelet-derived growth factor signalling and TGFβ signalling.

3.5.1 Introduction

The clinical use of genomics has advanced most rapidly in oncology, due in part to the advantage of direct access to neoplastic tissue. Another field involved in transcriptional profiling has been the discipline of infectious diseases using the potential of genomic tests to predict response of HIV and hepatitis C therapies. In the cardiovascular area, genomic research in humans has progressed more slowly, owing to the supposed inability to access informative tissue. Still, in the past 5 years, genomic investigations have been performed in the field of electrophysiology, arterial hypertension, congestive heart failure, cardiac transplantation and atherosclerosis using human atrial, ventricular respectively aortic tissue refs.[100–102] Aside from aortic tissue reflecting the extent of atherosclerotic burden, and thus, offering insight into gene expression phenotypes of atherosclerosis,[103] peripheral blood mononuclear cells may provide a diagnostic signature for atherosclerosis due to their role in inflammatory pathways leading to this systemic disease.[104] Given the sample size of five individuals who underwent serial analysis of CD14$^+$ monocyte gene expression in the study by Patino et al.,[104] it was meant to explore the role of peripheral blood mononuclear cells as reporters for the process of atherosclerosis.

As in atherosclerosis, circulating monocytes are considered the key element in its own natural repair mechanism, i.e. the development of a conductive collateral circulation or arteriogenesis.[2]

A further argument in favour of gene expression analysis in the context of the coronary collateral circulation is the following: The interindividual variability of collateral flow for a given coronary stenosis severity is very large (see Fig. 3.29), and accordingly, there is a chance in one out of four that well-developed collaterals are present even in the absence of coronary stenoses (see Fig. 3.13). Because of several dozens of clinical factors potentially determining the degree of collateral function in CAD patients with coronary stenosis severity as the only variable consistently reported as a determinant, it can be speculated that genetic influences on collateral preformation as well as on the growth response to atherosclerotic lesions must be substantial.

3.5.2 Evidence from Experimental Studies

Genes may determine the presence and extent of coronary collateral vessels principally in two ways, namely by determining the innate collateral network from which functioning collaterals arise, i.e. the state of preformed collaterals. The animal studies outlined below are related exclusively to this aspect, and not to the second, i.e. collateral growth in the presence of coronary atherosclerotic lesions or diffuse atherosclerosis as it is the case in humans. Thus, evidence from experimental animal models for the existence of a genetic programme during collateral growth is likely not representative for the situation in human CAD. Additionally, genetic determinants of collateral development in animals have, often, not been investigated in the presence of coronary artery but femoral artery ligation.

In order to analyse the differential gene expression in arteriogenesis of rabbits, cDNA of collateral arteries 24 hours after femoral artery occlusion or sham operation was subjected to suppression subtractive hybridization in a study by Boengler et al.[105] An upregulation was detected in the U6 snRNA binding protein Lsm5, cytochrome *b*, an expressed sequence tag and the actin-depolymerizing factor cofilin2 mRNA in collateral arteries, 24 hours after femoral ligation. For cofilin2, an increase in the protein level and a localization predominantly in smooth muscle cells of collaterals were also observed.[105]

Lee et al. elucidated the genomic programme leading to collateral vessel formation in a murine model of acute hindlimb ischaemia.[71] DNA array expression profiling was employed to determine the time course of differential expression of 12,000 genes after femoral artery ligation in C57BL/6 mice. In that model, development of an extensive collateral circulation has been well documented.[106] In the study by Lee et al.,[71] ribonucleic acid was extracted from the adductor muscle, which showed no signs of ischaemia (no elevation of hypoxia inducible factor 1-α protein level). Sampling was at baseline, 6 hours, and 1, 3, 7 and 14 days after femoral artery ligation or sham operation.[71] Femoral artery ligation caused a ≥2-fold differential expression of 783 genes at one or multiple time points: 518 were induced and 265 were repressed. Cluster analysis revealed four temporal patterns: (a) early upregulated genes (6–24 hours) – immediate early transcriptional factors, angiogenesis, inflammation and stress-related genes; (b) mid-phase upregulated genes (day 3) – cell cycle and cytoskeletal and inflammatory genes; (c) late upregulated genes (days 7–14) – angiostatic, anti-inflammatory and extracellular matrix-associated genes and (d) downregulated genes involved in energy metabolism, water channel and muscle contraction (Fig. 3.53).[71]

Lohr et al. investigated the temporal progress of gene *products* (proteomics) and not the genes themselves (genomics) involved in canine coronary collateral growth following repetitive arterial occlusions.[107] The acute-phase protein

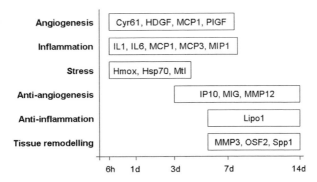

Fig. 3.53 Time course diagram of the expression of selected gene groups after femoral artery ligation in mice. Abbreviation: IL = interleukin; IP = interferon-gamma-inducible protein; MCP = monocyte chemoattractant protein; MIP = macrophage inflammatory protein; MMP = matrix metalloproteinase; PlGF = placenta growth factor

haptoglobin was identified in the group subjected to repetitive occlusion. Enzyme-linked immunosorbent assay of myocardial interstitial fluid showed haptoglobin to be elevated at all time points of collateral development compared with sham, with maximal production on day 7.

In the above-mentioned arterio-venous shunt model of femoral artery occlusion among rabbits,[7] expression profiling showed an upregulation of members of the Rho-pathway (RhoA, cofilin, focal adhesion kinase and vimentin) and the Rho-antagonist fasudil markedly inhibited arteriogenesis. The activities of Ras and ERK-1,-2 were markedly increased in collateral vessels of the shunt experiment.

3.5.3 Genetic Markers of Human Coronary Collaterals

Cross-cultural epidemiological studies of incident cardiovascular disease in the diabetic patient have demonstrated marked differences in susceptibility that may be due to a genetic factor.[108] The coronary artery collateral circulation is the chief determinant of the size of myocardial infarction and is highly variable between patients. It has been recently demonstrated that a functional allelic polymorphism in the haptoglobin gene is correlated with a number of diabetic vascular complications such as diabetic retinopathy, nephropathy and restenosis following angioplasty.[109,110] In man, there are two common alleles for the haptoglobin gene manifesting as three major phenotypes 1–1, 2–1 and 2–2. The distribution of these alleles differs substantially among different ethnic groups.[111] In the study by Hochberg et al.,[112] the haptoglobin phenotype (1–1, 2–1 or 2–2) as determined by polyacrylamide electrophoresis was correlated with the presence or absence of coronary collaterals by angiography in 82 consecutive diabetic patients and 138 consecutive non-diabetic patients who underwent catheterization. It was observed that diabetic patients with the haptoglobin phenotype 2–1 were more likely to have collaterals than diabetic patients with the haptoglobin phenotype 2–2 ($p = 0.007$). There was no correlation between haptoglobin phenotypes and the presence of collaterals in non-diabetic patients. Haptoglobin phenotype thus appears to be associated with the development of the coronary collateral circulation in diabetic patients with CAD. Haptoglobin 2–2 may predispose to less compensation for coronary artery stenosis in diabetic patients, and thereby portend a worse prognosis.[112]

Along the same line and in an American Indian population of 206 patients with cardiovascular disease and 206 matched controls aged 45–74 years, Levy et al. found that the odds ratio of having cardiovascular disease in patients with diabetes mellitus with the haptoglobin 2–2 phenotype was 5.0 times greater than in patients with diabetes mellitus with the haptoglobin 1–1 phenotype ($p = 0.002$).[113] An intermediate risk of cardiovascular disease was associated with the haptoglobin 2–1 phenotype.

A clinical study by Chittenden et al. was carried out in a small population of eight patients with angiographically poorly visible and of eight patients with well-visible collaterals in order to determine transcriptional profiles of circulating monocytes.[114] Monocyte transcriptomes from CAD patients with and without collateral vessels were obtained by use of high-throughput expression profiling. Using a newly developed redundancy-based data mining method, the authors identified a set of molecular markers characteristic of a 'noncollateralogenic' phenotype. Moreover, these transcriptional abnormalities were shown to be independent of the severity of CAD or any other known clinical parameter that was thought to affect collateral development, and they correlated with protein expression levels in monocytes and plasma.[114] Schirmer et al. hypothesized that circulating cell transcriptomes would provide mechanistic insights and new therapeutic strategies to stimulate arteriogenesis.[115] CFI was measured in 45 patients with single-vessel CAD, separating collateral responders (CFI, >0.21) and non-responders (CFI≤0.21). Isolated monocytes were stimulated with lipopolysaccharide. Genome-wide mRNA expression analysis revealed 244 differentially expressed genes in stimulated monocytes. Interferon-β and several interferon-related genes showed increased mRNA levels in three of four cellular phenotypes from non-responders.[115]

It is our experience that gene expression analysis in a setting of CAD requires exact coronary collateral quantification and a minimum sample size of 50–100 individuals in order to detect true genetic profiles and not 'data noise'. In this context, the above-cited study by Chittenden et al. is absolutely underpowered. Alternatively to increasing the sample size of a study, the pathophysiologically reasonable method of monocyte stimulation by lipopolysaccharide may require a smaller study population.[115] In our clinical investigation on differential gene expression, CFI was obtained invasively by angioplasty pressure sensor guide wire in 160 individuals (110 patients with CAD and 50 individuals without CAD).[116] RNA was extracted from monocytes, and analysis of 14,500 genes by microarray technology was performed. Seventy-six genes found by microarray analysis were analysed by real-time polymerase chain reaction. Receiver operating characteristics analysis based on differential gene expression was then performed to separate individuals with poor (CFI < 0.21) and well-developed collaterals (CFI≥0.21). The expression of 203 genes significantly correlated with CFI (p = 0.000002–0.00267; false discovery rate, FDR < 0.3) in patients with CAD. In individuals without CAD, the expression of 56 genes correlated with CFI at an FDR < 0.7 (Figs. 3.54 and 3.55). Biological pathway analysis revealed 76 of those genes belonging to four different pathways: angiogenesis, integrin signalling, platelet-derived growth factor signalling and TGFβ signalling. By polymerase chain reaction, 8 genes in patients with CAD and 13 in individuals without CAD could be confirmed. Three genes in each

Coronary artery disease

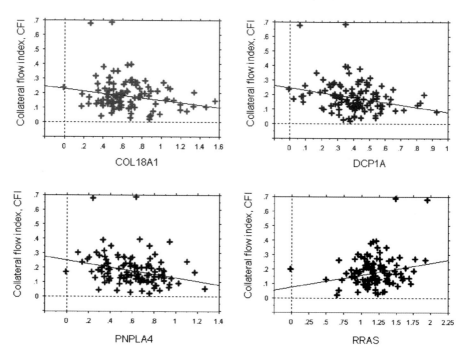

Fig. 3.54 Correlations between the expression of four different marker genes (*horizontal axis*; log2 fold change of the minimum expression) identified by microarray analysis and confirmed by polymerase chain reaction and the respective value of collateral flow index (*vertical axis*) in patients with coronary artery disease

subgroup differentiated with high specificity among individuals with low and high CFI ($\geq$0.21).

Preliminary data in patients with CAD from the group by Regieli et al. indicated that polymorphisms of the TNFα gene promoter region is related to the extent of collateral circulation as visible by angiography.[117]

Abbreviations

bFGF	basic fibroblast growth factor
CAD	coronary artery disease
CFI	collateral flow index (no unit)
CVP	central venous pressure (mmHg)
DNA	deoxyribonucleic acid

No coronary artery disease

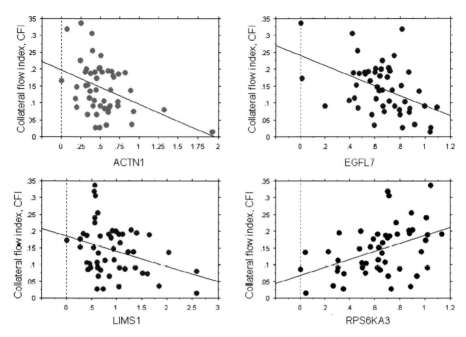

Fig. 3.55 Correlations between the expression of four different marker genes (*horizontal axis*; log2 fold change of the minimum expression) identified by microarray analysis and confirmed by polymerase chain reaction and the respective value of collateral flow index (*vertical axis*) in individuals without coronary artery disease

GM-CSF	granulocyte–macrophage colony-stimulating factor
ICAM	intercellular adhesion molecule
IS	infarct size
P_{ao}	mean aortic pressure (mmHg)
PCI	percutaneous coronary intervention
PlGF	placental growth factor
P_{occl}	mean coronary occlusive or wedge pressure (mmHg)
MCP-1	monocyte chemoattractant protein-1
MMP	matrix metallo proteinase
RNA	ribonucleic acid
TNFα	tumour necrosis factor-α
VCAM	vascular cell adhesion molecule
VEGF	vascular endothelial growth factor
V_{occl}	intracoronary occlusive blood flow velocity (cm/s)
$V_{\varnothing\text{-occl}}$	intracoronary non-occlusive blood flow velocity (cm/s)

References

1. Carmeliet P. Angiogenesis in life, disease and medicine. *Nature*. 2005;438:932–936.
2. Heil M, Eitenmüller I, Schmitz-Rixen T, Schaper W. Arteriogenesis versus angiogenesis: similarities and differences. *J Cell Mol Med*. 2006;10:45–55.
3. Risau W. Mechanisms of angiogenesis. *Nature*. 1997;386:671–674.
4. Ito W, Arras M, Winkler B, Scholz D, Schaper J, Schaper W. Monocyte chemotactic protein-1 increases collateral and peripheral conductance after femoral artery occlusion. *Circ Res*. 1997;80:829–837.
5. Zoll PM, Wessler S, Schlesinger MJ. Interarterial coronary anastomoses in the heart, with particular reference to anemia and relative cardiac anoxia. *Circulation*. 1951;4:797–815.
6. Fulton WFM. Arterial anastomoses in the coronary circulation. II. Distribution, enumeration and measurement of coronary arterial anastomoses in health and disease. *Scott Med J*. 1963;8:466–474.
7. Eitenmüller I, Volger O, Kluge A, et al. The range of adaptation by collateral vessels after femoral artery occlusion. *Circ Res*. 2006;99:656–662.
8. Lazarous D, Shou M, Scheinowitz M, et al. Comparative effects of basic fibroblast growth factor and vascular endothelial growth factor on coronary collateral development and the arterial response to injury. *Circulation*. 1996;94:1074–1082.
9. Wustmann K, Zbinden S, Windecker S, Meier B, Seiler C. Is there functional collateral flow during vascular occlusion in angiographically normal coronary arteries? *Circulation*. 2003;107:2213–2220.
10. Meier P, Gloekler S, Zbinden R, et al. Beneficial effect of recruitable collaterals: a 10-year follow-up study in patients with stable coronary artery disease undergoing quantitative collateral measurements. *Circulation*. 2007;116:975–983.
11. Feldman R, Pepine C. Evaluation of coronary collateral circulation in conscious humans. *Am J Cardiol*. 1984;53:1233–1238.
12. Rentrop K, Cohen M, Blanke H, Phillips R. Changes in collateral channel filling immediately after controlled coronary artery occlusion by an angioplasty balloon in human subjects. *J Am Coll Cardiol*. 1985;5:587–592.
13. Meier B, Luethy P, Finci L, Steffenino G, Rutishauser W. Coronary wedge pressure in relation to spontaneously visible and recruitable collaterals. *Circulation*. 1987;75:906–913.
14. Piek J, van Liebergen R, Koch K, Peters R, David G. Comparison of collateral vascular responses in the donor and recipient coronary artery during transient coronary occlusion assessed by intracoronary blood flow velocity analysis in patients. *J Am Coll Cardiol*. 1997;29:1528–1535.
15. Seiler C, Fleisch M, Garachemani A, Meier B. Coronary collateral quantitation in patients with coronary artery disease using intravascular flow velocity or pressure measurements. *J Am Coll Cardiol*. 1998;32:1272–1279.
16. Pijls NH, Bech GJ, el Gamal MI, et al. Quantification of recruitable coronary collateral blood flow in conscious humans and its potential to predict future ischemic events. *J Am Coll Cardiol*. 1995;25:1522–1528.
17. van Liebergen RA, Piek JJ, Koch KT, de Winter RJ, Schotborgh CE, Lie KI. Quantification of collateral flow in humans: a comparison of angiographic, electrocardiographic and hemodynamic variables. *J Am Coll Cardiol*. 1999;33:670–677.
18. Pohl T, Seiler C, Billinger M, Herren E, Wustmann K, Mehta H, Windecker S, Eberli FR, Meier B. Frequency distribution of collateral flow and factors influencing collateral channel development. Functional collateral channel measurement in 450 patients with coronary artery disease. *J Am Coll Cardiol*. 2001;38:1872–1878.
19. Schwartz H, Leiboff R, Bren G, et al. Temporal evolution of the human coronary collateral circulation after myocardial infarction. *J Am Coll Cardiol*. 1984;4:1088–1093.

20. Waldecker B, Waas W, Haberbosch W, Voss R, Wiecha J, Tillmanns H. Prevalence and significance of coronary collateral circulation in patients with acute myocardial infarct. *Z Kardiol*. 2002;91:243–248.

21. Vanoverschelde JLJ, Wijns W, Depré C, et al. Mechansims of chronic regional postischemic dysfunction in humans. New insights from the study of non-infarcted collateral-dependent myocardium. *Circulation*. 1993;87:1513–1523.

22. Vogel R, Indermühle A, Seiler C. Determination of the absolute perfusion threshold preventing myocardial ischemia in humans. *Heart*. 2007;93:115–116.

23. Werner G, Ferrari M, Heinke S, et al. Angiographic assessment of collateral connections in comparison with invasively determined collateral function in chronic coronary occlusions. *Circulation*. 2003;107:1972–1977.

24. Fulton W, van Royen N. Morphology of the collateral circulation in the human heart. In: Schaper W, Schaper J, eds. *Arteriogenesis*. Boston, Dirdrecht, London: Kluwer Academic Publishers; 2004:298–297.

25. Reiner L, Molnar J, Jimenez F, Freudenthal R. Interarterial coronary anastomoses in neonates. *Arch Pathol*. 1961;71:103–112.

26. Bloor C, Keefe J, Browne M. Intercoronary anastomoses in congenital heart disease. *Circulation*. 1966;33:227–231.

27. Pepler W, Meyer B. Interarterial coronary anastomoses and coronary arterial pattern. A comparative study of South African Bantu and European hearts. *Circulation*. 1960;22:14–24.

28. Goldstein RE, Michaelis LL, Morrow AG, Epstein SE. Coronary collateral function in patients without occlusive coronary artery disease. *Circulation*. 1975;51.118–125.

29. Cohen M, Sherman W, Rentrop K, Gorlin R. Determinants of collateral filling observed during sudden controlled coronary artery occlusion in human subjects. *J Am Coll Cardiol*. 1989;13:297–303.

30. Piek J, Koolen J, Hoedemaker G, David G, Visser C, Dunning A. Severity of single-vessel coronary arterial stenosis and duration of angina as determinants of recruitable collateral vessels during balloon angioplasty occlusion. *Am J Cardiol*. 1991;67:13–17.

31. Fujita M, Nakae I, Kihara Y, et al. Determinants of collateral development in patients with acute myocardial infarction. *Clin Cardiol*. 1999;9:595–599.

32. Nakae I, Fujita M, Miwa K, et al. Age-dependent impairment of coronary collateral development in humans. *Heart Vessels*. 2000;15:176–180.

33. Piek J, van Liebergen R, Koch K, Peters R, David G. Clinical, angiographic and hemodynamic predictors of recruitable collateral flow assessed during balloon angioplasty coronary occlusion. *J Am Coll Cardiol*. 1997;29:275–282.

34. Grundmann S, Piek J, Pasterkamp G, Hoefer I. Arteriogenesis: basic mechanisms and therapeutic stimulation. *Eur J Clin Invest*. 2007;37:755–766.

35. Juillière Y, Danchin N, Grentzinger A, et al. Role of previous angina pectoris and collateral flow to preserve left ventricular function in the presence or absence of myocardial infarction in isolated total occlusion of the left anterior descending coronary artery. *Am J Cardiol*. 1990;65:277–281.

36. Murry C, Jennings R, Reimer K. Preconditioning with ischemia: a delay of lethal cell injury in ischemic myocardium. *Circulation*. 1986;74:1124–1136.

37. Koerselman J, de Jaegere P, Verhaar M, Grobbee D, der Graaf Y, Group SS. Cardiac ischemic score determines the presence of coronary collateral circulation. *Cardiovasc Drugs Ther*. 2005;19:283–289.

38. Kurotobi T, Sato H, Kinjo K, et al. Reduced collateral circulation to the infarct-related artery in elderly patients with acute myocardial infarction. *J Am Coll Cardiol*. 2004;44:28–34.

39. Abaci A, Oguzhan A, Kahraman S, et al. Effect of diabetes mellitus on formation of coronary collateral vessels. *Circulation*. 1999;99:2239–2242.

40. Yilmaz M, Caldir V, Guray Y, et al. Relation of coronary collateral vessel development in patients with a totally occluded right coronary artery to the metabolic syndrome. *Am J Cardiol*. 2006;97:636–639.
41. Kyriakides Z, Kremastinos D, Michelakakis N, Matsakas E, Demovelis T, Toutouzas P. Coronary collateral circulation in coronary artery disease and systemic hypertension. *Am J Cardiol*. 1991;67:687–690.
42. Kilian J, Keech A, Adams M, Celermajer D. Coronary collateralization: determinants of adequate distal vessel filling after arterial occlusion. *Coron Artery Dis*. 2002;13:155–159.
43. Koerselman J, de Jaegere P, Verhaar M, Grobbee D, van der Graaf Y, Group SS. Coronary collateral circulation: the effects of smoking and alcohol. *Atherosclerosis*. 2007;191:191–198.
44. Zbinden R, Zbinden S, Billinger M, Windecker S, Meier B, Seiler C. Influence of diabetes mellitus on coronary collateral flow: an answer to an old controversy. *Heart*. 2005;91:1289–1293.
45. Olijhoek J, Koerselman J, de Jaegere P, et al. Presence of the metabolic syndrome does not impair coronary collateral vessel formation in patients with documented coronary artery disease. *Diabetes Care*. 2005;28:683–689.
46. Koerselman J, de Jaegere P, Verhaar M, van der Graaf Y, Grobbee D, Group SS. High blood pressure is inversely related with the presence and extent of coronary collaterals. *J Hum Hypertens*. 2005;19:809–811.
47. Van Belle E, Rivard A, Chen D, et al. Hypercholesterolemia attenuates angiogenesis but does not preclude augmentation by angiogenic cytokines. *Circulation*. 1997;96:2667–2274.
48 Zbinden S, Brunner N, Wustmann K, Billinger M, Meier B, Seiler C. Effect of statin treatment on coronary collateral flow in patients with coronary artery disease. *Heart*. 2004;90:448–449.
49. Kornowski R. Collateral formation and clinical variables in obstructive coronary artery disease: the influence of hypercholesterolemia and diabetes mellitus. *Coron Artery Dis*. 2003;14:61–64.
50. Heeschen C, Weis M, Cooke J. Nicotine promotes arteriogenesis. *J Am Coll Cardiol*. 2003;41:489–496.
51. Patel S, Breall J, Diver D, Gersh B, Levy A. Bradycardia is associated with development of coronary collateral vessels in humans. *Coron Artery Dis*. 2000;11:467–472.
52. Weis M, Heeschen C, Glassford A, Cooke J. Statins have biphasic effects on angiogenesis. *Circulation*. 2002;105:739–745.
53. Pourati I, Kimmelstiel C, Rand W, Karas R. Statin use is associated with enhanced collateralization of severely diseased coronary arteries. *Am Heart J*. 2004;146:876–881.
54. Fukuda D, Sata M, Tanaka K, Nagai R. Potent inhibitory effect of sirolimus on circulating vascular progenitor cells. *Circulation*. 2005;111:926–931.
55. Meier P, Zbinden R, Togni M, et al. Coronary collateral function long after drug-eluting stent implantation. *J Am Coll Cardiol*. 2007;49:15–20.
56. Hoefer I, Grundmann S, Schirmer S, et al. Aspirin, but not clopidogrel, reduces collateral conductance in a rabbit model of femoral artery occlusion. *J Am Coll Cardiol*. 2005;46:994–1001.
57. Klauber N, Browne F, Anand-Apte B, D'Amato R. New activity of spironolactone. Inhibition of angiogenesis in vitro and in vivo. *Circulation*. 1996;94:2566–2571.
58. Deindl E, Buschmann I, Hoefer I, et al. Role of ischemia and of hypoxia-inducible genes in arteriogenesis after femoral artery occlusion in the rabbit. *Circ Res*. 2001; 89:779–786.
59. Kamiya A, Togawa T. Adaptive regulation of wall shear stress to flow change in canine carotid artery. *Am J Physiol*. 1980;239:H14–H21.
60. Seiler C, Kirkeeide RL, Gould KL. Basic structure-function relations of the epicardial coronary vascular tree. Basis of quantitative coronary arteriography for diffuse coronary artery disease. *Circulation*. 1992;85:1987–2003.

61. Windecker S, Allemann Y, Billinger M, et al. Effect of endurance training on coronary artery size and function in healthy men: an invasive followup study. *Am J Physiol Heart Circ Physiol.* 2002;282:H2216–H2223.

62. Zbinden R, Zbinden S, Meier P, et al. Coronary collateral flow in response to endurance exercise training. *Eur J Cardiovasc Prev Rehabil.* 2007;14:250–257.

63. Schaper J, König R, Franz D, Schaper W. The endothelial surface of growing coronary collateral arteries. Intimal margination and diapedesis of monocytes. A combined SEM and TEM study. *Virchows Arch A Pathol Anat Histol.* 1976;370:193–205.

64. Davies P, Barbee K, Volin M, et al. Spatial relationships in early signaling events of flow-mediated endothelial mechanotransduction. *Annu Rev Physiol.* 1997;59:527–549.

65. Topper J, Gimbrone MJ. Blood flow and vascular gene expression: fluid shear stress as a modulator of endothelial phenotype. *Mol Med Today.* 1999;5:40–46.

66. Ingber D. Cellular basis of mechanotransduction. *Biol Bull.* 1998;194:323–325.

67. Cai W, Kocsis E, Luo X, Schaper W, Schaper J. Expression of endothelial nitric oxide synthase in the vascular wall during arteriogenesis. *Mol Cell Biochem.* 2004;264:193–200.

68. Mees B, Wagner S, Ninci E, et al. Endothelial nitric oxide synthase activity is essential for vasodilation during blood flow recovery but not for arteriogenesis. *Arterioscler Thromb Vasc Biol.* 2007;27:1926–1933.

69. Gimbrone MJ, Nagel T, Topper J. Biomechanical activation: an emerging paradigm in endothelial adhesion biology. *J Clin Invest.* 1997;99:1809–1813.

70. Barakat A. Responsiveness of vascular endothelium to shear stress: potential role of ion channels and cellular cytoskeleton. *Int J Mol Med.* 1999;4:323–332.

71. Lee C, Stabile E, Kinnaird T, et al. Temporal patterns of gene expression after acute hindlimb ischemia in mice: insights into the genomic program for collateral vessel development. *J Am Coll Cardiol.* 2004;43:474–482.

72. Werner G, Jandt E, Krack A, et al. Growth factors in the collateral circulation of chronic total coronary occlusions: relation to duration of occlusion and collateral function. *Circulation.* 2004;110:1940–1945.

73. Scholz D, Ito W, Fleming I, et al. Ultrastructure and molecular histology of rabbit hind-limb collateral artery growth (arteriogenesis). *Virchows Arch.* 2000;436: 257–270.

74. Pipp F, Heil M, Issbrücker K, et al. VEGFR-1-selective VEGF homologue PlGF is arteriogenic: evidence for a monocyte-mediated mechanism. *Circ Res.* 2003;92:378–385.

75. van Royen N, Hoefer I, Buschmann I, et al. Exogenous application of transforming growth factor beta 1 stimulates arteriogenesis in the peripheral circulation. *FASEB J.* 2002;16:432–434.

76. Kusch A, Tkachuk S, Lutter S, et al. Monocyte-expressed urokinase regulates human vascular smooth muscle cell migration in a coculture model. *Biol Chem.* 2002;383:217–221.

77. Menshikov M, Elizarova E, Plakida K, et al. Urokinase upregulates matrix metalloproteinase-9 expression in THP-1 monocytes via gene transcription and protein synthesis. *Biochem J.* 2002;367:833–839.

78. Arras M, Ito W, Scholz D, Winkler B, Schaper J, Schaper W. Monocyte activation in angiogenesis and collateral growth in the rabbit hindlimb. *J Clin Invest.* 1998;101:40–50.

79. Heil M, Ziegelhoeffer T, Pipp F, et al. Blood monocyte concentration is critical for enhancement of collateral artery growth. *Am J Physiol.* 2002;283:H2411–2419.

80. Zbinden R, Vogel R, Meier B, Seiler C. Coronary collateral flow and peripheral blood monocyte concentration in patients treated with granulocyte-macrophage colony stimulating factor. *Heart.* 2004;90:945–946.

81. Lee S, Wolf P, Escudero R, Deutsch R, Jamieson S, Thistlethwaite P. Early expression of angiogenesis factors in acute myocardial ischemia and infarction. *N Engl J Med.* 2000;342:626–633.

82. Hojo Y, Ikeda U, Zhu Y, et al. Expression of vascular endothelial growth factor in patients with acute myocardial infarction. *J Am Coll Cardiol.* 2000;35:968–973.
83. Heeschen C, Dimmeler S, Fichtlscherer S, et al. Prognostic value of placental growth factor in patients with acute chest pain. *JAMA.* 2004;291:435–441.
84. de Lemos J, Morrow D, Blazing M, et al. Serial measurement of monocyte chemoattractant protein-1 after acute coronary syndromes: results from the A to Z trial. *J Am Coll Cardiol.* 2007;50:2117–2124.
85. Fujita M, Ikemoto M, Kishishita M, et al. Elevated basic fibroblast growth factor in pericardial fluid of patients with unstable angina. *Circulation.* 1999;94:610–613.
86. Fleisch M, Billinger M, Eberli F, Garachemani A, Meier B, Seiler C. Physiologically assessed coronary collateral flow and intracoronary growth factor concentrations in patients with 1- to 3-vessel coronary artery disease. *Circulation.* 1999;100:1945–1950.
87. Lambiase P, Edwards R, Anthopoulos P, et al. Circulating humoral factors and endothelial progenitor cells in patients with differing coronary collateral support. *Circulation.* 2004;109:2986–2992.
88. Seiler C, Pohl T, Billinger M, Meier B. Tumour necrosis factor alpha concentration and collateral flow in patients with coronary artery disease and normal systolic left ventricular function. *Heart.* 2003;89:96–97.
89. Zbinden S, Zbinden R, Meier P, Windecker S, Seiler C. Safety and efficacy of subcutaneous-only granulocyte-macrophage colony-stimulating factor for collateral growth promotion in patients with coronary artery disease. *J Am Coll Cardiol.* 2005;46:1636–1642.
90. Khmelewski E, Becker A, Meinertz T, Ito W. Tissue resident cells play a dominant role in arteriogenesis and concomitant macrophage accumulation. *Circ Res.* 2004;95:E56–E64.
91. Stabile E, Burnett M, Watkins C, et al. Impaired arteriogenic response to acute hindlimb ischemia in CD4-knockout mice. *Circulation.* 2003;108:205–210.
92. van Weel V, Toes R, Seghers L, et al. Natural killer cells and CD4+ T-cells modulate collateral artery development. *Arterioscler Thromb Vasc Biol.* 2007;27:2310–2318.
93. Asahara T, Murohara T, Sullivan A, et al. Isolation of putative progenitor endothelial cells for angiogenesis. *Science.* 1997;275:964–967.
94. Asahara T, Masuda H, Takahashi T, et al. Bone marrow origin of endothelial progenitor cells responsible for postnatal vasculogenesis in physiological and pathological neovascularization. *Circ Res.* 1999;85:221–228.
95. Caplice N, Doyle B. Vascular progenitor cells: origin and mechanisms of mobilization, differentiation, integration, and vasculogenesis. *Stem Cells Dev.* 2005;14:122–139.
96. Ziegelhoeffer T, Fernandez B, Kostin S, et al. Bone marrow-derived cells do not incorporate into the adult growing vasculature. *Circ Res.* 2004;94:230–238.
97. Hill J, Syed M, Arai A, et al. Outcomes and risks of granulocyte colony-stimulating factor in patients with coronary artery disease. *J Am Coll Cardiol.* 2005;46:1643–1648.
98. Schächinger V, Erbs S, Elsässer A, et al. Intracoronary bone marrow-derived progenitor cells in acute myocardial infarction. *N Engl J Med.* 2006;355:1210–1221.
99. Assmus B, Honold J, Schächinger V, et al. Transcoronary transplantation of progenitor cells after myocardial infarction. *N Engl J Med.* 2006;355:1222–1232.
100. Ohki R, Yamamoto K, Ueno S, et al. Gene expression profiling of human atrial myocardium with atrial fibrillation by DNA microarray analysis. *Int J Cardiol.* 2005;102:233–238.
101. Mehra M, Uber P, Walther D, et al. Gene expression profiles and B-type natriuretic peptide elevation in heart transplantation: more than a hemodynamic marker. *Circulation.* 2006;114 (suppl I):I21–I26.
102. Karra R, Vemullapalli S, Dong C, et al. Molecular evidence for arterial repair in atherosclerosis. *Proc Natl Acad Sci USA.* 2005;102:16789–16794.

103. Seo D, Wang T, Dressman H, et al.. Gene expression phenotypes of atherosclerosis. *Arterioscler Thromb Vasc Biol.* 2004;24:1922–1927.
104. Patino W, Mian O, Kang J, et al. Circulating transcriptome reveals markers of atherosclerosis. *Proc Natl Acad Sci USA.* 2005;102:3423–3428.
105. Boengler K, Pipp F, Broich K, Fernandez B, Schaper W, Deindl E. Identification of differentially expressed genes like cofilin2 in growing collateral arteries. *Biochem Biophys Res Commun.* 2003;300:751–756.
106. Couffinhal T, Silver M, Zheng L, Kearney M, Witzenbichler B, Isner J. Mouse model of angiogenesis. *Am J Pathol.* 1998;152:1667–1679.
107. Lohr N, Warltier D, Chilian W, Weihrauch D. Haptoglobin expression and activity during coronary collateralization. *Am J Physiol.* 2005;288:H1389–1395.
108. Group UPDS. UK Prospective Diabetes Study 32. Ethnicity and cardiovascular disease. The incidence of myocardial infarction in white, South Asian, and Afro-Caribbean patients with type 2 diabetes. *Diabetes Care.* 1998;21:1271–1277.
109. Levy A, Roguin A, Hochberg I, et al. Haptoglobin phenotype and vascular complications in patients with diabetes. *N Engl J Med.* 2000;343:969–970.
110. Nakhoul F, Marsh S, Hochberg I, Leibu R, Miller B, Levy A. Haptoglobin genotype as a risk factor for diabetic retinopathy. *JAMA.* 2000;284:1244–1245.
111. Langlois M, Delanghe J. Biological and clinical significance of haptoglobin polymorphism in humans. *Clin Chem.* 1996;42:1589–1600.
112. Hochberg I, Roguin A, Nikolsky E, Chanderashekhar P, Cohen S, Levy A. Haptoglobin phenotype and coronary artery collaterals in diabetic patients. *Atherosclerosis.* 2002;161:441–446.
113. Levy A, Hochberg I, Jablonski K, et al. Haptoglobin phenotype is an independent risk factor for cardiovascular disease in individuals with diabetes: The Strong Heart Study. *J Am Coll Cardiol.* 2002;40:1984–1990.
114. Chittenden T, Sherman J, Xiong F, et al. Transcriptional profiling in coronary artery disease: indications for novel markers of coronary collateralization. *Circulation.* 2006;114:1811–1820.
115. Schirmer S, Fledderus J, Bot P, et al. Interferon-beta signaling is enhanced in patients with insufficient coronary collateral artery development and inhibits arteriogenesis in mice. *Circ Res.* 2008;102:1286–1294.
116. Meier P, Antonov J, Zbinden R, et al. Non-invasive gene-expression-based detection of well developed collateral function in individuals with and without coronary artery disease. *Heart.* 2008 Aug 26. [Epub ahead of print].
117. Regieli J, Nathoe H, Koerselman J, van der Graaf Y, Grobbee D, Doevendans P. Coronary collaterals – insights in molecular determinants and prognostic relevance. *Int J Cardiol.* 2007;116:139–143.
118. Fulton W. Anastomotic enlargement and ischaemic myocardial damage. *Br Heart J.* 1964;26:1–15.

Chapter 4
Pathophysiology of the Human Coronary Collateral Circulation

4.1 Introduction

The term pathophysiology relates to the Greek, πάθος, *pathos* (disease); φυσις, *physis* (nature, origin) and λόγος (speech), literally, the 'talk about the nature of diseased things', which is the study of the mechanical, physical and biochemical dysfunctions of living organism or organs. Focusing on the collateral circulation, pathophysiology has to be defined alternatively, because collaterals cannot be regarded as a disease but rather as its inherent repair mechanism: pathophysiology is the study of the physical and biochemical functions resulting from a disease, i.e. atherosclerosis.

4.2 Fluid Shear Stress and Vasomotor Function

As in arteriogenesis, vascular fluid shear stress plays an eminent role in the acute coronary adaptation to varying coronary flow demands. Accordingly, there is the concept of chronic *adaptive* shear stress control with vascular remodelling in response to chronic alteration of fluid shear stress as opposed to the concept of acute *limited* shear stress control, which prevents endothelial damage in response to acute flow increases, and implies shear stress adapted acute changes of vascular calibre. The principle of limited tangential wall shear stress states that arterial lumen is in such a size as to prevent coronary blood flow rate from causing endothelial damage during a short-term, acute maximum flow state. This is reasonable, given the pivotal role of the endothelium in vasomotor function. When blood flow increases in a vessel, the vessel dilates. This phenomenon has been coined as flow-mediated dilation. Tangential arterial wall shear stress is considered the primary stimulus for the endothelial-dependent flow-mediated vasodilator response.

In the past, it was proposed that coronary collateral vessels are able to maintain resting myocardial blood supply, but not the demands of an increased workload. Yet, in the canine coronary collateral circulation, structurally well-developed anastomoses with a muscular media capable of vasomotor activity have been documented. In humans without beta blockers, dynamic handgrip

C. Seiler, *Collateral Circulation of the Heart*, DOI 10.1007/978-1-84882-342-6_4,
© Springer-Verlag London Limited 2009

exercise induces an increase in collateral relative to normal antegrade flow by a factor of 1.75. Earlier clinical studies on the acute effect of isometric dynamic exercise on collateral function have employed nuclear perfusion imaging in patients with entirely collateralized, viable myocardial regions. Generally, it has been concluded in those studies that 'coronary collateral vessels may help maintain relative myocardial perfusion during exercise'. Supine bicycle exercise in humans with simultaneous assessment of coronary collateral function seems to have an effect similar to the more isotonic form of handgrip exercise, i.e. it induces a collateral flow reserve of approximately 1.9.

Adenosine is known to cause profound microvascular coronary dilation mediated by adenosine receptor on the cell membrane of resistance vessel smooth muscle cells. As a consequence, the flow in the upstream epicardial conductance arteries increases with augmented fluid shear stress and flow-mediated vasodilation. The observation of minimal or no coronary collateral function changes during hyperaemia in the absence of well-developed collaterals seems to be consistent. Coronary pressure-derived collateral flow index (CFI) remains practically unchanged on average under adenosine in the absence of angiographic collaterals, whereas it increases by a factor of 1.21 in the group with spontaneoulsy visible collaterals. However, the variability of collateral function responses in patients with well-developed collaterals is high.

4.2.1 Introduction

In humans, a situation of chronically augmented fluid shear stress in a coronary artery similar to that in the experimental model of a rabbit femoral artery-to-vein-shunt[1] can be encountered in congenital coronary artery malformations with a steep pressure gradient such as in a coronary-to-pulmonary-artery fistula (Fig. 4.1). Eitenmüller et al. investigated the range of structural and functional adaptation of collateral arteries in response to femoral artery occlusion with distal arterial stump-to-vein anastomosis.[1] After temporary reclosure of the shunt, collateral flow was measured at maximum vasodilatation, and maximum conductance reached the value of the non-ligated vessel at day 7 and had, after 4 weeks, surpassed the value before occlusion by a factor of 2. The 'natural experiment' of a human coronary artery fistula between the right coronary artery (RCA) and the proximal pulmonary artery (Fig. 4.1) illustrates several aspects of the relationship between chronically elevated vascular fluid shear stress and structural vascular remodelling as described in Section 4.4 (pathogenesis of coronary collateral growth): a chronically remodelled coronary collateral artery can be as large as the so called 'native' vessel, but it usually has a corkscrew-like appearance, since remodelling occurs in calibre as well as in length (Fig. 4.1). Immediately beyond the entrance of the coronary collateral artery into the pulmonary artery, a jet of radiographic contrast is visible (Fig. 4.1) indicating the presence of a stenosis between the systemic high- and

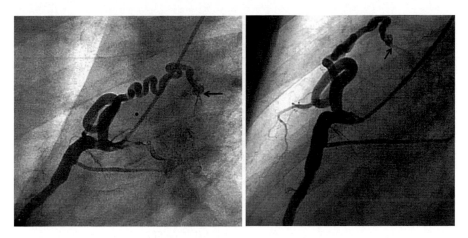

Fig. 4.1 Right coronary angiogram of a patient with a fistula of a conal branch to the pulmonary artery. Remodelling of the conal branch in response to the permanent pressure gradient between right coronary artery (RCA) and pulmonary artery (i.e. arteriogenesis) is visible by its corkscrew pattern and increased calibre. The pressure gradient is maintained by a narrowing at the orifice of the fistula (→). The stenosis can be appreciated by the presence of a contrast jet immediately downstream of the fistula orifice

the pulmonary low-pressure territories. This obstruction maintains the perfusion pressure gradient along the fistula, and the shunt flow is directly related to the perfusion pressure gradient and inversely proportional to the absolute size of the stenosis raised to the fourth power (Hagen-Poiseuille law). While Section 4.4 in this book on pathogenesis of the human coronary collateral circulation has focused on such *chronic* structural arterial response to permanently increased flow (collateral artery remodelling triggered by augmented shear force), this chapter relates to the *acute* vascular reactions to altering flow rates, i.e. one of the functional elements essential for coronary collateral physiology and pathophysiology. In the context of both chronically occurring collateral growth and acute coronary flow changes, vascular shear forces play an eminent role.

4.2.2   Limited and Adaptive Arterial Wall Shear Stress

4.2.2.1   Theoretical Considerations

According to the continuity equation of flow within a circulation, vascular flow rate (Q, cm^3/min) is the product of vascular cross-sectional area (A, cm^2) and the spatially averaged flow velocity (v_{mean}, cm/s): $Q = A \times v_{mean}$. Tangential vascular wall fluid shear stress τ (dyne/cm^2) is directly related to volume flow rate Q by the product of blood viscosity (μ, 0.03 dyne s/cm^2) and fluid shear rate dv/dr (s^{-1}; the change of flow velocity dv between different fluid layers of the

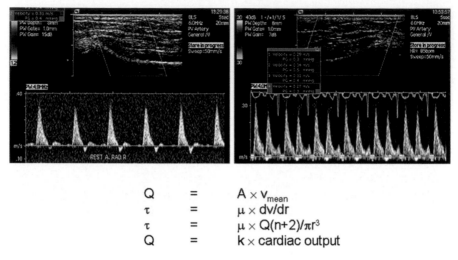

$$Q = A \times V_{mean}$$
$$\tau = \mu \times dv/dr$$
$$\tau = \mu \times Q(n+2)/\pi r^3$$
$$Q = k \times \text{cardiac output}$$

Fig. 4.2 Duplex sonographic images of the radial artery in a patient who underwent diastolic lower leg external counterpulsation at 300 mmHg (*right panel*) in comparison to the situation without counterpulsation (*left panel*). Right radial artery pulsed Doppler flow spectra are shown with a very low-diastolic flow velocity signal at rest (*left panel*), and with diastolic and systolic flow velocity signals at identical speeds during high pressure counterpulsation (*right panel*). Below, the fluid mechanic equations relevant for the relationship between blood volume flow rate (*Q*), vascular calibre (radius *r*, cross-sectional area *A*), cardiac output, blood flow velocity (*v*) and fluid shear stress (*τ*) are depicted. Abbreviations: k: constant; n: factor for the characterization of the flow velocity profile; V_{mean}: spatially averaged flow velocity; dv/dr: change of flow velocity between different fluid layers; μ = blood viscosity

thickness d*r* across the vascular lumen; Fig. 4.2). The fluid shear rate d*v*/d*r* at the endothelial surface can be given as: $Q(n+2)/\pi r^3$, whereby *Q* is the entire or a fraction of cardiac output, the value of n is dimensionless and dependent on the flow condition (n = 2 for laminar flow, n > 2 for turbulent flow) and *r* is the internal radius of the vessel (Fig. 4.2). A radial artery pulsed wave Doppler image from a patient with coronary artery disease (CAD) illustrates that during a 'regular' cardiac cycle (Fig. 4.2, left side), the fraction of cardiac output reaching the distal arm consists of the temporal average of the positive (= above the baseline) and negative, spatially averaged flow velocity signals (the positive fraction peaking during systole) multiplied by the temporal average of the radial artery calibre. During diastole, there is a second positive flow velocity peak reaching about 10% of the systolic peak flow velocity. The temporal average of forward flow velocity signals over the cardiac cycle is much augmented by adding a diastolic 'offbeat' (Fig. 4.2, right side) as generated by a cardiac assist device (external or internal counterpulsation). With regard to the above-described direct relationship between fluid shear rate and *Q*, the 'offbeat' doubles the fluid shear stress at the vessel wall over the cardiac cycle unless there is vascular enlargement in the sense of a constant shear stress regulation. As evidenced by data from the literature (see below and also in Section 4.4 of this book), constant vascular shear stress regulation occurs in the peripheral as well as in the coronary circulation in the sense of not only chronic *adaptive* shear stress control, but likely also as acute *limited* shear stress control. Chronic *adaptive* shear stress control has been reported to occur in response to physical endurance exercise training and in direct association with the level of fitness reached among healthy individuals (Fig. 4.3).[2] More importantly, it has been observed to be related to total or regional left ventricular (LV) mass (M) supplied by the entire or a fraction of the coronary artery tree according to the following equation: arterial cross-sectional area $= k \times M^{2/3}$.[3–5] A functional consequence of chronic adaptive shear stress control according to the just-mentioned design principle of vascular tree structures is that blood-flow velocity potentially harmful to the endothelium decreases on average by a factor of 1.25 at every downstream bifurcation as the summed cross-sectional areas of the two respective daughter vessels increase by the same factor.[6] In a broader sense, also arteriogenesis (remodelling of preformed coronary collateral vessels) is triggered by augmented fluid shear stress and can be regarded as chronic *adaptive* shear stress control,[7] whereby shear stress augmentation along a

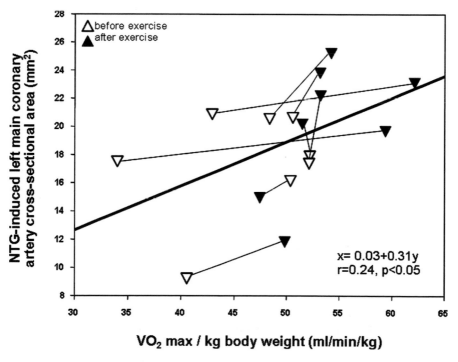

Fig. 4.3 Relationship between nitroglycerine (NTG)-induced left main coronary artery calibre (*vertical axis*) as assessed by quantitative coronary angiography before and after an endurance exercise training in healthy volunteers and peak oxygen uptake (VO$_2$max; *horizontal axis*) as obtained during spiroergometry

preformed collateral artery is caused by a pressure gradient between the collateral supplying and receiving arteries. The pressure gradient can be principally due to a flow limiting stenosis in the collateral receiving artery, and alternatively or in addition, to a proximal collateral origin from the collateral supplying artery with a distal collateral connection at the receiving artery, thus creating a certain imbalance between perfusion pressures in the contra- and ipsilateral artery. During hyperaemia, i.e. during elevated cardiac output or Q values, such small perfusion pressure imbalances between different coronary territories could be augmented and elevated values of shear rates and shear stress could trigger arteriogenesis even in the absence of relevant CAD. At the beginning of collateral remodelling in response to augmented fluid shear stress, the capacity for acute endothelial nitric oxide synthase dependent vasodilation has been described to precede arteriogenesis, which does, however, not appear to be essential for the chronic adaptation of the collateral circulation in a mouse hind limb ischaemia model.[8]

4.2.2.2 Fluid Shear Stress and Endothelial Damage

For *acute* functional changes of 'native' or collateral coronary artery calibres, the concept of *limited* wall shear stress regulation is more important than the chronic adaptive shear stress control. The principle of limited tangential wall shear stress states that arterial lumen would be in such a size as to prevent coronary blood flow rate from causing endothelial damage during a short-term, acute maximum flow state.[3] Limited shear stress determines the coronary 'native' or collateral artery calibre such that during acute increases to maximum flow rate, the endothelial wall shear stress does not exceed a level destructive to the endothelium, which starts to occur beyond about 300 dynes/cm^2.[9–11]

The study by Fry aimed at quantifying the acute changes in endothelial histology related to an increase in blood flow velocity.[9] For that purpose, an intraaortic device was designed to produce a convergence of the aortic blood stream into a narrow channel of the thoracic aorta in dogs. The endothelial surface overlying this channel was exposed to a broad range of shear stress values by the accelerated blood flow. The resulting distribution of shear stress at every point to which the endothelial surface was exposed within the channel was determined. Histological analysis of the endothelial cell layers was performed in order to determine states of injury relative to the applied shear stress. Exposure to shear stress beyond an average value of 380 dynes/cm^2 for periods as short as 1 hour resulted in marked deterioration of the endothelial surface consisting of endothelial cytoplasmatic swelling, cell deformation, cell disintegration and dissolution and erosion of cell substance.[9]

Kamiya and Togawa investigated the adaptive response of the vascular wall to blood flow changes in an arterio-venous shunt model that was constructed between the common carotid artery and the external jugular vein in 12 dogs.[10] Six to eight months post-operatively (i.e. chronic adaptive shear stress control), the arterial internal radius was determined. The results showed that the radius

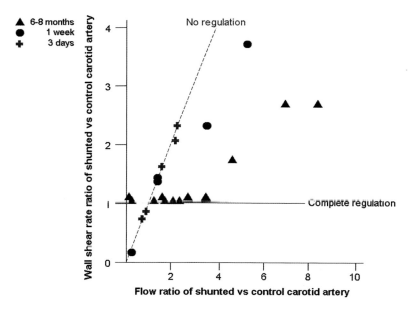

Fig. 4.4 Regulation of vascular wall shear rate by adaptive changes in arterial radius. Correlation of shear rate ratio of the shunted to the control side (*vertical axis*) versus the respective flow rate ratio (*horizontal axis*) in acute experiments (3 days after shunt operation), in subacute (1 week) and chronic experiments (6 8 months). The shunt operation consisted of a connection between the common carotid artery and the external jugular vein in 12 dogs.[10] Acutely, there is a direct and close association between the degree of flow and shear rate (regulation of vascular calibre to flow not yet achieved), whereas the correlation tends to disappear chronically (complete regulation)

had increased with increased flow load and vice versa. The shear rate, initially proportional to Q (no shear stress regulation; Fig. 4.4), had recovered almost to the control level due to vessel dilatation during the chronic experiment, when Q was less than 4 times the control. In the acute vascular response phase, the values of wall shear stress as obtained in the study by Kamiya and Togawa[10] were at least one order of magnitude lower than the values obtained in the study by Fry causing endothelial damage.[9]

4.2.2.3 Limited Shear Stress Control in the Human Epicardial Coronary Circulation

Based on the equation describing the shear rate being directly determined by Q and inversely by r^3 (Fig. 4.2), the results of the study by Kamiya and Togawa indicated a complete absence of acute vasodilatory regulation up to a fourfold increase of flow (Fig. 4.4). This is not in agreement with the concept of flow-mediated vasodilation,[12] and the absence of limited wall shear stress regulation is also challenged by recent findings in healthy individuals undergoing a physical endurance exercise programme with a chronic adaptation of epicardial coronary artery sizes[2]; the same individuals have also elicited an improved *acute* response of their coronary artery calibres to the flow-mediated stimulus of intracoronary adenosine (proximal left anterior descending coronary artery (LAD) without adenosine before and after the exercise period: 9.5±2.9 and 10.1±3.3 mm^2, respectively; proximal LAD with intracoronary adenosine before and after the exercise period: 10.1±3.5 and 11.0±3.9 mm^2, respectively, p = 0.03).[2] The coronary flow velocity reserve, in the study by Windecker et al. that included eight healthy volunteers, increased from a value of 3.8±0.8 before the exercise programme to 4.5±0.7 after the 9-month training programme (Fig. 4.5).[2] Considering the fact that resting heart rate was 63±13 beats/min before and 63±15 after the exercise programme, maximum hyperaemic coronary flow velocity was significantly higher following the exercise programme, and this was related to an augmented acute vasodilatory capacity. Since in these individuals,[2] tangential fluid shear rate had, thus, increased during hyperaemia and the corresponding vasodilatory capacity of epicardial coronary arteries had improved, the principle of limited acute shear stress regulation in the sense of flow-mediated dilation appears to be valid in the human 'native' epicardial coronary circulation.

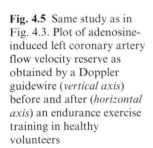

Fig. 4.5 Same study as in Fig. 4.3. Plot of adenosine-induced left coronary artery flow velocity reserve as obtained by a Doppler guidewire (*vertical axis*) before and after (*horizontal axis*) an endurance exercise training in healthy volunteers

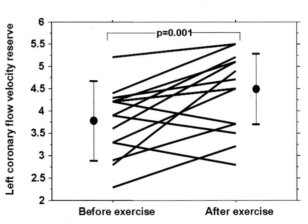

4.2.3 Flow-Mediated Vascular Function in 'Native' and Collateral Arteries

4.2.3.1 Flow-Mediated Vascular Function in 'Native' Arteries

The endothelium is of essential importance for the maintenance of vascular tone. It participates in the regulation of blood flow in response to changes in tissue and organ perfusion requirements. When blood flow increases through a vessel, the vessel dilates. This phenomenon has been coined as flow-mediated dilation. Schretzenmayer was the first to describe this physiological response,[13] and flow-mediated dilation has been demonstrated subsequently in a number of conduit arteries in vitro and in vivo, in animals and in humans. An intact endothelium is crucial for flow-dependent dilation of conduit arteries. This has first been demonstrated in femoral arteries[14] and epicardial arteries.[15,16] Only in some resistance arteries is flow-dependent dilation mediated, at least in part, independent from the endothelium.[17] Celermajer et al. introduced a unique setup to study the flow-dependent dilation non-invasively and reliably in the human forearm circulation.[18] An increase in flow through the brachial artery is induced by causing post-ischaemic dilation (normally reaching +7 to +10% of baseline diameter) in the downstream vascular bed of the distal forearm. Tangential arterial wall shear stress is considered to be the primary stimulus for the endothelial-dependent flow-mediated vasodilator response.[19]

However, the relationship between *directly obtained* shear stress and flow-mediated dilation has been studied in humans only rarely. In order to substantiate the concept of flow-mediated vascular function, Silber et al., using phase-contrast magnetic resonance imaging, studied the relationship between vascular wall shear stress and flow-mediated dilation in human radial arteries, and investigated whether this relationship could explain why flow-mediated dilation is greater in small than large arteries.[20] Post-ischaemic hyperaemic wall shear stress and flow-mediated dilation in the right brachial artery of 18 healthy volunteers were measured (hyperaemia induced by sphygmomanometry). Wall shear rate was calculated as the product of spatially averaged blood-flow velocity divided by the vessel diameter times 8 (assuming a parabolic flow velocity profile). Figure 4.6 illustrates that the range of spatial flow velocity profiles varies substantially between and within individuals, the fact of which translates into varying velocity profile 'bluntness' factors (see the above-mentioned factor 'n' for computing shear rates). As a consequence, the error in calculating fluid shear rates assuming an entirely parabolic flow velocity profile ($n = 2$) instead of obtaining it directly may be substantial. The 'bluntness' factor n is equal to $2([V_c/V_{mean}]-1)^{-1}$, whereby V_c is the centerline velocity and V_{mean} the spatially averaged velocity. In the study by Silber et al., flow-mediated dilation was directly proportional to hyperaemic peak systolic wall shear stress ($r = 0.79$, $p = 0.0001$), and hyperaemia-induced change in wall shear stress also correlated directly with the respective vasodilatory capacity (Fig. 4.7).[20] Flow-mediated dilation was inversely related to baseline diameter ($r = -0.62$, $p = 0.006$), but the hyperaemic peak wall shear stress stimulus was also inversely related to baseline diameter ($r = -0.47$, $p = 0.049$).

Dilatation of coronary resistance vessels to induce increases in wall shear stress in the upstream epicardial coronary arteries can be achieved by metabolic stimuli such as exercise or pacemaker stimulation. Alternatively, this can be mimicked by selective infusion of adenosine[21] or papaverine[22] into the midportion of the epicardial artery and simultaneous quantification of flow-mediated dilation in the proximal segment of the artery under investigation.

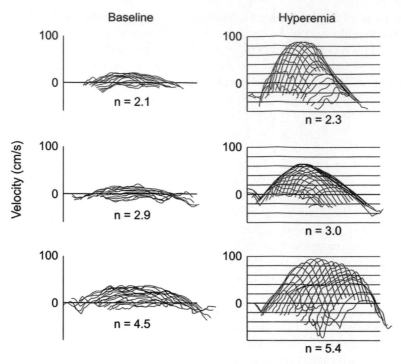

Fig. 4.6 Cross-sectional brachial artery blood flow velocity (*vertical axis*; obtained by phase-contrast magnetic resonance angiography) profiles at baseline and during peak hyperaemia for three healthy subjects with different flow velocity bluntness factors n. The smaller the n the lower the flow velocity profile.[20] For a fully developed parabolic velocity profile, $n = 2$

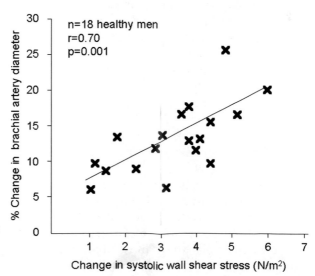

Fig. 4.7 Correlation between percent change in brachial artery diameter from baseline to hyperaemia (*vertical axis*) and the respective change in systolic wall shear stress[20]

4.2.3.2 Flow-Mediated Vascular Function in Coronary Collateral Arteries

Since functioning collateral arteries and arterioles are a constituent of the coronary circulation in a substantial proportion of individuals with and without CAD (54% of 1,069 individuals have a value of collateral relative to normal antegrade flow of $\geq 15\%$[23]), the above-described evidence of endothelium dependent, flow-mediated vasomotor function can be expected to be present also in coronary anastomoses of arteriolar or arterial size. On the other hand, Blumgart et al. proposed, almost 70 years ago, that coronary collateral vessels are able to maintain the resting myocardial requirement of blood supply, but not the demands of an increased workload.[24] Yet, in the canine coronary collateral circulation, Hautamaa et al. demonstrated the existence of structurally well-developed anastomoses with a muscular media capable of vasomotor activity in response to nitroglycerine.[25] Other experimental studies have illustrated collateral functional capacity by demonstrating that physical exercise induces a more than two- to threefold perfusion increase in collateral-dependent myocardium via β-adrenergic and nitric oxide mechanisms.[26–29] In light of the latter studies and the fact that coronary arteriolar dilation with increases in wall shear stress in the upstream epicardial coronary arteries can be achieved by stimuli such as exercise, Pohl et al. performed a study in 50 patients with CAD who underwent a 3-minute dynamic handgrip exercise protocol with quantitative collateral assessment during the last minute.[30] Specifically, CFI was determined at the start and the end of two 1-minute coronary occlusions, *randomly* accompanied by a resting state or the 3-minute dynamic handgrip exercise in order to account for possible collateral recruitment during repetitive occlusions. There was a statistically relevant haemodynamic response of heart rate and blood pressure to dynamic handgrip exercise (Fig. 4.8). When comparing CFI without and with dynamic handgrip exercise at the start as well as at the end of balloon occlusions, a significant increase was observed with dynamic handgrip exercise.[30] However, this was observed only in patients without β-blocker treatment (Fig. 4.9; coronary collateral flow reserve = 1.75 vs. 1.1 with β-blockers,

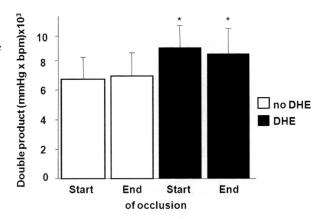

Fig. 4.8 Box plot of heart rate–systolic blood pressure double product (*vertical axis*) at the start and at the end of a 1-minute coronary balloon occlusion for the assessment of collateral function without (*hatched bars*) and with (*white bars*) dynamic handgrip exercise (DHE for 3 minutes). *p < 0.01 as compared to without DHE. *Error lines*: standard deviation

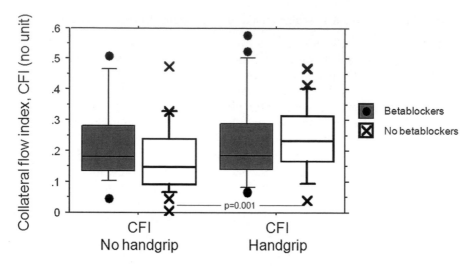

Fig. 4.9 Box plot with values of collateral flow index (CFI; *vertical axis*) obtained in 25 CAD patients with beta-blockers and in 25 CAD patients without beta-blockers. CFI obtained at the end of a 1-minute coronary balloon occlusion in the absence (*left side*) and presence (*right side*) of dynamic handgrip exercise. Error lines indicate mean, 25th and 75th percentile of confidence interval; 5th and 95th percentile of confidence interval

p < 0.01), and the maximum degree of contraction force reached during dynamic handgrip exercise was directly related to the change of CFI in response to exercise as compared with the resting condition (Fig. 4.10).[30]

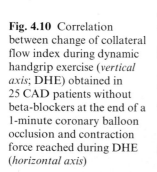

Fig. 4.10 Correlation between change of collateral flow index during dynamic handgrip exercise (*vertical axis*; DHE) obtained in 25 CAD patients without beta-blockers at the end of a 1-minute coronary balloon occlusion and contraction force reached during DHE (*horizontal axis*)

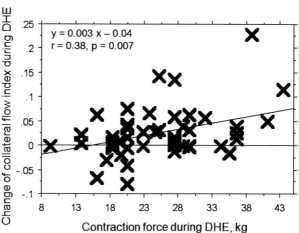

4.2.3.3 Isometric Physical Exercise and Coronary Collateral Function

In case of the just-mentioned dynamic handgrip exercise, it is probably more the sympathetic stimulus related to the isotonic phase at maximum force that affects coronary collateral function than an isometric feature as it occurs in treadmill or cycling exercise. The latter forms of exercise are more 'physiologic' and representative for daily physical activities. Therefore, this paragraph focuses on dynamic isometric physical exercise and its effect on collateral function. The physical exercise model is selected here to illustrate proof of principle of coronary collateral vascular function for two reasons: it is undisputable that physical exercise increases cardiac output, respectively the fraction of it supplying the myocardium, and that physical exercise heightens myocardial oxygen demand. The first response to exercise leads *directly* to an augmented coronary artery shear rate and thus to a flow-mediated dilation of the epicardial coronary arteries. The second response *indirectly* causes macrovascular flow-mediated dilation via the demand-related myocardial microvascular dilation, the latter of which being principally caused by the release and action of intramyocardial adenosine. Since the increase in cardiac output during exercise is related to both augmented ventricular stroke volume and tachycardia, the effect of the latter with particular focus on coronary collateral fluid shear rate can be discussed. Coronary flow is impeded during systole due to cardiac contraction, and it occurs during diastole in the absence of coronary obstructions. In the presence of stenoses and in the poorly developed collateral circulation, diastolic flow is reduced, which is more pronounced in the presence of a shortened diastole during tachycardia.[31] The potentially occurring reduced epicardial supply in CAD during exercise-induced tachycardia may or may not be corrected by an augmented microvascular dilation due to aggravated ischaemia. Earlier clinical studies on the acute effect of exercise on collateral function have employed thallium-201 perfusion imaging in patients with entirely collateralized, viable myocardial regions providing a qualitative, dichotomous measure of absent or present perfusion defects.[32–34] Rigo et al. concluded from their study that 'coronary collateral vessels may help maintain relative myocardial perfusion during exercise'.[32] Eng et al. studied collateral function by analysis of exercise thallium-201 myocardial perfusion images from 31 patients who had at least one non-infarcted, entirely collateralized myocardial region as documented during catheterization. Twenty-two of 41 of the collateralized regions manifested exercise-induced perfusion defects and 19 were normally perfused, whereby the latter 19 consisted of 13 with defects in other myocardial regions supplied by diseased vessels and were considered negative relative to other jeopardized regions.[34] Thus, only in about 1/7 of all collateralized regions (n = 6), perfusion was adequate during maximal exercise, whereas in about ½ exercise-induced coronary steal occurred. That the chronic total occlusion model may produce contradicting results with respect to exercise-induced collateral function has been illustrated even in the experimental setting. Whereas Schaper et al. observed a reduced hyperaemia-induced myocardial perfusion (steal) in the collateralized region among dogs 3–6 weeks after ameroid constriction,[35] Lambert et al. using the same model after 6 months of occlusion demonstrated a threefold exercise-induced flow augmentation (Fig. 4.11).[26]

Fig. 4.11 Line chart with individual values of myocardial blood flow (*vertical axis*) in a collateralized region of dogs that underwent ameroid constriction of the left circumflex coronary artery 6 months before the exercise test. Symbols and error lines: mean ± standard error[26]

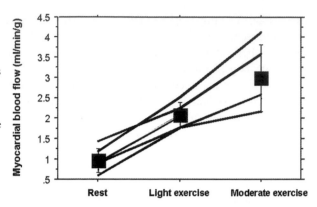

In the human coronary circulation without chronic total occlusion, it is technically challenging to obtain invasive collateral function measurements during supine bicycle exercise (Fig. 4.12). At present, quantitative collateral assessment can be performed only during coronary occlusion. Therefore, collateral measurement during bicycle exercise requires radial artery access percutaneous coronary intervention (PCI) in order to prevent the leg movements from pushing the angioplasty guiding catheter forcefully into the coronary

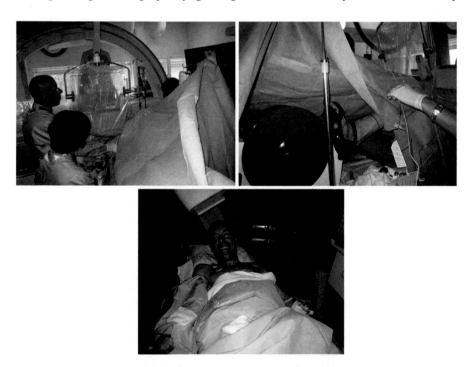

Fig. 4.12 Setting in the coronary catheterization laboratory for the assessment of collateral function in response to supine bicycle ergometry using 6-French right radial artery coronary angiography

ostium, which would substantially increase the risk of ostial coronary dissection. Preliminary data from our laboratory have demonstrated that a protocol with a 6-minute exercise period followed or preceded by a resting period with collateral function measurement during the last minute of each period is feasible. In order to measure collateral function during peak exercise, it has to be determined during the last minute of the bicycling period (Fig. 4.13). Figure 4.14 provides an example of simultaneously recorded phasic and mean aortic, distal coronary occlusive and central venous pressure during exercise and at rest, illustrating that the mean pressures during exercise are of sufficient signal quality for the calculation of CFI: $(P_{occl}-CVP)/(P_{ao}-CVP)$. Data obtained so far from 23 individuals have shown a statistically relevant increase in collateral function with a coronary collateral flow reserve amounting to 1.89 (Fig. 4.15).

Fig. 4.13 Scheme of the protocol employed during coronary collateral function assessment in response to supine bicycle ergometry. Collateral function measurement takes place during the last minute of the 6-minute exercise test by coronary balloon occlusion

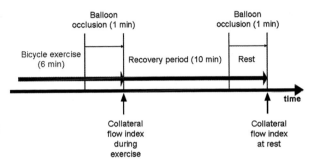

4.2.3.4 Adenosine and Flow-Mediated Coronary Vascular Function

Since the identification of nucleoside adenosine in the myocardium in 1929, many investigators have shown that it is synthesized in the myocardium and that the interstitial adenosine concentration rises in response to increased metabolic oxygen requirements and ischaemia.[36-38] Exogenously administered adenosine causes profound microvascular coronary dilation mediated by adenosine receptor on the cell membrane of resistance vessel smooth muscle cells.[39] As a consequence, the flow in the upstream epicardial conductance arteries increases with augmented fluid shear stress and flow-mediated vasodilation. Wilson et al. investigated, in humans, the effects of adenosine, administered by intracoronary bolus (2–16 µg), intracoronary infusion (10–240 µg/min) or intravenous infusion (35–140 µg/kg/min) on coronary and systemic haemodynamics and the electrocardiogram (ECG).[21] These authors found that maximal coronary vasodilation in comparison to papaverine (normal coronary blood flow velocity reserve, CRVR, of 4.5±0.2) could be achieved safely using intracoronary bolus administration of 12 µg for the RCA (n = 6; CFVR = 4.4±1.0) and 18 µg for the left coronary artery (LCA) (n = 20; CFVR = 4.6±0.7), and that intravenous infusion at a rate of 140 µg/kg/min caused near-maximal coronary hyperaemia in 84% of patients with CAD.[21]

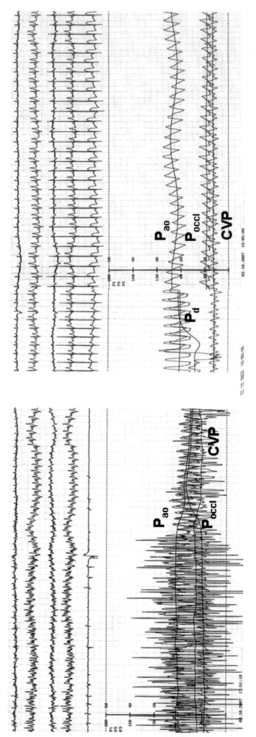

Fig. 4.14 Simultaneous ECG/pressure tracings obtained in the proximal left anterior descending coronary artery during supine bicycle exercise (*left side*) and at rest (*right side*). The lowest ECG lead is the intracoronary lead obtained via the pressure sensor guidewire (not attached during exercise due to motion artefacts). Abbreviations: CVP = central venous pressure (scale 50 mmHg); P_{ao} = aortic pressure (scale 200 mmHg); P_d = distal coronary pressure (scale 200 mmHg); P_{occl} = distal coronary occlusive pressure (scale 200 mmHg). Collateral flow index, CFI = $(P_{occl} - CVP)/(P_{ao} - CVP)$

Fig. 4.15 Line chart with
individual values of
collateral flow index
(*vertical axis*) obtained at
rest and during supine
bicycle ergometry
(*horizontal axis*) in patients
with CAD. Symbols and
error lines: mean ± standard
deviation

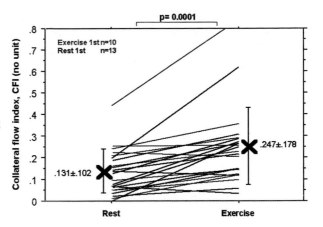

In this context, the purpose of the study by McFalls et al., using positron
emission tomography (PET) and oxygen-15-labelled water in five patients with
CAD, was to determine the vasodilator reserve in response to dipyridamole in
viable myocardium completely perfused by intramyocardial collateral blood
flow.[40] During resting conditions, myocardial blood flow in the control group
was 0.86±0.10 ml/min/g, 0.99±0.10 ml/min/g in the patients with normally
perfused myocardium and 0.86±0.14 ml/min/g in patients with collateral-
dependent myocardium. Absolute coronary flow reserve (dipyridamole blood
flow/resting blood flow) in the control group was 4.1±0.8 and 3.1±1.1 in
patients with normal regions and 1.9±1.0 (p < 0.001) in patients with collateralized regions (Fig. 4.16).[40] Since, dipyridamole inhibits the enzyme adenosine
deaminase, which normally breaks down adenosine to inosine, it leads to
a direct increase in the levels of extracellular adenosine. Similarly, Vanoverschelde et al. studied 26 anginal patients with chronic total coronary occlusion (CTO) of a major artery but without previous infarction.[41] PET was

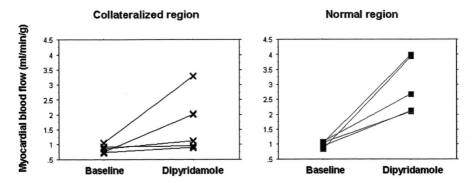

Fig. 4.16 Line chart with individual values of myocardial blood flow (*vertical axis*) to entirely
collateralized, viable myocardial regions (*black lines*) and to normal areas (*blue lines*) in five
patients with chronic total coronary occlusion at baseline and during dipyridamole-induced
hyperaemia (*horizontal axis*). On average coronary collateral flow reserve was 1.9[40]

performed to measure absolute regional myocardial blood flow with ^{13}N-ammonia at rest (n = 26) and after intravenous dipyridamole (n = 11). After intravenous dipyridamole, collateral-dependent myocardial blood flow increased from 0.78±0.05 to 2.38±0.54 ml/min/g in three patients with normal LV wall motion in the collateralized region, and from 0.88±0.17 to only 1.12±0.44 ml/min/g in eight patients with regional dysfunction.[41] Piek et al. used intracoronary adenosine injections in the collateral supplying artery of 38 CAD patients to induce flow-mediated vasomotion, while obtaining coronary flow velocity and wedge pressure during a brief occlusion of the collateral receiving artery.[42] The authors found that coronary collateral blood flow velocity as obtained by intracoronary Doppler could be increased with adenosine in patients with one-vessel disease and spontaneously visible collateral vessels on angiography, but not in patients with collateral vessels only recruitable upon vascular occlusion (Fig. 4.17).[42] However, on average, intracoronary blood flow velocity in response to adenosine increased much less (flow velocity reserve of 1.35) as compared with studies in patients with chronic occlusions cited just before. The fact that, in the study by Piek et al., no response of coronary collateral function to adenosine could be obtained in patients with less well-developed collaterals (not spontaneously visible on angiography) was possibly related to the route of injection via the falsely tagged *collateral supplying* artery rather than to an actual absence of collateral vasomotor function. Therefore, our laboratory performed a similar study in 50 CAD patients (29 without angiographic collaterals and 21 with spontaneously visible collaterals) applying intravenous adenosine (140 μg/kg/min) for inducing flow-mediated dilation.[43] Coronary pressure-derived CFI remained practically unchanged on average under adenosine in the absence of angiographic collaterals, whereas it increased by a factor of 1.21 in the group with spontaneously visible collaterals (Fig. 4.18).[43] Figure 4.18 illustrates that in the group with good collaterals, their function was highly variable in response to adenosine ranging between a CFI change of –0.3 to +0.3 (6 of 21 patients with a decrease). Such a high variability in adenosine-induced coronary collateral function among patients with well-developed collaterals cannot only be observed within but even more so

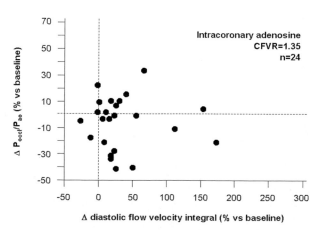

Fig. 4.17 Scatter plot of adenosine-induced change of mean coronary occlusive to mean aortic pressure (*vertical axis*; $\Delta P_{occl}/P_{ao}$) and of the respective occlusive coronary flow velocity change (*horizontal axis*). Average coronary flow velocity reserve (CFVR) is 1.35

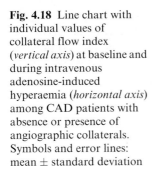

Fig. 4.18 Line chart with individual values of collateral flow index (*vertical axis*) at baseline and during intravenous adenosine-induced hyperaemia (*horizontal axis*) among CAD patients with absence or presence of angiographic collaterals. Symbols and error lines: mean ± standard deviation

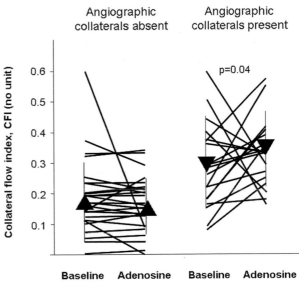

between investigations. A recent study by Perera et al., in 33 patients with one-vessel CAD who underwent coronary pressure-derived collateral assessment at rest and during intravenous adenosine (140 µg/kg/min), found no change in CFI among patients with poorly developed anastomoses (n = 18), but an overall decrease during hyperaemia with increasing collateral flow at rest (Fig. 4.19).[44]

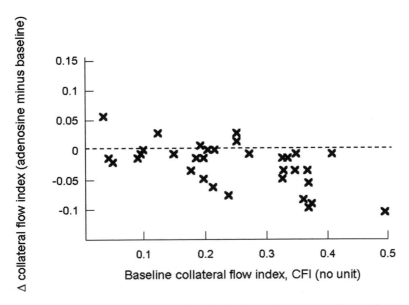

Fig. 4.19 Scatter plot of intravenous adenosine-induced change of collateral flow index (*vertical axis*) and baseline collateral flow index (*horizontal axis*) in 18 patients with non-occlusive CAD ($r = -0.63$, $p < 0.01$)[44]

The observation of minimal or no coronary collateral function changes during hyperaemia in the absence of well-developed collaterals seems to be consistent. During coronary occlusion, the lack of good collateral supply to the occluded myocardial region is related to severe ischaemia as evidenced by large ST-segment elevation on intracoronary ECG (Fig. 4.20).[45] Myocardial ischaemia is known to have a very strong vasodilating effect on the microcirculation,[46] such that an additional hyperaemic stimulus like adenosine is unlikely to further lower microvascular resistance. However, in this context, it would have to be expected that increasing baseline collateral flow ought to be associated with augmented vasoreactivity. Perera et al. found the contrary, i.e. an inverse relationship between CFI and flow-mediated vasodilation,[44] whereas the above-cited studies have consistently documented a *direct* association, although the extent of coronary collateral flow reserve varied between 1.2 and 3.1.[40-43] Considering those partly underpowered investigations, which are not all representative for the entire group of CAD patients (chronic total occlusions), the principal questions are whether the conflicting results are a

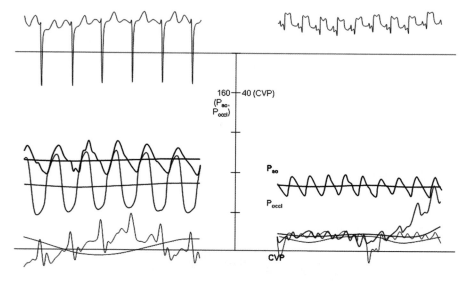

Fig. 4.20 Example of pressure/intracoronary ECG tracings from a patient with high collateral relative to normal antegrade flow (collateral flow index, CFI; left to the pressure scale) and without ECG signs of ischaemia during coronary occlusion. Right to the pressure scale: Example of pressure/ECG tracings from a patient with low CFI and severe ECG signs of ischaemia during coronary occlusion. Pressures are taken at two different scales: 160 mmHg for the phasic and mean aortic (*black thick curves*) and phasic and mean coronary (*red curves*) pressure, and 40 mmHg for phasic and mean central venous pressure (*black thin curves*). On the left side of each tracing, pressures and ECG are recorded before coronary occlusion; on the right side during occlusion. The distal coronary pressure (*red curve*) declines much less in response to the occlusion in the patient with high CFI as compared to that with low CFI. $CFI = (P_{occl}-CVP)/(P_{ao}-CVP)$; P_{occl} = coronary occlusive or wedge pressure; P_{ao} = aortic pressure; CVP = central venous pressure

statistical artefact or whether they are reflecting a biological phenomenon. The subsequent chapter is focusing on the biological phenomenon of a widely varying functional coronary collateral response to hyperaemia, which preferentially occurs in the presence of well-developed collaterals.

4.3   Vascular Resistance Distribution and the Collateral Network

Anastomoses between adjacent vascular territories together with spatially varying microvascular resistances to flow are the basis for pathophysiological aspects of collaterals, such as coronary steal, the decrease in collateral flow following recanalization of a chronic total occlusion and the enhanced risk of coronary restenosis after coronary intervention in the presence of high and competitive collateral flow to this area.

Coronary steal is defined as a decrease in coronary flow during hyperaemia as compared to the flow to a certain myocardial region at rest. Steal is hyperaemic redistribution of blood away from a territory in need due to unbalanced regional microvascular resistances. The uneven resistance distribution relates to the co-existence at rest of post-stenotic exhausted and normally functioning resistances. Well-functioning collaterals may contribute to precipitation of myocardial ischaemia due to their facilitating coronary steal. The prevalence of coronary steal in patients with non-occlusive CAD examined invasively is approximately 10%, whereas that in patients with chronic total occlusion is one-third to one-half. The unequivocal conditions for coronary steal are the presence of a severely ischaemic, viable myocardial region, which is well collateralized.

The most likely explanation for the decrease in collateral function following recanalization of chronic occlusion relates to 'redistribution' of blood due to altering *macrovascular* resistances, i.e. a heightened perfusion pressure at the orifice of the collaterals into the recanalized artery. Generally, functional collateral support declines following coronary intervention of an atherosclerotic lesion but does not regress completely.

Evidence in favour of high functional collateral flow being a risk factor for restenosis following balloon angioplasty as well as bare-metal stenting has not remained undisputed.

4.3.1   Introduction

Functional, haemodynamic or biophysical aspects of collateral vessels relate to the fact that they constitute a network within the coronary circulation (Fig. 4.21). Such connections between adjacent vascular territories together with spatially varying microvascular resistances to flow are the basis for pathophysiological aspects of collaterals rarely considered, such as the redistribution of blood during vasodilation away from a region in need, i.e. coronary steal,[47,48] the decrease in collateral flow following recanalization of a chronic total

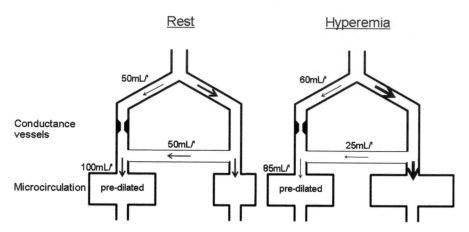

Fig. 4.21 Schematic drawing of a two-branch coronary circulation at rest (*left panel*) and during hyperaemia (*right panel*) with a stenotic and a non-stenotic vessel, both connected via a collateral vessel. The microcirculation is indicated by two rectangles. The red arrows show the direction and give an estimate of the amount of flow. The post-stenotic flow rate values during hyperaemia versus those at rest exemplify coronary steal with a coronary flow reserve of 0.85

occlusion[49] and the enhanced risk of coronary restenosis after PCI in the presence of high and competitive collateral flow to this area.[50] These manifestations of interacting myocardial or epicardial coronary resistances as mediated predominantly by well-developed collaterals are apparently all related to negative aspects of the collateral circulation. In part, they can explain the unpredictable functional response of collateral flow to hyperaemia as described in the previous chapter. Since the subgroup of patients with CAD having a CTO has, on average, systematically better-developed collaterals compared to a group of individuals with non-occlusive CAD, the former is a methodologically favourable 'model' for studying regional vascular resistance interactions.

4.3.2 Redistribution of Blood due to Altering Microvascular Resistances

4.3.2.1 Biophysical Mechanisms

In the normal heart, e.g. *exercise* -induced increase in myocardial contractile function is associated with heightened metabolic demands, and they are met, to a very small extent, by augmented oxygen extraction and predominantly by an increase in myocardial blood flow.[51] Within physiological ranges of systemic blood pressure, myocardial blood flow is regulated by altering coronary microvascular resistance (autoregulation[51,52]). This autoregulation of coronary blood flow occurs in a spatially orchestrated way in the normal coronary circulation, but in an uncoordinated fashion among patients with CAD. The functional disorder in the presence of ≥1 coronary epicardial stenotic lesions consists of an uneven distribution of microvascular resistances between different coronary territories. From Fig. 4.21, it becomes intuitively evident that an altered, hyperaemia-induced balance of microvascular resistances between two adjacent myocardial regions has an influence on regional blood flow even in the case, if the resistance to flow in one territory remains constant. Such a redistribution of flow may become effective via coronary arterial bifurcations, but more importantly in the presence of sizeable intercoronary anastomoses. Since the territorial unbalance of microvascular resistances may be any continuous number and not just take on discrete 'jumps', the consequences on regional myocardial flow are fluent ranging from an almost undetectable impairment in the capacity to augment flow during hyperaemia to an actual change in flow direction away from a certain territory to an adjacent one ('real steal'). Figure 4.21 does not depict a situation of 'real steal' during hyperaemia, but one of a flow deficit as compared to baseline to the area downstream of a coronary obstruction, i.e. coronary flow or myocardial perfusion reserve <1, which is the conventional definition of coronary steal (Figs. 4.22 and 4.23).

Specifically, the mechanism leading to an uneven flow distribution during increased myocardial demand can be described as follows: In the presence of a flow limiting coronary artery stenosis, perfusion into the ischaemic terminal vascular bed is the sum of epicardial arterial inflow through the stenosis and collateral inflow from adjacent non- or less-ischaemic areas (Fig. 4.24).[53] Collateral inflow depends on the pressure gradient between the origin of collaterals in the haemodynamically normal donor artery and their orifice into the ischaemic recipient artery (driving pressure $\Delta P = P1-P2$). In case the microvascular dilator capacity of the ischaemic collateral receiving vessel is exhausted and

Upstream of stenosis   **Downstream of stenosis**

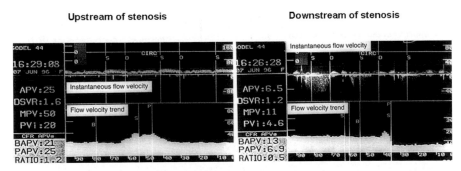

Fig. 4.22 Intracoronary Doppler guidewire–obtained documentation of coronary steal, i.e. coronary flow velocity reserve (CFVR) <1. Both panels show instantaneous flow velocity spectra (*top*) at the time indicated in upper left column and flow velocity trends over 90 s (*bottom*). Adenosine-induced CFVR measurements (18 and 12 μg intracoronary bolus for left and right coronary arteries respectively) are shown proximal (*left panel*; CFVR = 1.2) and distal (*right panel*; CFVR = 0.5) to an left circumflex coronary artery stenotic lesion to be dilated. APV indicates average peak flow velocity (cm/s, i.e. maximum flow velocity during a cardiac cycle averaged over three cardiac cycles); B, baseline flow velocity (cm/s) at rest; S, search mode for peak flow velocity and P, peak flow velocity during hyperaemia

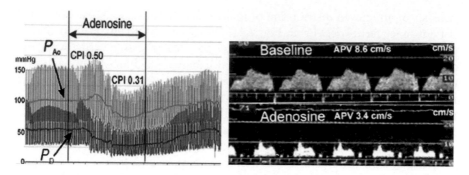

Fig. 4.23 Intravenous adenosine-induced coronary collateral steal in a patient with chronic total occlusion of the left anterior descending coronary artery as documented by pressure (*left panel*) and by Doppler flow velocity measurements (*right panel*). Collateral pressure index (CPI identical to pressure-derived collateral flow index $=[P_d-CVP]/[P_{ao}-CVP]$; see also Fig. 4.20). Distal coronary occlusive pressure (in chronic occlusion, P_d is identical to P_{occl}) as well as aortic pressure (P_{ao}) drop during adenosine infusion. Intracoronary Doppler flow velocity measurement obtained distal to the occlusion also shows a decrease in flow velocity during adenosine

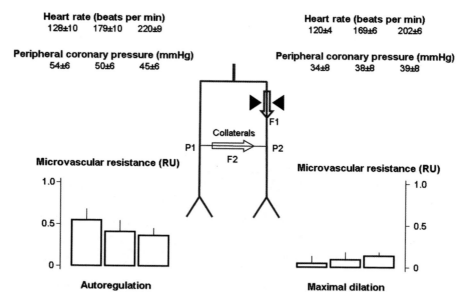

Fig. 4.24 Scheme of coronary steal via collaterals (*left*; 'horizontal' steal) and at the transmural level (*right*; 'vertical' steal). P1 is the pressure at the origin of collaterals, P2 the pressure at the orifice of collaterals into the ischaemic myocardial bed downstream of a coronary stenosis with the flow F1. Unilateral dilation of the normal microvascular bed decreases P1, and thus, the gradient between P1 and P2, and therefore also collateral flow F2. Increased heart rate decreases microvascular resistance and pressure at the origin of collaterals in normal myocardium (*left*), but increases microvascular resistance and pressure at the orifice of collaterals in post-stenotic myocardium (*right*). The driving pressure for collateral flow (P1–P2) is reduced[53]

flow is, therefore, pressure-dependent, any dilation, i.e. resistance decrease of the non-ischaemic collateral supplying terminal vascular bed during enhanced metabolic demand or in response to dilator agents reduces the pressure gradient across the collaterals, and hence, collateral flow. As soon as the net flow to the area of interest during hyperaemia is less than the flow at rest, the phenomenon of redistribution of blood away from the ischaemic region in need is called coronary steal.[54] A similar situation occurs with respect to the transmural distribution of myocardial blood flow when the subendocardial autoregulatory reserve or capacity is exhausted but the subepicardial reserve is maintained. The dilation of subepicardial vessels during hyperaemia does then impair subendocardial blood flow, a phenomenon called vertical or transmural steal (as opposed to the above-described 'horizontal' steal). Transmural steal can be regarded as the major cause of the *first* manifestation of myocardial ischaemia and infarction preferentially at the subendocardial region. That the subendo-cardial vasodilator capacity is exhausted before the subepicardial reserve is likely related to extracoronary physical determinants of coronary flow see Chapter 4, i.e. increased wall stress close as compared to farther away from the LV cavity. A well-developed collateral circulation salvages myocardium in case of a coronary occlusion,[23] but functioning collaterals may contribute to precipitation of myocardial ischaemia due to their facilitating coronary steal. Since in about two-thirds of the patients with CAD, the collateral circulation is rather poorly developed with collateral relative to normal antegrade flow values less than ¼, the clinical relevance of coronary steal in patients without coronary occlusion is probably not that important. The effects of tachycardia on the mechanisms leading to redistribution of coronary flow or even to coronary steal have to be considered in particular. Obviously, tachycardia increases myo-cardial oxygen demand per time and, via a contractile force-frequency effect, also due to an augmented myocardial inotropic state. In the normal coronary circula-tion, microvascular dilation serves to augment coronary blood flow to match the increased oxygen demand. Acceleration of heart rate also shortens diastolic duration and thus the period in the cardiac cycle, when almost all the coronary blood flow takes place. In the intact coronary circulation, metabolic vasodilation is strong enough to overcome the abridged coronary blood flow resulting from reduced diastolic duration. In the presence of a severe coronary stenosis, when the autoregulatory capacity of the area distal to the stenosis is exhausted in order to maintain resting perfusion, tachycardia with its reduction in diastolic duration compromises blood flow, so that it is reduced at higher heart rates. In terms of regional microvascular resistances, an uneven distribution takes place during increasing heart rates favouring the occurrence of coronary steal (Fig. 4.24). In the vascular area supplied by a normal coronary artery, microvascular resistance decreases with heart rate acceleration due to metabolic vasodilation, whereas in the region downstream of the stenotic artery, developing ischaemia due to the stenosis and to the shortened diastolic perfusion leads to worsened ischaemia with increasing transmural tension and, consequently, heightened microvascular resistance (Fig. 4.24).

4.3.2.2 Evidence for the Occurrence of Coronary Steal

The phenomenon of coronary steal has been recognized for more than 40 years.[54,55] Fam and McGregor studied the effects of nitroglycerin and dipyridamole on the coronary collateral flow in 12 dogs with chronic myocardial ischaemia of the left circumflex coronary artery (LCX).[55] Both nitroglycerin and dipyridamole caused a reduction in systemic blood pressure, but only dipyridamole was related to a decrease in retrograde collateral flow. Subsequently, coronary steal has been studied experimentally,[35,56,57] suspected clinically,[58,59] modelled theoretically[60] and demonstrated by PET[61] as well as invasively.[47,48,62–65] Thus, the occurrence of steal under certain coronary structural and haemodynamic conditions is unequivocally acknowledged. However, its prevalence and, thus, the clinical relevance have been reported variably, and even more so, the necessary conditions have been controversial. Data from the literature, on the pro-ischaemic effect of the calcium antagonist nifedipine due to suspected coronary steal, may serve to estimate the prevalence of this phenomenon. An increased nifedipine-induced exertional ECG ST segment depression or worsening of anginal symptoms was detected by Loos and Kaltenbach in 20%,[66] Stone et al. in 14%[67] and by Schulz et al. in 10–20% of their patients.[59] Of 1,100 cardiac positron emission studies in patients with collateralized, occluded vascular territories, 75 (7%) revealed coronary steal.[68] The prevalence of coronary steal among 100 patients with non-occlusive CAD examined invasively at our laboratory was 10%,[48] whereas that in a recent investigation by Werner et al. was 46% (26 of 56 patients with chronic total occlusion).[64] In a much smaller study using [13]ammonia PET, coronary steal was observed in 8 of 18 patients with multivessel CAD (chronic total occlusions in 10 cases), whereby myocardial perfusion in the collateralized region decreased from 90 ± 18 ml/min/100 g at rest to 68 ± 27 ml/min/100 g during hyperaemia induced by dipyridamole.[69] The functional reserve of collaterals supplying long-term CTO in 62 patients without prior myocardial infarction was studied by Werner et al. using intravenous adenosine for hyperaemia induction.[70] Figure 4.25

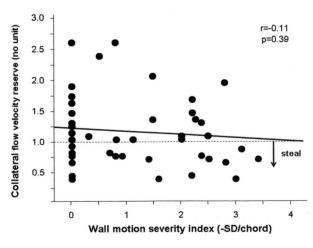

Fig. 4.25 Scatterplot of coronary collateral flow velocity reserve (*vertical axis*) obtained in 62 patients with chronic total occlusion and left ventricular wall motion severity index (*horizontal axis*). Normal wall motion severity index (WMSI) is defined as >−1 standard deviation (SD) change/chord[119]

illustrates that the collateral flow velocity reserve was not related to LV wall motion abnormalities, flow reserve values as high as 2.6 were reached (with 7% >2.0) and coronary steal occurred in one-third of the patients.[70]

Clinically, coronary steal as manifested by chest pain and ECG ST segment depression predominantly during adenosine or dipyridamole stress testing is a sign of severe CAD with viable myocardium in the ischaemic region, and it is a sign for well-developed coronary collaterals.[71] Pathophysiologically, the occurrence of coronary steal via collaterals draws attention to the dynamic nature of the collateral circulation and to the issue that the large variability of responses to different vasodilator stimuli (see also below) is due, in part, to the interaction of resistances to coronary flow beyond that of the occluded or severely stenotic bed alone.

4.3.2.3   Conditions for Coronary Steal

Recently, it has been stated by Kern[72] that 'there are three critical conditions needed for coronary steal in man as previously postulated by Gould et al.,[68] Schaper et al.[35] and Becker,[56] namely, that: (1) the epicardial donor artery resistance is high (with low post-stenotic pressure proximal to the collateral origin during hyperaemia); (2) the collateral pathway resistance is not negligible and (3) the microvasculature distal to the total occlusion is maximally dilated, with exhaustion of vasodilatory reserve, thus producing a shift of flow away from the collateral bed with the potential for inducible ischaemia' Close scrutiny of the investigations cited by Kern and older works as well as more recent work on coronary steal indicates the following: (a) The three 'candidate'. conditions for coronary steal are a stenosis in the contralateral (collateral supplying or donor) artery, anastomoses between the less and the more severely stenotic artery and a very severely stenotic or occluded collateral recipient or ipsilateral artery; (b) the sequence of the conditions cited is inversely related to their importance; and (c) the definition of steal as given by Kern ('a shift of flow away from the collateral bed'[72]) is erroneous. Coronary steal is defined as a fall in coronary perfusion of collateralized myocardium after arteriolar vasodilation.[71] Theoretically, 'a shift of flow away from the collateral bed' may be part of the conventional definition, but practically, a change in the vector of flow has not been documented in coronary steal so far. Thus, the term 'steal' does not indicate that blood is 'stolen' from the collateralized bed by backward flow ('real steal') through collateral channels. It merely reflects a fall in collateral flow during hyperaemia below resting conditions.[71]

The condition for coronary steal most intensely debated is the mandatory presence of a coronary artery stenotic lesion proximal to the origin of the collateral vessels in the contralateral artery. Schaper et al. investigated coronary steal in seven dogs that underwent an ameroid constriction of the LCX with the other arteries left intact.[35] The average myocardial perfusion reserve in the collateralized region was 1.70 and in the normal LAD area it was 2.54 (hyperaemia induced by lidoflazine), without information on the individual values. A mathematical model on the basis of a Wheatstone bridge showed the largest degree of uneven coronary flow distribution between the normal and the collateralized myocardial areas being present in case of the collaterals behaving as rigid tubes (Fig. 4.26).[35] Thus, the study by Schaper et al. did not examine the influence on steal of a contralateral stenosis.[35] Yet, they found that in the presence of a collateralized viable myocardial bed and in response to a vasodilator drug, the regional imbalance of normal and collateral flow increased with decreasing collateral vasodilator capacity. On the other hand, Becker

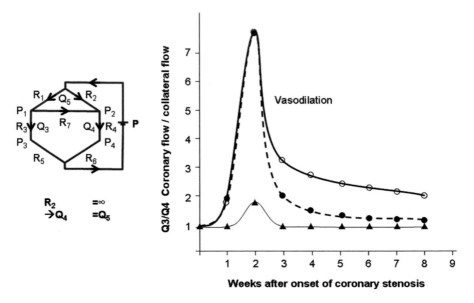

Fig. 4.26 Wheatstone-bridge electrical analogue modelling (*left scheme*) of the degree of imbalance between coronary and coronary collateral flow (*right scheme; vertical axis*) as a function of time (*horizontal axis*). In this model, the resistance of the left circumflex coronary artery (LCX; R2) increases progressively over a period of 3 weeks to a value approaching infinity so as to simulate stenosis development to chronic total occlusion. Simultaneously with increase in R2, collateral resistance (R7) decreases as a function of time due to collateral growth (arteriogenesis). Once every week after the onset of LCX stenosis, hyperaemia is induced, i.e. R3 and R4 are lowered to their minimal possible value. Solid squares: Degree of imbalance between coronary and collateral flow in the absence of hyperaemia (baseline or resting flow). During the period of increasing stenosis severity and collateral growth, there is unequal flow to the normal versus the post-stenotic, collateralized region even at rest. The degree of separation between the hyperaemic curves (*circles*) and the baseline curve (*squares*) gives an estimate of collateral steal. Collateral steal is greater in case of the collaterals behaving as rigid tubes during hyperaemia (R4 constant; *open circles*) as compared to the situation when they dilate to the same extent as other resistance vessels (R2 and R3; *solid circles*). Note that in this model there is no stenosis in the collateral supplying artery, the left anterior descending coronary artery (LAD), and during collateral growth, steal may develop even at rest. Abbreviations: R1 = resistance of the LAD; R2 = resistance of the LCX; R3 and R4 = arteriolar resistances; R5 and R6 = capillary resistances; R7 = collateral resistance; P_{ao} = aortic pressure; P1 = pressure at the origin of collaterals; P2 = pressure at the orifice of collaterals; Q = coronary flow over respective resistances[35]

exclusively focused on the experimental model with a contralateral stenosis (n = 26 dogs, no control group without a stenosis in the collateral supplying artery).[56] Thus strictly speaking, the conclusion could not be drawn that a stenosis of the artery supplying the collaterals to the occluded region is a necessary condition for coronary steal. Patterson and Kirk demonstrated in dogs with an occluded LAD collateralized by the LCX that increments of vascular resistance proximal to the origin of the collaterals caused an increase in the magnitude of steal.[57] However, a certain degree of steal could be observed even in the absence of a stenotic lesion upstream in the contralateral artery. In their analysis of a general network model simulating the collateralized coronary circulation similar to the model by Schaper et al., [35] Demer et al. predicted the occurrence of steal in case that collaterals originating from the LCX (with a 60% proximal cross-sectional area stenosis) to an occluded LAD conducted >1% of blood relative to normal maximal conductance (equal to a CFI value of 0.01).[61] Assuming a much higher collateral conductance sufficient to provide normal resting perfusion of the LAD territory, i.e. 20%, steal was predicted to take place already in the presence of a much less severe contralateral proximal stenosis (cross-sectional area reduction $\geq$20%).[61] In a study performed by our laboratory,[48] 100 patients with a coronary artery stenosis to be dilated were examined with intracoronary Doppler guidewires. Intracoronary adenosine-induced coronary flow velocity reserve <1 obtained distal to the stenosis was defined as steal. Coronary steal occurred in 10 of 100 patients (Fig. 4.27).

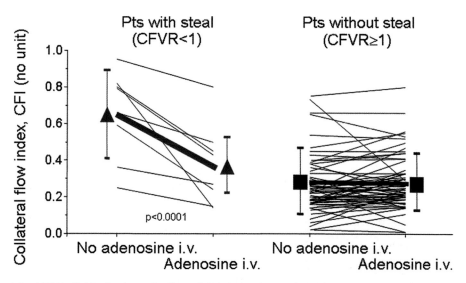

Fig. 4.27 Individual values of collateral flow index (*vertical axis*) in 100 patients with CAD at rest and during intravenous adenosine at 140 mg/kg/min according to the presence or absence of intracoronary Doppler-derived coronary flow velocity reserve of <1 (steal) in the collateral receiving, non-occluded artery (*horizontal axis*). Symbols and error lines: mean $\pm$ standard deviation

Patients with steal showed superior collaterals compared with those without steal: CFI was equal to 0.65 ± 0.24 in patients with steal vs. 0.29 ± 0.18 in those without steal ($p = 0.0001$). In all patients with steal, there was a reduction in collateral flow during intravenous adenosine-induced hyperaemia, whereas in the majority (70%) of patients without steal, collateral flow increased or remained unchanged during hyperaemia.[48] Coronary steal was observed in both situations with and without stenoses in the contralateral vessel. It was more prevalent with increasing CFI (Fig. 4.28). In a more elaborated investigation by our group,[65] the influence of hyperaemic ipsilateral, collateral and contralateral vascular resistance changes on the coronary flow velocity reserve of the collateral receiving (i.e. ipsilateral) artery was examined, thus testing the validity of a model describing the development of coronary steal. During stenosis occlusion, simultaneous intracoronary distal ipsilateral flow velocity and pressure using a pressure guidewire as well as contralateral flow velocity measurements via a third intracoronary wire were performed before and during intravenous adenosine (Fig. 4.29). These measurements plus the recording of mean aortic pressure provided the basis for calculating regional coronary resistances. In the group with high collateral flow, the flow reserve of the collateral receiving artery was directly and inversely associated with the collateral resistance and the contralateral resistance, respectively. It was concluded that the coronary flow velocity reserve of a collateralized region could be more dependent on hyperaemic vascular resistance changes of the collateral and collateral supplying area than on the ipsilateral stenosis severity, and could even fall below 1.[65] Werner et al. studied the determinants of coronary steal in CTO of 56 patients who underwent recanalization of the lesion.[64] It was documented that coronary steal in man not only occurred preferentially in the context of a haemodynamically significant donor artery lesion, but could also

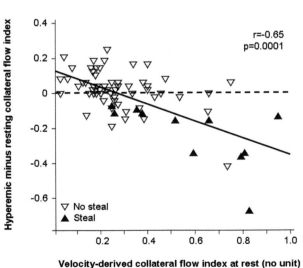

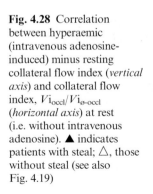

Fig. 4.28 Correlation between hyperaemic (intravenous adenosine-induced) minus resting collateral flow index (*vertical axis*) and collateral flow index, $Vi_{occl}/Vi_{\varnothing\text{-}occl}$ (*horizontal axis*) at rest (i.e. without intravenous adenosine). ▲ indicates patients with steal; △, those without steal (see also Fig. 4.19)

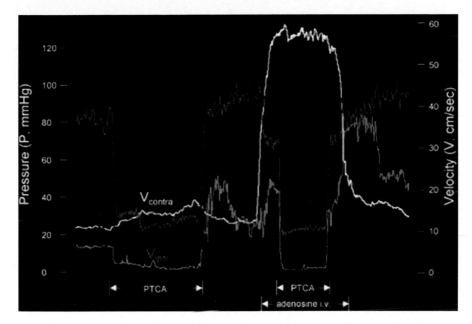

Fig. 4.29 Tracing of temporally recorded, simultaneous intracoronary (i.c.) pressure and velocity measurements in the collateral-receiving, ipsilateral (suffix 'ipsi') and collateral-supplying, contralateral (suffix 'contra') coronary arteries before and during (suffix 'occl') two stenosis occlusions. *Pink line*: i.c. distal ipsilateral pressure; *red line*: mean aortic pressure obtained via the guiding catheter (P_{ao}); *blue line*: i.c. distal ipsilateral blood flow velocity; *white line*: i.c. contralateral blood flow velocity. The two stenosis occlusions (PTCA) were performed without and with intravenous adenosine (140 µg/kg/min). The scale for pressure is depicted on the left (*vertical axis*), the scale for velocity on the right hand side (*vertical axis*)[65]

be observed due to an impaired vasodilatory reserve of the microcirculation in the absence of a donor artery lesion.

Thus, the unequivocal conditions for coronary steal are first the presence of a severely ischaemic, viable myocardial region, which is, second, well collateralized.

4.3.3 'Redistribution' of Blood due to Altering Macrovascular Resistances

Coronary perfusion across an occlusion is 0 ml/min/g of myocardium, and the respective conductance is equal to 0 ml/min/mmHg (Fig. 4.30). Since flow conductance is the inverse of resistance, the macrovascular or epicardial coronary resistance in this particular situation is infinitely high. During the development of an epicardial coronary occlusion from a haemodynamically irrelevant atherosclerotic obstruction to the total occlusion, the rising resistance to antegrade coronary flow is progressively related to a perfusion pressure drop

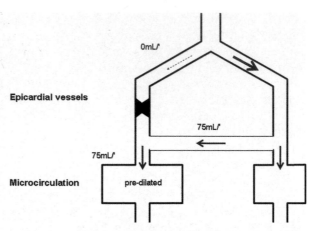

Fig. 4.30 Schematic drawing of a two-branch coronary circulation with a chronic total occlusion (*left*) and a non-stenotic vessel (*right*), both connected via a collateral vessel. The microcirculation is indicated by two rectangles. The red arrows show the direction and give an estimate of the amount of flow. The post-stenotic myocardial region is entirely collateralized

across the stenosis. Preformed intercoronary anastomoses are obviously also subjected to this pressure drop, respectively to the uneven distribution of *macrovascular* resistances between the collateral supplying and receiving arteries (Fig. 4.30). Assuming a situation with one-vessel CAD, it is the micro-vascular resistance governing flow in the collateral supplying artery, whereas in the collateral-dependent artery, it is the upstream occlusion, i.e. the macrovas-cular resistance with its pressure drop and the ensuing drop in collateral resistance determining flow (microvascular resistance minimal and constant due to the occlusion). In the pathogenesis of well-conducting coronary collat-eral arteries (arteriogenesis), the pressure drop across a total coronary occlusion or severe stenosis is considered *the* biophysical trigger initiating collateral growth via augmented fluid shear stress acting at the endothelial cell layer of preformed small collaterals.[7] In case of a sudden coronary occlusion, the preformed collateral vessels are not given the required time of several weeks to enlarge, and therefore, myocardial tissue is not salvaged. In a consecutive series of CTO, Werner et al. found that the process of lowering collateral vascular resistance to compensate for the perfusion pressure drop across the occlusion was obviously not fast enough to prevent transmural myocardial infarction in 70 of 208 patients (33%).[70] The issues just mentioned relate to pathogenesis of collateral vessels. However, the situation of the change of a very high to a negligible marcovascular resistance as it occurs routinely during PCI affects functional and thus physiological aspects of collaterals.

4.3.3.1 Recanalization of CTO

There have been anecdotal reports documenting a possible negative effect of recanalizing CTO on collateral flow.[73,74] In an uncontrolled study that included 18 patients, a reduction in myocardial perfusion in collateralized segments has been found after recanalization.[75] Collateral perfusion has been assessed using semi-quantitative intracoronary contrast echocardiography (visual score for video-density), an imprecise method for determining collateral flow. It has been speculated on the reason for a negative effect of recanalization on collateral flow: thrombotic material may be mobilized by the procedure to disturb the downstream circulation[73] or vasoactive substances may be released through the intervention to cause reduction of collateral flow.[73] However, the more likely explanation for the evident decrease in collateral function following recanalization of chronic occlusion relates to 'redistribution' of blood due to altering macrovascular resistances, i.e. a heightened, close to aortic perfusion pressure at the orifice of the collaterals into the recanalized artery. The study by Werner et al. provided evidence for the occurrence of immediate changes of collateral function after successful recanalization of CTO.[49] In 21 patients with chronic total occlusions, intracoronary Doppler recordings of basal collateral flow were obtained before the first balloon inflation. Angioplasty was performed with stent implantation in all lesions. At the end of the procedure, recruitable collateral flow was measured during a repeat balloon inflation. After recanalization, Doppler-derived CFI fell from 0.48 ± 0.25 to 0.21 ± 0.16 (p $<$ 0.001). There was no further change in CFI during the following 24 hours.[49] A similar study by Pohl et al. compared 27 patients with a chronic total occlusion (occlusion group) with 27 patients without occlusion (stenosis group) matched for age, sex and CFI at the first occlusion.[76] Following revascularization, i.e. during the second as compared to the first balloon occlusion, CFI decreased in 17 of the patients in the occlusion group (63%) and in eight of the patients in the stenosis group (30%) (Fig. 4.31).[76] Focusing on the intraindividual change of collateral function between the first and the second balloon occlusions (Fig. 4.32), a trend to collateral de-recruitment could be observed in patients who underwent recanalization of chronic total occlusion, while collateral recruitment occurred between the first and the second balloon occlusions among patients with non-occlusive CAD.[76] In the non-occlusive group, the very forceful hyperaemic stimulus of ischaemia and, even more so, repetitive ischaemia can be interpreted here as the cause for further lowering microvascular resistance in the terminal bed of the collateralized myocardial area. In

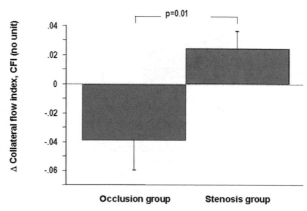

Fig. 4.31 Difference in collateral flow index ($\triangle$CFI) between the first and the second balloon occlusion. Unpaired comparison of $\triangle$CFI (value of collateral flow index at second balloon occlusion minus value at first balloon occlusion) with a significant difference between the occlusion group (n = 27) and the stenosis (n = 27) group (p = 0.01)

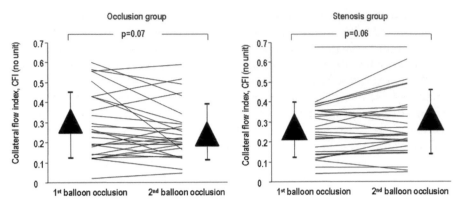

Fig. 4.32 Individual values with mean and standard deviation for collateral flow index (CFI; *vertical axis*) at the end of the first two vessel occlusions in patients with chronic total occlusions and in patients with coronary stenoses

contrast, the PCI induced lowering of the macrovascular resistance upstream of the collateral orifice in the occlusion group removed much if not all of the pressure gradient across the collateral path. In the situation of an acutely occluded coronary artery, unpublished data from our group indicate that between two immediately subsequent coronary balloon occlusions, collateral function becomes impaired following primary PCI in the absence ($n = 29$), but not in the presence ($n = 18$) of a distal coronary embolization protection device (Fig. 4.33). In the setting of acute thrombotic coronary occlusion, the above-mentioned mechanism of distal microembolization with increasing peripheral microvascular resistance and low flow may be more relevant for collateral function disturbance than in chronic occlusions.

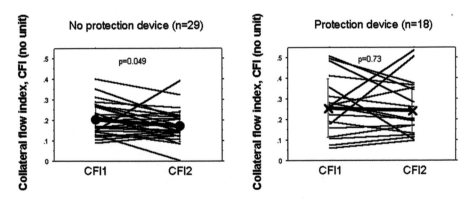

Fig. 4.33 Individual changes of collateral flow index between the first (CFI1) and the second coronary balloon occlusion (CFI2) following recanalization of the lesion responsible for the acute myocardial infarction in 47 patients. The changes are depicted for the group without (*left panel*) and for that with (*right panel*) distal embolization protection device. The blue symbols and error lines indicate mean values ± standard error

In the context of the finding by Werner et al. that 24 hours after recanalization, there was no further change of collateral function relative to the initial drop, the question on the long-term plasticity or functional recruitability of collaterals is virulent. Perera et al. focused on that problem by determining the baseline CFI and by reassessing it during transient balloon occlusion 5 minutes and 24 hours after PCI in the first 29 patients and at 6 months in the subsequent 25 patients.[77] Overall, CFI at baseline was 0.23±0.10, with no change 5 minutes and 1 day later (0.21±0.12 and 0.22±0.11). At 6 months, CFI was 0.14±0.07 or 63±27% of the baseline value (p < 0.001). The drop in collateral function following recanalization of a chronic total occlusion was more pronounced than after PCI of a non-occlusive coronary stenosis (Fig. 4.34).[77] Thus, functional collateral support declines following PCI of an atherosclerotic lesion but does not regress completely.

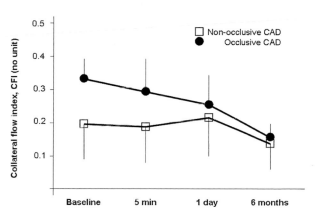

Fig. 4.34 Coronary collateral flow index (CFI, *vertical axis*) plasticity in patients with chronic total occlusions (CTO) and non-occlusive coronary artery disease. Patients with CTO have a higher collateral flow index at baseline and a steeper decline in CFI over time than patients with non-occlusive stenotic lesions. *Error lines*: standard deviation[77]

4.3.3.2 Revascularization of Stenotic Lesions

Assuming a case with very well-developed collateral arteries to a stenotic coronary artery, it is conceivable that this anastomosis poses a negligible resistance to flow in relation to the epicardial, macrovascular resistance of the stenosis upstream of the collateral orifice (see also Fig. 4.30). Furthermore, it may be plausible that following PCI of that stenosis with macrovascular resistance decrease to a negligible value, both the epicardial antegrade and the collateral resistance to flow differ only minimally, and that the antegrade and collateral perfusion pressure may compete with each other. Such a coronary pressure equilibrium may be dynamic and delicate depending on resting or hyperaemic flow conditions and on the occurrence of arterial recoil following PCI, the latter of which would turn the tip of the balance towards collateral perfusion pressure, impede antegrade coronary flow and, thus, create a risk for restenosis of the stenosis treated by PCI. With this background, Urban et al. hypothesized that an elevated coronary pressure as obtained during balloon occlusion, i.e. coronary wedge pressure, was a risk factor for restenosis following coronary angioplasty.[78] In 100 consecutive vessels (91 patients) for which coronary wedge pressure had been measured at the time of angioplasty, the angiographic results at 7±3 months follow-up were evaluated. The overall angiographic restenosis rate was 37%. It was 52% (25 of 48) in arteries with a coronary wedge pressure ≥30 mmHg and 23% (12 of 52) in arteries with a coronary wedge pressure <30 mmHg (p < 0.01).[78] It was concluded that a high collateral perfusion pressure above 30 mmHg indicated a negative influence of competitive collateral flow on long-term results after balloon angioplasty. In an investigation with invasive assessment of collateral relative to normal antegrade coronary flow (CFI), among 64 patients with angiographic follow-up at least 2 months after an initial balloon angioplasty, Wahl et al. found that patients with restenosis (>50% diameter stenosis, n = 34) had a significantly higher CFI at the initial coronary angiography than patients without restenosis (0.26±0.14 vs. 0.12±0.09).[50] In the same context, the aim of Jansen et al. was to assess the influence of recruitable collateral blood flow on restenosis in patients who underwent PCI with bare-metal stents and using optimal antithrombotic treatment.[79] Compared to patients with poorly developed collaterals (CFI < 0.25), patients with well-developed collaterals had a higher binary restenosis rate (54.2% vs. 19.4, p = 0.003). The described evidence in favour of high functional collateral flow being a risk factor for restenosis following balloon angioplasty as well as bare-metal stenting has not remained undisputed.[80] Using quantitative coronary angiography as well as intravascular ultrasound for the assessment of stenotic lesions 6 months after stenting, Perera et al. observed similar restenosis rates in poor (n = 33) and good (n = 25) collateral groups (35% vs. 43%, p = 0.76 for diameter restenosis, 27% vs. 45%, p = 0.34 for area restenosis and 23% vs. 24%, p = 0.84 for volumetric restenosis; Fig. 4.35 depicting the extent of restenosis).[80]

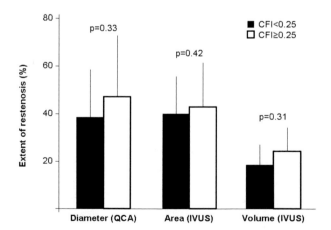

Fig. 4.35 Bar graph of the extent of restenosis (*vertical axis*) 6 months following percutaneous coronary intervention in 58 patients with CAD according to the presence of well-developed (*white bars*, collateral flow index, CFI≥0.25) or poorly developed (CFI < 0.25) collaterals (*horizontal axis*). Extent of restenosis was assessed using quantitative coronary angiography (QCA) or intravascular ultrasound (IVUS)[80]

4.4 Stimuli for Lowering Coronary Collateral Resistance

In humans, stimulation of peripheral cold receptors have been shown to strongly activate the sympathetic nervous system and also to increase coronary collateral function in the absence of beta-blocker treatment (flow reserve of ~1.2).

In the setting of human coronary collateral function assessment, the following pharmacological substances have been employed: ergonovine, isoproterenol, dipyridamole, adenosine and nitroglycerin. The clinical relevance of vasopressin and ergonovine as collateral vasoconstricting agents is questionable as opposed to that of the ubiquitously used beta-blockers, which appear to impede collateral function. On average, the capacity to increase collateral flow acutely in response to the mentioned substances in humans is better in well than poorly developed collaterals, and it amounts to a factor of 1.4.

In the past, the peak hyperaemic response after a brief coronary artery occlusion was thought to be indicative for maximum dilatory capacity. This notion has been challenged by demonstrating that coronary pharmacological vasodilator reserve was larger than that observed at the peak of reactive hyperaemia. Assuming a uniform occlusion time, the degree of ischaemia is not identical between individuals. The level of myocardial ischaemia is equal to the product of occlusion time, the inverse of collateral flow, the ischaemic bed size, the absence of preconditioning and oxygen consumption during occlusion. Repetitive arterial occlusions have a less-pronounced effect on ischaemia than a single occlusion, because of the combined result of ischaemic preconditioning and collateral recruitment, the latter of which is a feature of coronary collateral vasomotor function.

4.4.1 Introduction

As outlined above in this section on the pathophysiology of the human coronary collateral circulation, altering tangential fluid shear stress plays an important role as stimulus for coronary collateral vasomotion. The purpose of this chapter is to discuss stimuli of collateral vasomotion other than those involved in fluid shear stress-mediated collateral function changes. However, and in particular, adenosine's role as pharmacological instead of fluid shear stress mediating stimulus and of the physiological stimulus of dynamic isometric exercise (bicycle exercise) will be reviewed here again from another perspective.

4.4.2 Neurohumoral and Pharmacological Stimuli

From the previous chapter on the distribution of vascular resistances between adjacent myocardial areas, it has become evident that collateral perfusion must traverse not just collateral vessels but also vessels up- and downstream of them. This sequence of resistances results in a unique situation, in which regulation of collateral blood flow is subject to control mechanisms not present in normally perfused myocardium. In order to discriminate between alterations in true collateral vascular tone and in the vasomotor tone of up- or downstream resistances, special experimental preparations suitable only in the animal model have to be used. Specifically and in the context of studies focusing on neurohumoral or pharmacological stimuli of collateral function, heart rate, LV diastolic pressure and contraction ought to be held constant, because these variables are known to influence collateral flow.[81–84]

4.4.2.1 Neurohumoral Stimuli

Histologically, one aspect of coronary collateral development is the formation of a medial layer.[25] This newly grown vascular smooth muscle provides a substrate for collateral vasomotion, and the regulation of collateral blood flow by neurohumoral influences. However by 6 months following epicardial coronary artery ligation with collateral development, mature canine collateral arteries appear quite similar to epicardial vessels of equivalent size, except for the fact that the internal elastic lamina is not continuous and adrenergic nerves are sparse.[85] To determine if mature coronary collateral vascular smooth muscle contains functioning α-adrenergic receptors, Harrison et al. studied 13 dogs, 6–10 months after circumflex ameroid occlusion.[86] Regional myocardial blood flow was measured with radioactive microspheres in a blood-perfused heart preparation at constant aortic pressure (80 mmHg). Normal zone and transcollateral resistance to flow were calculated. Flow and resistance were measured during adenosine vasodilation before and during graded doses of a constant infusion of the α-adrenergic agonist methoxamine (α1 selective agonist; n = 6) or the α2-adrenergic agonist clonidine (n = 7). In the hearts that received methoxamine, normal zone resistance increased during infusion of 10^{-5} M methoxamine (Fig. 4.36). In contrast, transcollateral resistance did not change during methoxamine infusion. In the hearts that received clonidine, normal zone resistance increased with the highest dose of clonidine administered (Fig. 4.37). Transcollateral resistance averaged 0.17±0.03 resistance units during control conditions and did not change with clonidine infusion.[86] In separate studies, Harrison et al. examined isometric tension development in organ baths by the LAD and coronary collateral vessels.[86] The LAD demonstrated dose-dependent constriction to phenylephrine (peak response 22±5% of the response to 100 mM KCl). Clonidine produced weak constrictor responses in the LAD (5±2.5% maximal KCl response). In contrast, neither phenylephrine nor clonidine produced responses in mature collaterals (Fig. 4.37). The experiments performed by Harrison et al. on intact hearts and *isolated* vascular rings demonstrated that mature coronary collaterals do not contain functioning α-adrenergic receptors.[86] Studies of collateral perfusion in

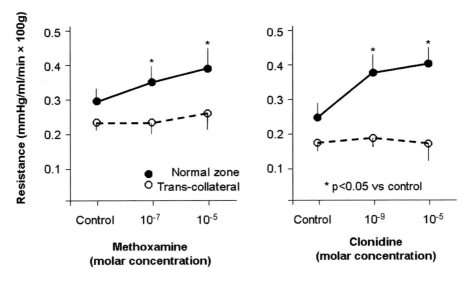

Fig. 4.36 Normal myocardial zone (*closed symbols*) and trans-collateral (*open symbols*) resistance (*vertical axes*) in response to different dosages of methoxamine and clonidine. Studies performed in isolated, blood-perfused dog hearts with well-developed collaterals. Symbols and error lines: mean ± standard error[86]

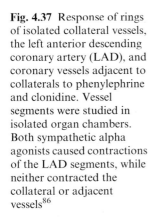

Fig. 4.37 Response of rings of isolated collateral vessels, the left anterior descending coronary artery (LAD), and coronary vessels adjacent to collaterals to phenylephrine and clonidine. Vessel segments were studied in isolated organ chambers. Both sympathetic alpha agonists caused contractions of the LAD segments, while neither contracted the collateral or adjacent vessels[86]

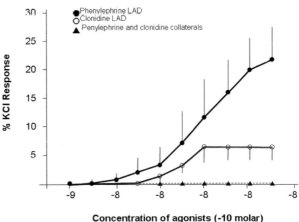

the *intact* animal (dog; 4–16 weeks after collateral growth stimulation by LAD embolization) were performed by Bache et al., whereby they examined the effect of nerve stimulation, the α1 adrenergic agonist phenyephrine, an α2 agonist BHT933 and ergonovine (serotonergic and α-adrenergic agonist) with respect to both retrograde collateral flow and microsphere-derived collateral perfusion.[87] Neither nerve stimulation nor phenylephrine altered collateral perfusion, but BHT933 and ergonivine decreased measures of collateral flow.[87] In these studies, neither norepinephrine nor direct nerve stimulation altered collateral resistance or flow, even in the presence of β-blockade.

For methodological reasons, similar studies in humans are very sparse and practically impossible to perform. The human 'model' of CTO without myocardial infarction in the dependent region is one akin to the setting in the intact animal. Pupita et al. observed, in patients with stable CAD, a quite variable ischaemic threshold for the production of effort-related angina.[88] They hypothesized that this could be caused not only by changes in the calibre of coronary arteries at the site of stenosis, but also by the constriction of distal vessels, collateral vessels or both. In order to test the hypothesis, they studied 11 patients with stable angina, total occlusion of a single coronary artery that was supplied by collateral vessels, normal ventricular function, no evidence of coronary artery spasm and no other coronary stenoses.[88] The ischaemic threshold, as assessed by multiplying the heart rate by the systolic blood pressure at a 0.1 mV depression of the ECG ST segment during exercise testing, increased by 19% after the administration of nitroglycerin and decreased by 18% after ergonovine.[88] In three patients, delayed and reduced filling of collateral and collateralized vessels associated with depression of the ECG ST segment similar to that observed during ambulatory monitoring was detected on angiographic evaluation after the intracoronary administration of ergonovine.[88] The authors proposed that the constriction of distal coronary arteries, collateral vessels, or both may cause myocardial ischaemia in patients with chronic stable angina.

In contrast to α-adrenergic receptors, mature canine collateral vessels contain a population of β-adrenergic receptors very similar to that in other native coronary arteries.[89] Feldman et al. used an autoradiographic technique to detect β-adrenergic receptors on the vascular smooth muscle of histological specimens of well-developed canine coronary collateral vessels, neighbouring, similarly sized vessels and the LAD artery.[90] β-Adrenergic relaxation of native coronary vessels and collateral vessels was studied in isolated organ chambers after pre-constriction with prostaglandin F2 α. Both native coronary arteries and collateral segments demonstrated β-adrenergic-mediated relaxation with affinities for both agonists and antagonists compatible with a mixed population of β1- and β2-adrenergic receptors.[90] In humans, stimulation of peripheral cold receptors has been shown to strongly activate the sympathetic nervous system.[91] Therefore, Uren et al. investigated the vasomotor response (cold pressor/ basal flow) in myocardium perfused entirely by collaterals, using the reflex sympathetic stimulation of cold pressor stress.[92] Nine patients with an occluded coronary artery supplied entirely by collaterals from other angiographically normal arteries were studied using PET with ^{15}O water at rest and at cold pressor stress. In remote myocardium, basal and cold pressor flows were 0.99 ± 0.26 and 1.46 ± 0.60 ml/min/g, respectively, and a myocardial vasomotor response of 1.46 ± 0.45. In collateral-dependent myocardium, basal and cold pressor flows were 0.91 ± 0.20 and 0.87 ± 0.35 ml/min/g (Fig. 4.38), respectively

Fig. 4.38 Individual values of myocardial blood flow (*vertical axis*) as assessed by positron emission tomography in collateralized and normal myocardial regions at baseline and during cold pressor test (*horizontal axis*). Error lines: mean ± standard deviation

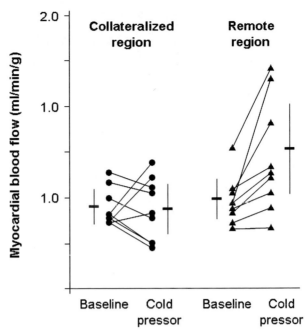

(the latter value, p < 0.05 vs. remote region), and a myocardial vasomotor response of 0.97±0.43).[92] The authors of that study concluded that in contrast to the vascular resistance decrease in remote myocardium with cold pressor, an increase was observed in collateral-dependent myocardium suggesting a vaso-constrictor response in resistive vessels without demonstrable myocardial ischaemia. In light of the above-cited experimental work, the results of the clinical study by Uren et al. may be interpreted as follows: collateral flow response to cold pressor showed an increase in three and a decrease in six patients, which may be related to either one or both the collateral and the downstream coronary microvascular resistance change. The animal studies with evidence of absence of α-adrenergic receptors in collateral vessels speak for peripheral vasoconstriction leading to a decrease in collateral flow. Our own study group examined 30 patients with chronic stable CAD exposed to two consecutive occlusive collateral flow measurements with or without randomly assigned preceding cold pressor test (3 minutes, the last 1 minute during coronary balloon occlusion).[93] During cold pressor test, collateral relative to normal antegrade flow was significantly higher at the beginning as well as at the end of the occlusion compared to identical instants without cold pressor test (Fig. 4.39). Cold pressor-induced coronary collateral flow reserve was 1.18. Focusing on the subgroup of patients on β-blocker treatment (n = 17), CFI did not change in response to cold pressor test.[93] The latter may be an argument in favour of β-adrenergic-mediated coronary collateral vasodilation.

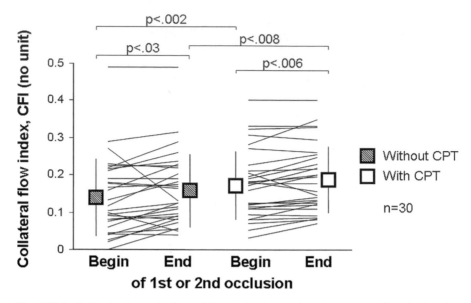

Fig. 4.39 Individual values of collateral flow index (*vertical axis*) as assessed invasively using coronary pressure measurements at the start and end of a 1-minute coronary occlusion without and with cold pressor test (CPT; *horizontal axis*). Symbols and error lines: mean ± standard deviation

4.4.2.2 Pharmacological Stimuli

As reviewed above and in the context of neurohumoral stimuli for collateral function response, the following substances have been studied in the experimental animal model: methoxamine ($\alpha 1$ agonist), clonidine ($\alpha 2$ agonist), phenyephrine (α agonist), ergonivine (α agonist and serotonergic agonist), prenalteral ($\beta 1$ agonist) and albuteral ($\beta 2$ agonist).[89] Also, chronically collateralized myocardium in dogs (n = 6) has been investigated with regard to the response of perfusion to vasopressin.[94] Peters et al. showed that at baseline, regional blood flow to the collateral-dependent myocardium and to the normally perfused myocardium was similar; however, during vasopressin infusion, collateral-dependent zone flow decreased by 49±14%, whereas normal zone flow decreased by only 9±9% (p < 0.0005, normal zone perfusion vs. collateral perfusion).[94] The contemporary clinical relevance of vasopressin and of ergonovine[88] as collateral vasoconstricting agents is questionable as opposed to that of the ubiquitously used β blockers, which appear to impede collateral function (see above; dynamic handgrip exercise, cold pressor test). Also based on experimental evidence in dogs, the activation of adenosine triphosphate (ATP)-sensitive K + channels appears involved in the coronary vascular response to decreases in perfusion pressure and ischaemia. In the beating heart of dogs, Lamping compared responses of non-collaterals less than 100 μm in diameter to collaterals of similar size using stroboscopic epi-illumination of the LV coupled to a microscope-video system.[95] Aprikalim, a selective activator of ATP-sensitive K+ channels (0.1–10 μM) produced similar dose-dependent dilation of non-collaterals and collaterals. Relaxation was decreased by inhibition of ATP-sensitive K+ channels with glibenclamide, but not by inhibition of nitric oxide synthase with nitro-l-arginine. Bradykinin (10–100 μM) produced similar dilation of non-collaterals and collaterals which was decreased by nitro-L-arginine but not by glibenclamide. Partly in contrast, Mees et al. showed, in mice deficient for endothelial nitric oxide synthase, that administration of a nitric oxide donor induced vasodilation in collateral vessels following chronic femoral artery ligation.[8] This study clearly demonstrated that endothelial nitric oxide synthase activity is crucial for nitric oxide-mediated vasodilation of peripheral collateral vessels but not for collateral artery growth. With regard to the clinical situation of an atherosclerotic patient with endothelial dysfunction and abrupt arterial occlusion, the mouse model deficient of endothelial nitric oxide synthase is relevant, because it highlights the importance of the acute vasodilatory reaction with its tissue salvaging effect. An intact collateral growth (arteriogenic) process which is time consuming is useless in the absence of an intact acute collateral dilatory response to sudden vascular occlusion.

In the setting of human coronary collateral function assessment, the following pharmacological substances have been employed aside from the above-mentioned ergonovine (Table 4.1): isoproterenol, dipyridamole, adenosine and nitroglycerin. Early attempts to measure myocardial blood flow before and after isoproterenol have shown only a small coronary flow reserve (flow during hyperaemia/flow at rest) in the distribution area of collateral vessels.[96] However, Knoebel et al. using [84]Rubidium as an indicator did not measure regional but only total myocardial blood flow (in ml/min) by the coincidence counting system.[96] Even more importantly, the study was not restricted to patients with chronic total occlusions and a downstream collateralized, viable myocardial region, but the entire range of CAD patients with non-occlusive and occlusive disease was included. Such a study design does not allow to differentiate between the contribution to hyperaemic flow of the diseased native coronary artery and the collateral vessel, thus measuring a fused or net coronary flow reserve between native and collateral vessels. Depending on the angiographic degree of collateral vessels (score 0–4), the myocardial blood flow reserve ranged between 1.05 and 1.4 (Table 4.1)[96]; in comparison, coronary flow reserve in individuals without CAD was 1.9±1.4, indicating that isoproterenol (β-adrenergic agonist) is not a substance for the induction of maximal hyperaemia. The methodological limitation just described is also inherent in the study by Demer et al. because among patients with angiographic coronary collaterals (n = 28), they studied both individuals with (n = 21) and without (n = 7) chronic total occlusions.[61] As a further limitation, half of the patients in the group with angiographic collaterals had previously suffered a myocardial infarction, the fact of which very likely impaired the vasodilatory capacity within the region of interest irrespective of the upstream collateral vasomotor function. In the study by Demer et al., regional myocardial activity of [82]Rubidium or ^{13}N-ammonia

Table 4.1 Pharmacological stimuli of human coronary collateral function

Author	Year	n	Substance	Method	Model	Coronary collateral flow reserve
Knoebel	1972	45	Isoproterenol	^{84}Rubidium	Non-occlusive and occlusive CAD	1.2 ± 1.2
Demer	1990	28	Dipyridamole	PET, ^{82}Rb or $^{13}NH_3$	Non-occlusive and occlusive CAD	1.1 ± 1.2
McFalls	1993	5	Dipyridamole	PET, $^{15}H_2O$	Chronic total occlusion	1.9 ± 1.0
Vanoverschelde	1993	11	Dipyridamole ammonia	PET, $^{13}NH_3$	Chronic total occlusion	2.2 ± 0.6
Sambuceti	1995	19	Dipyridamole ammonia	PET, $^{13}NH_3$	Chronic total occlusion	1.5 ± 1.0
Piek	1997	24*	Adenosine i.c.	Collateral flow velocity	Balloon occlusion	1.4 ± 1.0
Seiler	1999	21*	Adenosine i.v.	Collateral flow index	Balloon occlusion	1.2 ± 0.8
Billinger	2004	25	Adenosine i.v.	Collateral flow index	Balloon occlusion	1.1 ± 0.8
Werner	2006	62	Adenosine i.v.	Collateral flow index	Chronic total occlusion	1.1 ± 0.6
Total		240				1.4

Abbreviations: CAD = coronary artery disease; i.c. = intracoronary; i.v. = intravenous; NH3vN ammonia; PET = positron emission tomography; Rb = Rubidium.
Coronary flow reserve: flow during hyperaemia/flow at rest.
*Patients with angiographically well-developed collaterals.

was measured by PET at rest and with intravenous dipyridamole/handgrip stress in 28 patients with angiographic collaterals and in 25 control patients with similar CAD severity by angiography.[61] Regional myocardial activity decreased after dipyridamole, indicating coronary steal (i.e. coronary flow reserve <1), in 25 of 28 patients with angiographic collaterals and in only 4 of 25 control patients without angiographic collaterals. The range of coronary flow reserve to partially or entirely collateralized regions was 0.61–1.40 (including the three patients without steal; Table 4.1); remote region coronary flow reserve averaged 1.27.[61] Vanoverschelde et al. obtained much higher values of coronary flow reserve by ^{13}N-ammonia PET in patients with entirely collateralized and non-infarcted myocardium.[41] They averaged between 3.0±0.6 and 1.4±0.6 depending on whether the collateral artery was supplying a myocardial area without (n = 3) and with (n = 8) ventricular wall motion abnormalities, respectively (Table 4.1); the remote region coronary flow reserve was 3.1±1.0.[41] Microvascular function of entirely collateral dependent, non-infarcted myocardium was also investigated by Sambuceti et al. [97], whereby these authors employed the same technique as the previously described work. The coronary flow reserve in the collateralized region ranged between 0.75 and 3.05 and averaged 1.5 (<1 in 2 cases; Table 4.1); remote region coronary flow reserve = 2.2±1.0 (Fig. 4.40).[97] Aside from providing individual values of myocardial blood flow changes during hyperaemia versus resting conditions, Fig. 4.40 also illustrates that atrial pacing to a submaximal heart rate induces less myocardial

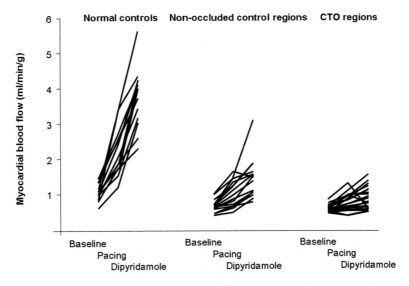

Fig. 4.40 Individual values of myocardial blood flow (*vertical axis*) as assessed by positron emission tomography in normal (*left*), post-stenotic, non-occluded (*middle*) and entirely collateralized myocardial regions (*right*; chronic total occlusions) at baseline, during atrial pacing and during dipyridamole infusion (*horizontal axis*)

hyperaemia than dipyridamole at an intravenous dose of 0.56 mg/kg. Piek et al. studied the responsiveness of the coronary collateral circulation to adenosine and nitroglycerin in humans using the angioplasty model of collateral assessment.[42] An index of collateral flow in the recipient coronary artery was determined with an angioplasty Doppler guidewire during balloon coronary occlusion and expressed as the diastolic blood flow velocity integral. Adenosine (12–18 µg) and nitroglycerin (0.2 mg) were injected as a bolus in the donor coronary artery during subsequent balloon inflations to assess their effect on these haemodynamic variables. In patients with spontaneously visible collateral vessels on angiography, the occlusive diastolic flow velocity integral increased from 8.0±4.5 to 10.8±8.0 cm after adenosine and from 7.4±4.5 to 10.3±6.9 cm after nitroglycerin (Table 4.1). The administration of adenosine or nitroglycerin in patients with collateral vessels recruitable in response to coronary occlusion (as opposed to spontaneously visible collaterals) did not induce a change in diastolic flow velocity integral.[42] Since in the study by Piek et al.,[42] coronary pressure distal to the balloon-occluded vessel was also obtained, an index for collateral as well as peripheral resistance to flow could be calculated, thus clarifying the open question in human investigations on collateral function, whether a change in flow is related to an alteration in peripheral or both collateral and peripheral vascular resistance. Collateral flow increase in response to adenosine and nitroglycerin was the result of both a reduction in the collateral vascular resistance and peripheral vascular resistance of the recipient coronary artery.[42] The principal drawback of that study is the route of administration of adenosine and nitroglycerin from the collateral supplying artery, which results in a systematically higher dose administered in the group with spontaneously visible collaterals as compared to that with low collateral flow (recruitable collaterals). In a group of patients with CAD and angiographically present collaterals from our laboratory, administration of intravenous adenosine during artificial coronary occlusion increased collateral relative to normal antegrade flow (pressure-derived CFI) by a factor of 1.2 (Table 4.1; see also Fig. 4.18).[43] However, patients with no angiographic collaterals (n = 29) manifested on average a decrease in hyperaemic versus resting CFI. A further investigation performed at our laboratory found that in 25 patients with CAD who underwent PCI, administration of metoprolol not only abolished a slight increase in CFI in response to intravenous adenosine (Table 4.1), but also resulted in a significant decrease in collateral function.[98] Werner et al. performed adenosine-induced hyperaemia in 62 patients with completely collateralized, viable myocardium, and measured the capacity to increase CFI versus resting conditions.[70] Among patients without regional LV wall motion abnormalities in the region of interest, coronary collateral flow reserve was 1.20±0.58, whereas in patients with impaired regional systolic LV function (n = 23) it was 1.06±0.49 (Table 4.1; see also Fig. 4.25).

4.4.3 Single and Repetitive Bouts of Myocardial Ischaemia

4.4.3.1 Ischaemia Induced Myocardial Hyperaemia

Reactive hyperaemia is the term used to describe the transient increase in flow rate above the control level which follows an interval of arterial occlusion. A brief arterial occlusion was stated to be the greatest stimulus known to cause coronary vasodilation, and the peak hyperaemic response after 15–30 seconds of coronary artery occlusion was thought to be indicative of maximum dilatory capacity.[46] Warltier et al. challenged this notion by demonstrating that total coronary pharmacological vasodilator reserve was larger than that observed at the peak of reactive hyperaemia.[99] For that purpose, responses of total coronary and regional myocardial blood flow to ischaemia- or drug-induced coronary artery vasodilation were studied in open-chest anaesthetized dogs (n = 24; coronary blood flow measured by radioactive microspheres). Systolic, diastolic and mean coronary blood flows after addition of chromonar (8 mg/kg intravenous), ATP (400 µm/min intracoronary), or adenosine (500 µm/min intracoronary) exceeded the respective flow at the peak of reactive hyperaemia (90 seconds occlusion period).[99] In each animal preparation, the reactive hyperaemic response to a 10-, 30-, 60-, 75-, 90- and 120-seconds occlusion period of the LCX was determined, and the same peak coronary flow responses were observed following a 75- or a 90-s occlusion (Fig. 4.41).[99] The fact of a constant

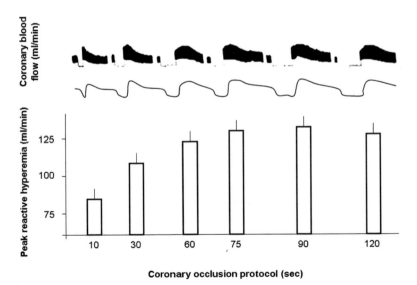

Fig. 4.41 Mean and phasic coronary blood flow tracings in a dog with coronary occlusions of different durations. Bars (*lower panel*) show the average ± standard error of peak reactive hyperaemic response in six dogs that underwent 10- 30-, 60-, 75-, 90- and 120-s coronary occlusions[99]

but individually variable increase in the reactive hyperaemic response with
occlusion periods extending from 10 to 75 seconds is important, because it
points to several methodological and biological issues related to coronary
occlusion as a stimulus for lowering microvascular resistance: the variable
'dose' of occlusion time applied in different studies, the variable effect of a
uniform occlusion time and the variable effect of repetitive as opposed to a
single bout of ischaemia.

In a recent study, VanTeeffelen et al. hypothesized that coronary reactive
hyperaemia is limited in comparison to hyperaemia in response to adenosine,
because of the presence of the glycocalyx lining the inner surface of the vascular
endothelium exerting its unrestricted effect on vascular resistance in reactive
hyperaemia but not in the presence of adenosine (Fig. 4.42).[100] In the cited
work, a coronary occlusion time of 15 seconds was employed, which was
methodologically flawed by a priori introducing a systematic disadvantage of
reactive hyperaemia versus the adenosine-induced degree of hyperaemia.

Assuming a uniform occlusion time of 75 seconds, the degree of ischaemia is
by no means identical between individuals, because occlusion time ≠ amount of
ischaemia. It has been known since the 1970s that the level of ischaemia as
determined by radioactive microspheres is equal to the product of occlusion
time, the inverse of collateral flow, the ischaemic bed size and myocardial
oxygen consumption during occlusion.[101,102] Later, the degree of myocardial
ischaemic preconditioning has been added to the list of determinants of ischaemia.[103] In clinical studies, the quantity of ECG ST segment shift during coronary occlusion has been employed as a measure of ischaemia severity.[104] Thus,

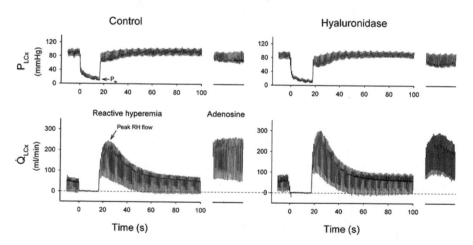

Fig. 4.42 Coronary pressure and blood flow tracings during reactive hyperaemia (RH) and
adenosine bolus. *Top*: left circumflex coronary artery pressure (P_{LCX}). *Bottom*: LCX blood
flow (Q_{LCX}). *Left*: control conditions. *Right*: after second infusion of active hyaluronidase.
Occlusion of LCX inflow starts at time = 0 s: Q_{LCX} decreases to almost 0 (*red line*) and P_{LCX}
drops to coronary occlusive or wedge pressure (P_w)[100]

depending on the variability of the determinants of ischaemia aside from occlusion time, substantially altering amounts of ischaemia can be expected. For example, more distally versus proximally located coronary occlusions have been shown to introduce a higher variability in ischaemia.[102] The vulnerability of the myocardium to ischaemia at identical durations of occlusion and with equal collateral flow is higher in LCA than RCA system (Fig. 4.43), the fact of which has been explained by the bradycardic effect of occlusion in RCA but not in LCA (Fig. 4.44).[45] Considering the large variability in collateral flow among patients with CAD and also in normal coronary arteries,[23] a similar distribution of collateral function can also be expected within an animal species such as the dog. Consequently, a uniform occlusion time of, e.g. 15 seconds as performed in the above-mentioned study by VanTeeffelen et al. does not imply a consistent

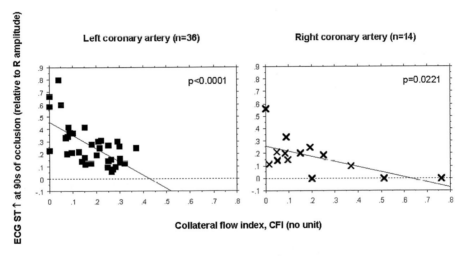

Fig. 4.43 Correlation between intracoronary ECG ST segment elevation (↑; *vertical axis*) normalized for ECG R amplitude and simultaneously obtained collateral flow index (*horizontal axis*) in the left (*left panel*) and right coronary artery (*right panel*). The relationship between the tow variables is much steeper in the left than in the right coronary artery

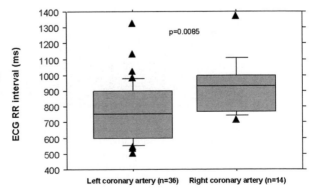

Fig. 4.44 Same study as in Fig. 4.43. Box plots of ECG RR intervals (*vertical axis*) as obtained during a 1-minute occlusion of the left and right coronary artery (*horizontal axis*). Error bars indicate mean values, 75 and 95% confidence interval

amount of ischaemia when different groups of animals are compared.[100] In the example of occlusive coronary pressure and flow tracings (Fig. 4.42),[100] coronary occlusive pressures (coronary wedge pressures) appear to be higher than central venous back pressure (5–10 mmHg), and there may be some residual, i.e. collateral flow in the recording on the right side. The amount of ischaemia developing during occlusion is lower in cases with more pronounced collateral flow to the occluded vascular region than given in the tracings.

Also, the variable effect of repetitive bouts as opposed to a single episode of ischaemia on its level has to be considered.

4.4.3.2 Repetitive Episodes of Ischaemia and Collateral Recruitment

The observation of lessening angina pectoris in the course of repeated episodes of physical exercise or continued exercise at a lower work load dates back to the first description of angina pectoris by William Heberden,[105] and it was called warm-up angina or walking through angina.[106] By that, the phenomenon of developing tolerance to repetitive episodes of myocardial ischaemia is described. The mechanisms involved in growing tolerance to ischaemia have been controversial, i.e. recruitment of collateral vessels (Fig. 4.45)[107,108] and

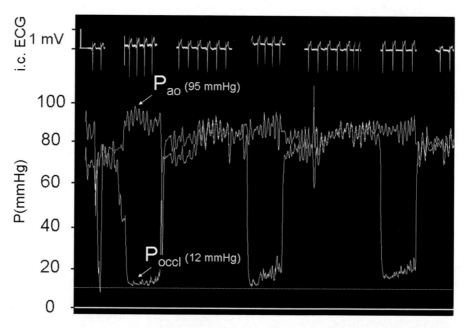

Fig. 4.45 Mean aortic (P_{ao}) and distal coronary pressure tracings during three consecutive 2-minute angioplasty balloon occlusions (P_{occl}) with corresponding intracoronary ECG recordings (*upper part*) showing diminishing ST-segment elevation with increasing P_{occl} during subsequent occlusions (coronary collateral recruitment). The time scale of the ECG is much shorter than that of the pressure tracings

ischaemic preconditioning,[103,109] or both have been described as factors responsible for warm-up angina. In an investigation by Sakata et al., the clinical,
electrocardiographic, haemodynamic and echocardiographic responses to three
150-s occlusions of the LAD were assessed in relation to collateral recruitment
in 18 patients with effort angina who underwent elective percutaneous transluminal coronary angioplasty.[107] The authors concluded that in the presence of
well-developed collaterals as imaged by myocardial contrast echocardiography
during occlusion, further collateral recruitment during subsequent occlusions
played a predominant role, whereas in the presence of poorly developed collaterals, ischaemic preconditioning primarily contributed to ischaemic tolerance.[107] In 30 patients who underwent PCI at our own laboratory, myocardial
adaptation to ischaemia was measured using intracoronary ECG ST segment
elevation changes obtained from an angioplasty pressure guidewire positioned
distal to the stenosis during three subsequent 2-min balloon occlusions.[108]
Simultaneously, pressure-derived CFI was determined as the ratio between
distal occlusive minus central venous pressure divided by the mean aortic
minus central venous pressure. The intracoronary ECG ST elevation (normalized for the QRS amplitude) at the first occlusion was equal to 0.25 ± 0.17, and it
decreased significantly during subsequent coronary occlusions to 0.20 ± 0.15
and to 0.17 ± 0.13, respectively (Fig. 4.46). There was a correlation between
the change in collateral function from the first to third occlusion and the

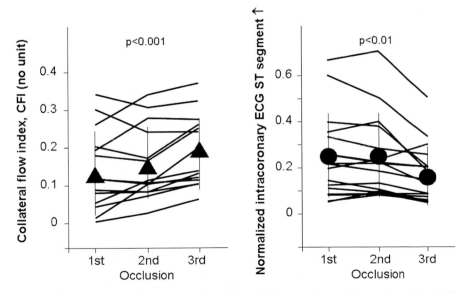

Fig. 4.46 Individual data of collateral flow index (CFI; *vertical axis, left panel*) and the ECG
ST segment elevation (intracoronary electrocardiographic ECG ST ↑ normalized for R
amplitude; *vertical axis, right panel*) during three subsequent 2-minute coronary artery occlusions (*horizontal axis*) for patients with non-occlusive CAD. The filled symbols with vertical
lines indicate mean values ± standard deviation

respective ECG ST elevation shift (Fig. 4.46; $r^2 = 0.29$, p = 0.002).[108] However, collateral recruitment accounted for only 30% of the observed variation in ECG ST segment shift during recurring episodes of ischaemia, indicating that ischaemic preconditioning likely was also a factor contributing to ischaemic tolerance. Edwards et al., using similar methods for collateral and ischaemia assessment, observed in 28 CAD patients who underwent a 3-min coronary occlusion that ventricular arrhythmias, ST deviation and angina were reduced during a second exertion or a second coronary occlusion, but that this protective effect could occur independently of collateral recruitment.[110]

4.5 Extracoronary Physical Determinants of Collateral Flow

Extracoronary physical determinants of collateral flow are myocardial contraction and contractility, LV filling pressure, LV distensibility and wall stress. End-diastolic LV wall stress is the reference parameter to describe LV preload. 'Transmission' of LV diastolic pressure to the collateral circulation as 'back pressure' in general terms or as 'surrounding pressure' in terms of a Starling resistor can advance pre-existing myocardial ischaemia in the sense of vicious cycle, by reducing collateral flow after an initiating event of ischaemia with a further increase in LV filling pressure.

In patients with ECG signs of ischaemia during coronary occlusion and beyond an occlusive LV filling pressure >27 mmHg, collateral and peripheral microvascular resistance increases as a function of LV end-diastolic pressure (LVEDP). Experimentally, the reduction in collateral flow with increased LV preload has been found to be mainly mediated by augmented extravascular pressure tending to collapse the collaterals in the sense of a Starling resistor, i.e. a phenomenon called vascular waterfall mechanism. At the 'waterfall pressure' for the collateral circulation (24–30 mmHg), flow is directly lowered depending on increasing myocardial tissue pressure.

In a broad sense, coronary perfusion pressure can be regarded as 'extracoronary' determinant of collateral flow. It has been demonstrated in open-chest dogs that flow to an entirely collateralized myocardial region increases with acutely augmented mean diastolic aortic pressure (MDP).

Because coronary collateral flow is a purely diastolic phenomenon, the duration of diastole plays a crucial role for collateral function.

In the beating heart at coronary perfusion pressures of 35–200 mmHg, coronary flow for a given perfusion pressure is impaired in comparison to the arrested situation. Hence, minimal coronary vascular resistance to flow is increased in the beating versus the arrested state due to intramyocardial compression of the coronary vessels.

There is no effect of LV afterload change on the coronary flow to a collateralized myocardial region.

4.5.1 Introduction

With regard to epicardially located coronary collaterals, extracoronary structures potentially influencing their function are the adjacent myocardium, the pericardial space and the LV cavity. For reasons of simplicity, the case of pericardial tamponade and its effect on collateral flow will not be discussed here. However, aside from the potential influence on collateral function of physical factors such as myocardial contraction and contractility, LV filling pressure, distensibility and wall stress, the effect of collateral function on some of these variables has, vice versa, also to be considered. In fact, there is a cross-talk between the more or less 'pressurized' coronary collateral network and the extracoronary physical determinants of collateral flow. The most widely appreciated effect of well 'pressurized', i.e. well-developed collateral arteries existing in advance of coronary occlusion is the salvage of contracting myocardium at and beyond the instant of occlusion. Salvage of myocardium is preservation of systolic function and, thus, of diastolic function. Conversely, the lack of collateral flow relates to more extended ischaemia with elevated LV filling pressure (Fig. 4.47).[111] The concept of an 'erectile' function of a well-developed collateral network to reduce diastolic expandibility or distensibility (corresponding to increased LV pressure change per volume change, $\uparrow dP/dV$; Fig. 4.47) and thus to lessen LV remodelling following infarction is less well known, but may even apply to the situation, when collaterals develop only after myocardial infarction.[112,113] On the basis of Laplace's law of wall stress (σ), it is evident that well 'pressurized' collaterals in the area of thin-walled myocardial scar must alleviate regional wall stress and thus the tendency to remodelling: $\sigma = \Delta P \times D/4h$, where D is LV cavity diameter and h the LV wall thickness. ΔP, usually inserted as single pressure value (LV pressure) instead of pressure difference, is the difference between the pressure in and 'around' the LV cavity. Epicardial coronary collateral vessels under perfusion pressure represent the pressure 'around' the LV, and thus, reduce the pressure drop at increasing level, thus mitigating the wall stress σ.

However, and among others, the focus of this chapter is on the reverse influence, namely that of the pressure within the LV cavity on flow or perfusion pressure in the collateral vessel (Figs. 4.48 and 4.49). Figure 4.48, i.e. the recording of phasic and mean aortic (P_{ao}), distal coronary (P_d, obtained via an angioplasty pressure sensor guidewire) and central venous pressure during accidental adenosine-induced ventricular arrest over 6 seconds, provides proof of principle that intracardiac pressures can be transmitted to the epicardial coronary circulation. During the episode of complete heart block, right atrial contraction waves appearing shortly after the ECG P waves are visible on the phasic central venous pressure curve. Below a mean coronary pressure of around 50 mmHg, brief coronary pressure signals simultaneous to right atrial contraction waves become visible, indicating transmission of atrial contraction via LV cavity to the epicardial coronary circulation. A similar phenomenon can be observed if LV pressure instead of atrial pressure and occlusive coronary pressure (coronary wedge pressure) are recorded simultaneously

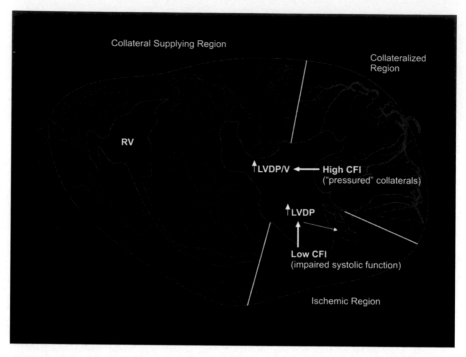

Fig. 4.47 Drawing of a short axis view of the left (LV) and right ventricle (RV) to illustrate the concept of a reciprocal relationship between LV diastolic pressure (LVDP) and the coronary collateral circulation (blue and black vessels). The black, straight lines mark the borders between three LV vascular territories, of which one is the collateral-supplying region (*red area*, patent left anterior descending coronary artery) to the second, collateral-receiving or collateralized area (*blue area*, occluded left circumflex coronary artery, LCX). The third region (*black area*, occluded right coronary artery) receives only minimal collateral flow and is ischaemic. The low collateral flow index (CFI) in the ischaemic area leads to increased LVDP via impaired systolic LV function of the inferior and posterior wall (*arrow*). The increased LVDP itself may influence the flow in the sparse collateral vessels of that area (*thin arrow*; waterfall phenomenon). In the collateralized LCX region, high CFI, or rather the 'pressurized' collaterals, may render the myocardial wall less distensible against diastolic filling (↑LVDP per volume of filling) when compared with the ischaemic region

(Fig. 4.49). The end-diastolic LV atrial contraction wave (A-wave) is reproduced on the occlusive coronary pressure tracing with absolute temporal agreement.

4.5.2 LV Preload, Diastolic Coronary Perfusion Pressure and Heart Rate

4.5.2.1 LV Preload

Left ventricular preload is characterized by LVEDP or volume or, more accurately, by LV wall stress at end-diastole, whereby LV wall stress is defined by the

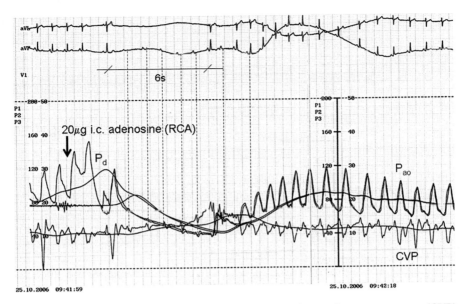

Fig. 4.48 ECG and aortic (P_{ao}), distal coronary (P_d) and central venous pressure (CVP) tracings before, during and after accidental ventricular cardiac arrest in response to right coronary artery (RCA) adenosine injection. P_d is obtained via a pressure sensor guidewire just positioned proximal to the RCA bifurcation of the posterolateral branch and ramus interventricularis posterior. See text for further details

Laplace's law ($\sigma = \Delta P \times D / 4h$; see below). Whether LVEDP influences collateral flow has been investigated infrequently.[111] However, this pathophysiological problem is similarly relevant as the ability of abundant collaterals to salvage myocardium, or their capacity to withhold remodelling of an infarcted ventricle.[112] This is because the transmission of LV diastolic pressure to the collateral circulation as 'back pressure' in general terms or as 'surrounding pressure' in terms of a Starling resistor could advance pre-existing myocardial ischaemia in the sense of vicious cycle, by reducing collateral flow after an initiating event of ischaemia with a further increase in LV filling pressure. The latter event would then further decrease collateral flow with resulting aggravation of ischaemia (Table 4.2). Accordingly, the aim of a study performed at our laboratory, in 50 patients with CAD and presence or absence myocardial ischaemia during coronary occlusion, was to test whether (a) LV filling pressure is influenced by the collateral circulation and (b) whether its resistance to flow is directly associated with LV filling pressure.[111] The following parameters were obtained before and during a 1 minute balloon occlusion: LV, aortic and coronary occlusive pressure, coronary flow velocity, central venous pressure and coronary flow velocity after coronary angioplasty. The following were the variables determined and analysed at 10-second intervals during occlusion and at 60 seconds of occlusion: LVEDP, velocity-derived and pressure-derived CFI, coronary collateral (R_{coll}) and peripheral resistance

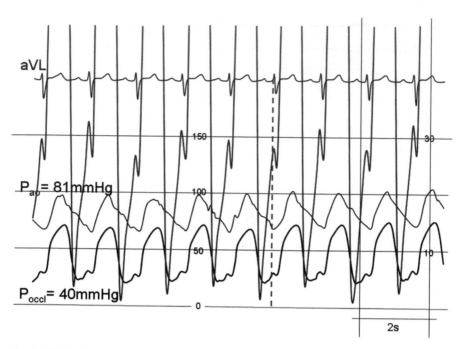

Fig. 4.49 Simultaneous recordings in a patient with insufficient collateral flow of ECG, left ventricular pressure (scale 40 mmHg), phasic aortic pressure (P_{ao}, scale 200 mmHg) and phasic coronary occlusive pressure (P_{occl}, scale 200 mmHg). ECG ST-segment elevations in lead II represent signs of ischaemia. Pressure-derived collateral flow index (CFI_p, no unit) is calculated as mean coronary occlusive pressure (P_{occl}) minus central venous pressure (CVP = 7 mmHg) divided by mean aortic pressure (P_{ao}) minus CVP. ECG P-waves are followed by pressure a-waves not only on the LV pressure curve but simultaneously also on the distal coronary curve

Table 4.2 Extracoronary physical determinants of collateral function

Extracoronary physical determinant	Effect on coronary collateral conductance (ml/min/g)
↑ Left ventricular preload	↓
↑ Mean diastolic coronary perfusion pressure	↑
↑ Heart rate	↓
Left ventricular contraction	**0** (Resistance $= \infty$)
↑ Left ventricular afterload	→

index to flow (R_{periph}). Focusing on the outward transmission of LV filling pressure, it was observed that in patients with ECG signs of ischaemia during occlusion, velocity-derived collateral function remained unchanged and pressure-derived collateral function increased during occlusion (Fig. 4.50). This 'cross-over' pattern

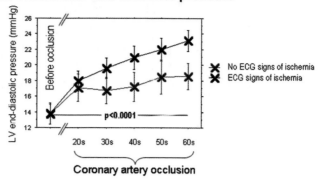

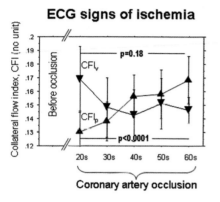

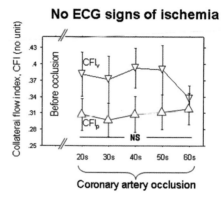

Fig. 4.50 Intra-individual changes before and during the first 60-s coronary balloon occlusion over time (*horizontal axis*). The *upper panel* shows changes in left ventricular end-diastolic pressure (LVEDP) in patients with insufficient collateral flow index ($CFI_v < 0.25$, *black symbols*) and sufficient collaterals ($CFI_v \geq 0.25$, *blue symbols*); the p value is identical for both groups. *Lower right panel*: Temporal changes of pressure-derived (CFI_p, upright triangles; lower p value) and velocity-derived collateral flow index (CFI_v, reversed triangles) in patients with insufficient collateral flow. *Lower left panel*: the respective values in patients with sufficient collaterals (significance level 'NS: not significant' is given for both CFIs). Error bars: standard error. All p values are given for repeated measures comparison

of the simultaneously recorded collateral function values could only be explained by a scenario in which there is outward transmission of LV diastolic pressure with steady increase in coronary wedge relative to aortic pressure and constant velocity-derived collateral function. Beyond an occlusive LVEDP>27 mmHg, R_{coll} and R_{periph} increased as a function of LVEDP (Fig. 4.51).[111]

With respect to physiological research in this field, there is precedence from experimental work in dogs. Almost 50 years ago, Kattus and Gregg reported an inhibition of collateral blood flow by distension of the LV in the open-chest dog.[114] Later, the reduction in collateral flow with increased LV preload has been found to be mediated by elongation of the collateral vessels as the

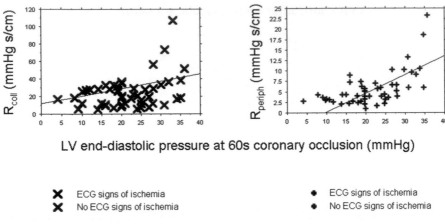

LV end-diastolic pressure at 60s coronary occlusion (mmHg)

✗ ECG signs of ischemia   ● ECG signs of ischemia
✗ No ECG signs of ischemia   ● No ECG signs of ischemia

Fig. 4.51 Correlation between left ventricular end-diastolic pressure (LVEDP; *horizontal axis*) and simultaneously obtained coronary collateral resistance index (R_{coll}; *left*) and coronary peripheral resistance index (R_{periph}; *right*) at 60 s of occlusion. Black symbols: insufficient collaterals; blue symbols: sufficient collaterals. $R_{coll} = 0.90$ LVEDP–5.24, $r = 37$, $P = 0.008$; $R_{periph} = 0.32$ LVEDP–1.35, $r = 61$, $P < 0.0001$. There was no association between the respective parameters in patients with sufficient collaterals[111]

ventricular size increases, but more importantly, by augmented extravascular pressure tending to collapse the collaterals in the sense of a Starling resistor, i.e. a phenomenon called vascular waterfall mechanism.[83] The haemodynamic criteria for waterfall behaviour were first described by Permutt et al.[115] It was elucidated for the pulmonary circulation supporting the claim that when alveolar pressure exceeds the pulmonary outflow pressure, pulmonary flow depends on the former and not on the latter.[115] Downey and Kirk extended these observations of the waterfall phenomenon to antegrade flow in the coronary circulation, considering the transmural gradient of extravascular pressure across the LV wall.[116] In the context of a collapsible vessel surrounded by tissue under a certain pressure, the following parameters decisive with regard to the collapse can be defined: inflow pressure at the origin of the vessel (P_i), surround pressure (P_s), outflow pressure (P_o) and the resistance to flow in the vessel (R).

Flow $= 0 \, (R = \infty)$ if $P_i < P_s$

Flow $= (P_i P_s)/R$ if $P_i > P_s > P_o$ (flow is independent of the outflow pressure)

Flow $= (P_i P_o)/R$ if $P_i > P_o > P_s$ (flow is independent of the surround pressure)

The waterfall behaviour is present if flow is independent of the outflow pressure, i.e. in a cataract the water falls irrespective of the 'back pressure' in the downstream portion of the river. In case of the normally perfused myocardium with normal LV systolic and diastolic function, coronary flow is independent of 'surround' pressure, i.e. LV filling pressure. At the 'waterfall pressure', which has been estimated to be 24–30 mmHg for the collateral circulation (assuming minimal and constant R),[83,117] flow is directly lowered in dependence of increasing myocardial tissue or surround pressure (directly influenced by the LV filling pressure), i.e. it is no longer dependent on the driving pressure ($P_i–P_o$). In accordance with the experimental observations, de Marchi et al. observed a sharp increase in the resistance to coronary flow (R_{coll} and R_{periph}) beyond an LV filling pressure of 25–27 mmHg.[111]

4.5.2.2 Diastolic Coronary Perfusion Pressure

Diastolic coronary perfusion pressure can be interpreted as an *extra*coronary physical determinant of collateral flow in the sense that it is diastolic *aortic* perfusion pressure at the coronary ostia representing the principal force of coronary perfusion. No studies in humans have investigated the relationship between *acutely* altered diastolic coronary perfusion pressure and simultaneously obtained coronary collateral flow to a region entirely supplied by collaterals either chronically or during a brief period of artificial vascular occlusion. However, a chronically recurring augmentation of diastolic aortic pressure by external counterpulsation appears to increase functional collateral flow. Preliminary data from our laboratory in 10 patients with chronic stable CAD who were randomly assigned to lower limb external counterpulsation at a pressure of 300 or 80 mmHg (total of 30 h) revealed a change in CFI from 0.143 ± 0.07 to 0.238 ± 0.08 (p $= 0.0049$) in the high-pressure group and from 0.179 ± 0.08 to 0.143 ± 0.06 in the low-pressure group (p $= 0.09$). Obviously, these are not data in support of collateral *function* but rather structural change in relation to diastolic perfusion pressure. Using a similar method for altering diastolic perfusion pressure, i.e. intra-aortic balloon counterpulsation, Brown et al. demonstrated, in 10 open-chest dogs, that flow in millilitre per minute to a collateralized LAD territory increased with MDP (mmHg) according to the following equation: 0.006 MDP $+ 0.00004$ MDP^2 (Fig. 4.52; Table 4.2).[81]

4.5.2.3 Heart Rate

Because coronary collateral flow is a purely diastolic phenomenon (ventricular contraction ceases collateral flow; see below), the duration of diastole plays a crucial role for collateral function. In the above-cited study by Brown et al.,[81] tachycardia induced by atrial pacing resulted in decreased flow to the entirely collateralized LAD region, the reduction correlating with a decrease in the diastolic fraction of the cardiac cycle (Table 4.2). Theoretically, the shortened diastolic duration can be compensated for by a reduced collateral and peripheral microvascular resistance to coronary flow. The study by Brown et al. documented an increase in collateral perfusion in response to β-adrenergic stimulation (isoproterenol; n $= 2$ experiments).[81] In humans, the net effect of bicycle exercise on collateral function appears to be positive, despite the negative consequence of exercise-induced tachycardia on diastolic duration (see also Fig. 4.15).

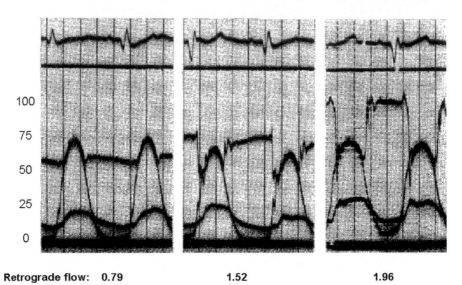

Retrograde flow: 0.79   1.52   1.96

Fig. 4.52 ECG and aortic, left ventricular and coronary pressure tracings in a dog with an entirely collateralized left anterior descending coronary artery that underwent internal aortic counterpulsation. When systolic pressure is held constant and diastolic pressure is increased, coronary occlusive pressure as well as retrograde, i.e. collateral flow, also increase [81]

4.5.3 LV Contraction

The majority of experimental studies on coronary pressure-flow relationships have been performed during asystole or cardiac arrest. The slope of the coronary flow relative to pressure is equal to coronary conductance, and principally, a similar conductance *index* can be obtained in humans using angioplasty Doppler guidewire and pressure sensors. The investigation of the influence of cardiac contraction on coronary conductance (i.e. the inverse of resistance) requires cardiac arrest, which, for obvious reasons, cannot be applied systematically in a human study, but may be encountered just accidentally (see Fig. 4.48). As evident from Fig. 4.49, the duration of cardiac arrest would possibly not be long enough to reach a coronary perfusion pressure, where the flow ceases. Therefore, data on the influence of cardiac contraction on coronary flow and, particularly, collateral flow have been performed experimentally.

Sabiston and Gregg were the first to observe an increase in coronary flow at constant pressure when the heart was arrested by inducing ventricular asystole (4–26 seconds duration) and fibrillation.[118] Downey and Kirk studied the *mechanism* of systolic inhibition of coronary blood flow.[116] A branch of the LCA was maximally dilated using adenosine infusion, and the pressure-flow relationship was obtained for the beating and arrested states of hearts. The relationship for the arrested state was linear from <20 mmHg to >200 mmHg. The curve for the beating state was shifted rightward to higher pressure values (Fig. 4.53). In the range below peak ventricular pressure, the pressure-flow

Fig. 4.53 Scatterplot of coronary blood flow (*vertical axis*) and coronary perfusion pressure (*horizontal axis*) from an individual dog for the beating heart (*right line*) and for the heart in the arrested state (*left line*; cardiac arrest induced for 5–7 s by vagal nerve stimulation)[116]

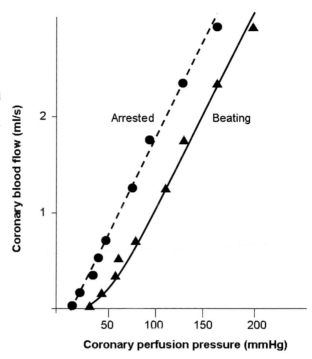

curve converged toward that for the arrested state. Figure 4.54 illustrates that between coronary perfusion pressures of 35–200 mmHg in the beating state, coronary flow for a given perfusion pressure (conductance) is impaired in comparison to the arrested situation (Table 4.2). Hence, minimal coronary vascular resistance to flow is increased in the beating versus the arrested state

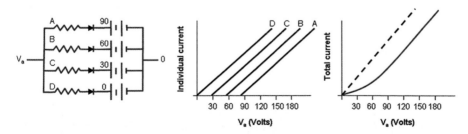

Fig. 4.54 Electrical analogue model of varying tissue pressures at different myocardial depths (A–D). *Left panel*: Coronary vessels at various depths in the ventricular wall are represented by parallel circuit elements, each with a different battery voltage. The voltage V_a is analogous to coronary inflow or aortic pressure P_a; P_t is analogous to tissue or coronary surround pressure P_t; the current in the circuits is analogous to coronary flow in the model. *Middle panel*: Individual leg currents at different tissue depths as a function of V_a. *Left panel*: The solid line corresponds to the total current for the network as a function of V_a, and the broken line indicates the current that occurs if the individual battery voltages are set to zero, representing a state of minimal tissue pressure, thus mimicking cardiac arrest[116]

due to intramyocardial compression of the coronary vessels (Starling resistor). Electrical analogue modelling of numerous parallel circuit elements (i.e. the branches of intramyocardial to epicardial vessels) with increasing individual voltages from the epicardial to the endocardial level allowed the interpretation that systole inhibits coronary perfusion by the formation of vascular waterfalls (Fig. 4.54), and that the intramyocardial pressure values responsible for the flow inhibition were close to peak ventricular pressures.[116]

The study by Russell et al. was performed to specifically determine the effect of cardiac contraction on coronary flow in a myocardial area entirely supplied by collateral vessels.[84] The results of the study comparing normally perfused and collateralized areas revealed that beating of the heart caused a gradient of blood flow inhibition from zero at the epicardium to about 50% at the endocardium in both normal and collateralized zones. Inhibition to flow at the mid wall of the collateralized zone was significantly greater than that seen at the corresponding depth in the normally perfused region.[84]

4.5.4 LV Afterload

Ventricular afterload is best defined according to Laplace's law as wall stress obtained at peak systole. Since collateral flow to subendocardial and mid-wall

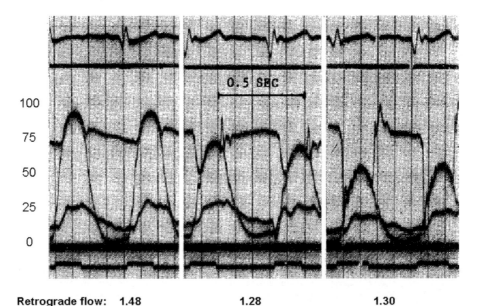

Retrograde flow: 1.48   1.28   1.30

Fig. 4.55 ECG and aortic, left ventricular and coronary pressure tracings in a dog with an entirely collateralized left anterior descending coronary artery that underwent internal aortic counterpulsation. When diastolic pressure is held constant and systolic pressure is lowered, retrograde, i.e. collateral flow, remains relatively unchanged[81]

myocardial regions is entirely blocked by ventricular contraction, it is logical that afterload increase does not alter this relationship, and respectively would 'vertically' extend the region of zero flow to epicardial areas, in case if there would have been some systolic flow before afterload increase. The above-cited study by Brown et al. investigated the effect of afterload change on collateral flow by applying intraaortic counterpulsation specifically during systole.[81] There was very little effect on the coronary flow to the collateralized LAD territory, when mean systolic pressure was varied while keeping mean diastolic pressure constant (Fig. 4.55; Table 4.2).[81]

Abbreviations

A	cross-sectional area (mm^2)
bFGF	basic fibroblast growth factor
CAD	coronary artery disease
CFI	collateral flow index (no unit)
CVP	central venous pressure (mmHg)
GM-CSF	granulocyte-macrophage colony-stimulating factor
IS	infarct size
LAD	left anterior descending coronary artery
LCX	left circumflex coronary artery
LV	left ventricle
P_{ao}	mean aortic pressure (mmHg)
PCI	percutaneous coronary intervention
P_{occl}	mean coronary occlusive or wedge pressure (mmHg)
Q	flow rate (ml/min)
RCA	right coronary artery
VEGF	vascular endothelial growth factor
V_{mean}	spatially
V_{occl}	intracoronary occlusive blood flow velocity (cm/s)
$V_{\emptyset\text{-}occl}$	intracoronary non-occlusive blood flow velocity (cm/s)

References

1. Eitenmüller I, Volger O, Kluge A, et al. The range of adaptation by collateral vessels after femoral artery occlusion. *Circ Res.* 2006;99:656–662.
2. Windecker S, Allemann Y, Billinger M, et al. Effect of endurance training on coronary artery size and function in healthy men: an invasive followup study. *Am J Physiol Heart Circ Physiol.* 2002;282:H2216–H2223.
3. Seiler C, Kirkeeide RL, Gould KL. Basic structure-function relations of the epicardial coronary vascular tree. Basis of quantitative coronary arteriography for diffuse coronary artery disease. *Circulation.* 1992;85:1987–2003.
4. Seiler C, Kirkeeide R, Gould K. Measurement from arteriograms of regional myocardial bed size distal to any point in the coronary vascular tree for assessing anatomic area at risk. *J Am Coll Cardiol.* 1993;21:783–797.

5. Choy J, Kassab G. Scaling of myocardial mass to flow and morphometry of coronary arteries. *J Appl Physiol*. 2008;Mar 6:Epub ahead of print.

6. Seiler C. Coronary velocity pressure tracings. *Eur Heart J*. 1997;18:697–699.

7. Heil M, Eitenmüller I, Schmitz-Rixen T, Schaper W. Arteriogenesis versus angiogenesis: similarities and differences. *J Cell Mol Med*. 2006;10:45–55.

8. Mees B, Wagner S, Ninci E, et al. Endothelial nitric oxide synthase activity is essential for vasodilation during blood flow recovery but not for arteriogenesis. *Arterioscler Thromb Vasc Biol*. 2007;27:1926–1933.

9. Fry D. Acute vascular endothelial changes associated with increased blood velocity gradients. *Circ Res*. 1968;22:165–197.

10. Kamiya A, Togawa T. Adaptive regulation of wall shear stress to flow change in canine carotid artery. *Am J Physiol*. 1980;239:H14–H21.

11. Saihara K, Hamasaki S, Okui H, et al. Association of coronary shear stress with endothelial function and vascular remodeling in patients with normal or mildly diseased coronary arteries. *Coron Artery Dis*. 2006;17:401–407.

12. Kelm M. Flow-mediated dilatation in human circulation: diagnostic and therapeutic aspects. *Am J Physiol*. 2002;282:H1–H5.

13. Schretzenmayer A. Ueber kreislaufregulatorische Vorgänge an den grossen Arterien bei der Muskelarbeit. *Pflügers Arch*. 1933;232:S743–S748.

14. Pohl U, Holtz J, Busse R, Bassenge E. Crucial role of endothelium in the vasodilator response to increased flow in vivo. *Hypertension*. 1986;8:37–44.

15. Holtz J, Förstermann U, Pohl U, Giesler M, Bassenge E. Flow-dependent, endothelium-mediated dilation of epicardial coronary arteries in conscious dogs: effects of cyclooxygenase inhibition. *J Cardiovasc Pharmacol*. 1984;6:1161–1169.

16. Inoue T, Tomoike H, Hisano K, Nakamura M. Endothelium determines flow-dependent dilation of the epicardial coronary artery in dogs. *J Am Coll Cardiol*. 1988;11:187–191.

17. Bevan J, Joyce E, Wellman G. Flow-dependent dilation in a resistance artery still occurs after endothelium removal. *Circ Res*. 1988;63:980–985.

18. Celermajer D, Sorensen K, Gooch V, et al. Non-invasive detection of endothelial dysfunction in children and adults at risk of atherosclerosis. *Lancet*. 1992;340: 1111–1115.

19. Busse R, Fleming I. Pulsatile stretch and shear stress: physical stimuli determining the production of endothelium-derived relaxing factors. *J Vasc Res*. 1998;35:73–84.

20. Silber H, Bluemke D, Ouyang P, Du Y, Post W, Lima J. The relationship between vascular wall shear stress and flow-mediated dilation: endothelial function assessed by phase-contrast magnetic resonance angiography. *J Am Coll Cardiol*. 2001;38:1859–1865.

21. Wilson R, Wyche K, Christensen B, Zimmer S, Laxson D. Effects of adenosine on human coronary arterial circulation. *Circulation*. 1990;82:1595–1606.

22. Wilson R, White C. Intracoronary papaverine: an ideal coronary vasodilator for studies of the coronary circulation in conscious humans. *Circulation*. 1986;73:444–451.

23. Meier P, Gloekler S, Zbinden R, et al. Beneficial effect of recruitable collaterals: a 10-year follow-up study in patients with stable coronary artery disease undergoing quantitative collateral measurements. *Circulation*. 2007;116:975–983.

24. Blumgart HL, Schlesinger MJ, Davis D. Studies on the relation of the clinical manifestations of angina pectoris, coronary thrombosis and myocardial infarction to the pathological findings. *Am Heart J*. 1940;19:1–91.

25. Hautamaa P, Dai X, Homans D, Bache R. Vasomotor activity of moderately well-developed canine coronary collateral circulation. *Am J Physiol*. 1989;256: H890–H897.

26. Lambert P, Hess D, Bache R. Effect of exercise on perfusion of collateral-dependent myocardium in dogs with chronic coronary artery occlusion. *J Clin Invest*. 1977;59:1–7.

27. Foreman B, Dai X, Bache R. Vasoconstriction of canine coronary collateral vessels with vasopressin limits blood flow to collateral-dependent myocardium during exercise. *Circ Res*. 1991;69:657–664.

28. Traverse J, Altman J, Kinn J, Duncker D, Bache R. Effect of beta-adrenergic receptor blockade on blood flow to collateral-dependent myocardium during exercise. *Circulation.* 1995;91:1560–1567.
29. Klassen C, Traverse J, Bache R. Nitroglycerin dilates coronary collateral vessels during exercise after blockade of endogenous NO production. *Am J Physiol.* 1999;277: H918–923.
30. Pohl T, Wustmann K, Zbinden S, et al. Exercise-induced human coronary collateral function: quantitative assessment during acute coronary occlusions. *Cardiology.* 2003;100:53–60.
31. Heusch G. Heart rate in the pathophysiology of coronary blood flow and myocardial ischaemia: benefit from selective bradycardic agents. *Br J Pharmacol.* 2008:[Epub ahead of print].
32. Rigo P, Becker L, Griffith L, et al. Influence of coronary collateral vessels on the results of thallium-201 myocardial stress imaging. *Am J Cardiol.* 1979;44:452–458.
33. Kolibash A, Bush C, Wepsic R, Schroeder D, Tetalman M, Lewis R. Coronary collateral vessels: spectrum of physiologic capabilities with respect to providing rest and stress myocardial perfusion, maintenance of left ventricular function and protection against infarction. *Am J Cardiol.* 1982;50:230–238.
34. Eng C, Patterson R, Horowitz S, et al. Coronary collateral function during exercise. *Circulation.* 1982;66:309–316.
35. Schaper W, Lewi P, Flameng W, Gijpen L. Myocardial steal produced by coronary vasocilation in chronic coronary artery occlusion. *Basic Res Cardiol.* 1973;68:3–20.
36. Klaubunde R. Dipyridamole inhibition of adenosine metabolism in human blood. *Eur J Pharmacol.* 1983;93:21–26.
37. Drury A, Szent-Györgyi A. The physiological activity of adenine compounds with especial reference to their action upon the mammalian hear. *J Physiol.* 1929;68:213–237.
38. Berne R. The role of adenosine in the regulation of coronary blood flow. *Circ Res.* 1980;47:807–813.
39. Olsson R, Davis C, Khouri E, Patterson R. Evidence for an adenosine receptor on the surface of dog coronary myocytes. *Circ Res.* 1976;39:93–98.
40. McFalls E, Araujo L, Lammertsma A, et al. Vasodilator reserve in collateral-dependent myocardium as measured by positron emission tomography. *Eur Heart J.* 1993;14:336–343.
41. Vanoverschelde JLJ, Wijns W, Depré C, et al. Mechansims of chronic regional postis-chemic dysfunction in humans. New insights from the study of non-infarcted collateral-dependent myocardium. *Circulation.* 1993;87:1513–1523.
42. Piek J, van Liebergen R, Koch K, de Winter R, Peters R, David G. Pharmacological modulation of the human collateral vascular resistance in acute and chronic coronary occlusion assessed by intracoronary blood flow velocity analysis in an angioplasty model. *Circulation.* 1997;96:106–115.
43. Seiler C, Fleisch M, Billinger M, Meier B. Simultaneous intracoronary velocity- and pressure-derived assessment of adenosine-induced collateral hemodynamics in patients with one- to two-vessel coronary artery disease. *J Am Coll Cardiol.* 1999;34:1985–1994.
44. Perera D, Patel S, Blows L, Tomsett E, Marber M, Redwood SR. Pharmacological vasodilatation in the assessment of pressure-derived collateral flow index. *Heart.* 2006; 92:1149–1150.
45. de Marchi S, Meier P, Oswald P, Seiler C. Variable ECG signs of ischemia during controlled occlusion of the left and right coronary artery in humans. *Am J Physiol.* 2006;291:H351–356.
46. Olsson R. Myocardial reactive hyperemia. *Circ Res.* 1975;37:263–270.
47. Seiler C, Kaufmann U, Meier B. Intracoronary demonstration of adenosine-induced coronary collateral steal. *Heart.* 1997;77:78–81.
48. Seiler C, Fleisch M, Meier B. Direct intracoronary evidence of collateral steal in humans. *Circulation.* 1997;96:4261–4267.

49. Werner G, Richartz B, Gastmann O, Ferrari M, Figulla HR. Immediate changes of collateral function after successful recanalization of chronic total coronary occlusions. *Circulation.* 2000;102:2959–2965.
50. Wahl A, Billinger M, Fleisch M, Meier B, Seiler C. Quantitatively assessed coronary collateral circulation and restenosis following percutaneous revascularization. *Eur Heart J.* 2000;21:1776–1784.
51. Feigl E. Coronary physiology. *Physiol Rev.* 1983;63:1–205.
52. Rouleau J, Boerboom L, Surjadhana A, Hoffman J. The role of autoregulation and tissue diastolic pressures in the transmural distribution of left ventricular blood flow in anesthetized dogs. *Circ Res.* 1979;45:804–815.
53. Heusch G, Schulz R. The role of heart rate and the benefits of heart rate reduction in acute myocardial ischemia. *Eur Heart J.* 2007;9 (supplement F):F8–F14.
54. Rowe G. Inequalities of myocardial perfusion in coronary artery disease ("coronary steal"). *Circulation.* 1970;42:193–194.
55. Fam W, McGregor M. Effect of coronary vasodilator drugs on retrograde flow in areas of chronic myocardial ischemia. *Circ Res.* 1964;15:355–365.
56. Becker L. Conditions for vasodilator-induced coronary steal in experimental myocardial ischemia. *Circulation.* 1978;57:1103–1110.
57. Patterson R, Kirk E. Coronary steal mechanism in dogs with one-vessel occlusion and other arteries normal. *Circulation.* 1983;67:1009–1015.
58. Egstrup K, Andersen PJ. Transient myocardial ischemia during nifedipine therapy in stable angina pectoris, and its relation to coronary collateral flow and comparison with metoprolol. *Am J Cardiol.* 1993;71:177–183.
59. Schulz W, Jost S, Kober G, Kaltenbach M. Relation of antianginal efficacy of nifedipine to degree of coronary arterial narrowing and to presence of coronary collateral vessels. *Am J Cardiol.* 1985;55:26–32.
60. Demer L, Gould K, Kirkeeide RL. Assessing stenosis severity: coronary flow reserve, collateral function, quantitative coronary arteriography, positron imaging, and digital subtraction angiography. A review and analysis. *Prog Cardiovasc Dis.* 1988;30:307–322.
61. Demer L, Gould K, Goldstein R, Kirkeeide R. Noninvasive assessment of coronary collaterals in man by PET perfusion imaging. *J Nucl Med.* 1990;31:259–270.
62. Kern M, Wolford T, Donohue T, et al. Quantitative demonstration of dipyridamole-induced coronary steal and alteration by angioplasty in man: analysis by simultaneous, continuous dual Doppler spectral flow velocity. *Catheter Cardiovasc Diagn.* 1993;29:329–334.
63. Werner G, Figulla H. Direct assessment of coronary steal and associated changes of collateral hemodynamics in chronic total coronary occlusions. *Circulation.* 2002;106:435–440.
64. Werner GS, Fritzenwanger M, Prochnau D, et al. Determinants of coronary steal in chronic total coronary occlusions donor artery, collateral, and microvascular resistance. *J Am Coll Cardiol.* 2006;48:51–58.
65. Billinger M, Fleisch M, Eberli F, Meier B, Seiler C. Collateral and collateral-adjacent hyperemic vascular resistance changes and the ipsilateral coronary flow reserve. Documentation of a mechanism causing coronary steal in patients with coronary artery disease. *Cardiovasc Res.* 2001;49:600–608.
66. Loos A, Kaltenbach M. Die Wirkung von Nifedipin auf das Belastungs-EKG von Angina-pectoris-Kranken. *Drug Res.* 1972;22:358–362.
67. Stone P, Muller J, Turi Z, Geltman E, Jaffe A, Braunwald E. Efficacy of nifedipine therapy in patients with refractory angina pectoris: significance of the presence of coronary vasospasm. *Am Heart J.* 1983;106:644–652.
68. Gould K. *Coronary Collateral Function Assessed by PET.* New York: Elsevier Science Publishing Co Inc; 1991.
69. Akinboboye O, Idris O, Chou R, Sciacca R, Cannon P, Bergmann S. Absolute quantitation of coronary steal induced by intravenous dipyridamole. *J Am Coll Cardiol.* 2001;37:109–116.

70. Werner G, Surber R, Ferrari M, Fritzenwanger M, Figulla H. The functional reserve of collaterals supplying long-term chronic total coronary occlusions in patients without prior myocardial infarction. *Eur Heart J*. 2006;27:2406–2412.

71. Gould K. Coronary steal. Is it clinically important? *Chest*. 1989;96:227–228.

72. Kern M. Walking with Sir William: reflections on collateral steal, recruitment, and ischemic protection. *J Am Coll Cardiol*. 2006;48:66–69.

73. Pijls N, Bracke F. Damage to the collateral circulation by PTCA of an occluded coronary artery. *Catheter Cardiovasc Diagn*. 1995;34:61–64.

74. Waser M, Kaufmann U, Meier B. Mechanism of myocardial infarction in a case with acute reocclusion of a recanalized chronic total occlusion: A case report. *J Interven Cardiol*. 1999;12:137–140.

75. Petronio A, Baglini R, Limbruno U, et al. Coronary collateral circulation behaviour and myocardial viability in chronic total occlusion treated with coronary angioplasty. *Eur Heart J*. 1998;19:1681–1687.

76. Pohl T, Hochstrasser P, Billinger M, Fleisch M, Meier B, Seiler C. Influence on collateral flow of recanalising chronic total coronary occlusions: a case-control study. *Heart*. 2001;86:438–443.

77. Perera D, Kanaganayagam G, Saha M, Rashid R, Marber M, Redwood S. Coronary collaterals remain recruitable after percutaneous intervention. *Circulation*. 2007;115:2015–2021.

78. Urban P, Meier B, Finci L, de Bruyne B, Steffenino G, Rutishauser W. Coronary wedge pressure: a predictor of restenosis after coronary balloon angioplasty. *J Am Coll Cardiol*. 1987;10:504–509.

79. Jensen L, Thayssen P, Lassen J, et al. Recruitable collateral blood flow index predicts coronary instent restenosis after percutaneous coronary intervention. *Eur Heart J*. 2007;28:1820–1826.

80. Perera D, Postema P, Rashid R, et al. Does a well developed collateral circulation predispose to restenosis after percutaneous coronary intervention? An intravascular ultrasound study. *Heart*. 2006;92:763–767.

81. Brown B, Gundel W, Gott V, Covell J. Coronary collateral flow following acute coronary occlusion: a diastolic phenomenon. *Cardiovasc Res*. 1974;8:621–631.

82. Kjekshus J. Mechanism for flow distribution in normal and ischemic myocardium during increased ventricular preload in the dog. *Circ Res*. 1973;33:489–499.

83. Conway R, Kirk E, Eng C. Ventricular preload alters intravascular and extravascular resistances of coronary collaterals. *Am J Physiol*. 1988;254:H532–541.

84. Russell R, Chagrasulis R, Downey J. Inhibitory effect of cardiac contraction on coronary collateral blood flow. *Am J Physiol*. 1977;233:H541–546.

85. Schaper W, Schaper J, Xhonneux R, Vandesteene R. The morphology of intercoronary anastomoses in chronic coronary artery occlusion. *Cardiovasc Res*. 1969;3:315–323.

86. Harrison D, Chilian W, Marcus M. Absence of functioning alpha-adrenergic receptors in mature canine coronary collaterals. *Circ Res*. 1986;59:133–142.

87. Bache R, Foreman B, Hautamaa P. Response of canine coronary collateral vessels to ergonovine and alpha-adrenergic stimulation. *Am J Physiol*. 1991;261:H1019–H1025.

88. Pupita G, Maseri A, Kaski J, et al. Myocardial ischemia caused by distal coronary-artery constriction in stable angina pectoris. *N Engl J Med*. 1990;323:514–520.

89. Harrison D. Neurohumoral and pharmacologic regulation of collateral perfusion. In: Schaper W SJ, ed. *Collateral Circulation*. Boston: Kluwer Academic Publishers; 1993: 329–336.

90. Feldman R, Christy J, Paul S, Harrison D. Beta-adrenergic receptors on canine coronary collateral vessels: characterization and function. *Am J Physiol*. 1989;275: H1634–1639.

91. Victor R, Leimbach WJ, Seals D, Wallin B, Mark A. Effects of the cold pressor test on muscle sympathetic nerve activity in humans. *Hypertension*. 1987;9:429–436.

92. Uren N, Crake T, Tousoulis D, Seydoux C, Davies G, Maseri A. Impairment of the myocardial vasomotor response to cold pressor stress in collateral dependent myocardium. *Heart.* 1997;78:61–67.
93. de Marchi S, Schwerzmann M, Billinger M, Windecker S, Meier B, Seiler C. Sympathetic stimulation using the cold pressor test increases coronary collateral flow. *Swiss Med Wkly.* 2001;131:351–356.
94. Peters K, Marcus M, Harrison D. Vasopressin and the mature coronary collateral circulation. *Circulation.* 1989;79:1324–1331.
95. Lamping K. Collateral response to activation of potassium channels in vivo. *Basic Res Cardiol.* 1998;93:136–142.
96. Knoebel S, McHenry P, Phillips J, Pauletto F. Coronary collateral circulation and myocardial blood flow reserve. *Circulation.* 1972;46:84–94.
97. Sambuceti G, Parodi O, Giorgetti A, et al. Microvascular dysfunction in collateral-dependent myocardium. *J Am Coll Cardiol.* 1995;26:615–623.
98. Billinger M, Raeber L, Seiler C, Windecker S, Meier B, Hess O. Coronary collateral perfusion in patients with coronary artery disease: effect of metoprolol. *Eur Heart J.* 2004;25:565–570.
99. Warltier D, Gross G, Brooks H. Pharmacologic- vs. ischemia-induced coronary artery vasodilation. *Am J Physiol.* 1981;240:H767–H774.
100. VanTeeffelen J, Dekker S, Fokkema D, Siebes M, Vink H, Spaan J. Hyaluronidase treatment of coronary glycocalyx increases reactive hyperemia but not adenosine hyperemia in dog hearts. *Am J Physiol.* 2005;289:H2508–2513.
101. Schaper W, Frenzel H, Hort W. Experimental coronary artery occlusion. I. Measurement of infarct size. *Basic Res Cardiol.* 1979;74:46–53.
102. Reimer KA, Ideker RE, Jennings RB. Effect of coronary occlusion site on ischemic bed size and collateral blood flow in dogs. *Cardiovasc Res.* 1981;15:668–674.
103. Murry C, Jennings R, Reimer K. Preconditioning with ischemia: a delay of lethal cell injury in ischemic myocardium. *Circulation.* 1986;74:1124–1136.
104. Macdonald R, Hill J, Feldman R. ST segment response to acute coronary occlusion: coronary hemodynamic and angiographic determinants of direction of ST segment shift. *Circulation.* 1986;74:973–979.
105. Heberden W. Commentaries on the history and cure of diseases. In: Wilius F, Kays T, eds. *Classics of cardiology.* New York: Dover; 1961:220–224.
106. MacAlpin R, Weidner W, Kattus AJ, Hanafee W. Electrocardiographic changes during selective coronary cineangiography. *Circulation.* 1966;34:627–637.
107. Sakata Y, Kodama K, Kitakaze M, et al. Different mechanisms of ischemic adaptation to repeated coronary occlusion in patients with and without recruitable collateral circulation. *J Am Coll Cardiol.* 1997;30:1679–1686.
108. Billinger M, Fleisch M, Eberli FR, Garachemani AR, Meier B, Seiler C. Is the development of myocardial tolerance to repeated ischemia in humans due to preconditioning or to collateral recruitment? *J Am Coll Cardiol.* 1999;33:1027–1035.
109. Tomai F. Warm up phenomenon and preconditioning in clinical practice. *Heart.* 2002;87:99–100.
110. Edwards RR, Little WC. Coronary collaterals in acute myocardial infarction without underlying coronary stenosis. *Am Heart J* 1990;120:424–427.
111. de Marchi S, Oswald P, Windecker S, Meier B, Seiler C. Reciprocal relationship between left ventricular filling pressure and the recruitable human coronary collateral circulation. *Eur Heart J.* 2005;26:558–566.
112. Kodama K, Kusuoka H, Sakai A, et al. Collateral channels that develop after an acute myocardial infarction prevent subsequent left ventricular dilation. *J Am Coll Cardiol.* 1996;27:1133–1139.
113. Remah H, Asanoi H, Joho S, et al. Modulation of left ventricular diastolic distensibility by collateral flow recruitment during balloon coronary occlusion. *J Am Coll Cardiol.* 1999;34:500–506.

114. Kattus A, Gregg D. Some determinants of coronary collateral blood flow in the open-chest dog. *Circ Res.* 1959;7:628–642.
115. Permutt S, Riley R. Hemodynamics of collapsible vessels with tone: the vascular water-fall. *J Appl Physiol.* 1963;18:924–932.
116. Downey J, Kirk E. Inhibition of coronary blood flow by a vascular waterfall mechansim. *Circ Res.* 1975;36:753–760.
117. Eng C, Kirk E. Flow into ischemic myocardium and across coronary collateral vessels is modulated by a waterfall mechansom. *Circ Res.* 1984;55:10–17.
118. Sabiston DJ, Gregg D. Effect of cardiac contraction on coronary blood flow. *Circulation.* 1957;15:14–20.
119. Sheehan F, Bolson E, Dodge H, Mathey D, Schofer J, Woo H. Advantages and applications of the centerline method for characterizing regional ventricular function. *Circulation.* 1986;74:293–305.

Chapter 5
Therapeutic Promotion of the Human Coronary Collateral Circulation

5.1 Introduction

Coronary artery disease (CAD) is the leading cause of morbidity and mortality in industrialized countries. Annual mortality rate from cardiovascular causes across Europe amounts to 5.4 people per 1000 inhabitants (49% of all deaths), and 2.4 deaths per 1000 inhabitants occur due to ischaemic heart disease (22%).[1] In 10–20% of patients with CAD, a treatment strategy alternative to conventional revascularization like percutaneous coronary intervention (PCI) or coronary bypass grafting is warranted, because the extent of coronary atherosclerosis is too severe.[2,3] Therapeutic angiogenesis/arteriogenesis are new approaches for revascularizing ischaemic myocardial tissue by formation of 'natural bypasses', i.e. collateral vessels. The current interest in this field is reflected in the number of publications. From a total of 1,468 articles found under the keywords 'angiogenesis OR arteriogenesis AND heart NOT cancer' published between 1967 and 2008, 782 articles were published in the last 5 years (Fig. 5.1). The respective number of publications with the limitation 'humans' adds up to 746, whereby 404 articles were published in the last 5 years. For reasons of simplicity, a focus on *human* aspects of the coronary collateral circulation in this section on therapeutic promotion will be maintained.

Aside from a review article on cardiac embryology first mentioning the term 'angiogenesis',[4] Fujita et al. published in 1988, the results of a first small clinical 'angiogenic' trial using heparin for the treatment of patients with stable effort angina.[5] Repeat coronary angiography in 10 patients who underwent intravenous heparin treatment revealed an increase in the extent of opacification of collaterals to the jeopardized myocardium. Also, exercise with heparin pretreatment increased the total exercise duration from 6 to 9 minutes and the maximal heart rate–blood pressure product (Fig. 5.2).[5] The authors concluded that 'heparin accelerates exercise-induced coronary collateral development by promoting angiogenesis', and that 'the development of such a therapeutic modality will open a new field for the treatment of patients with ischaemia'. Subsequently and starting with small open label trials of pro-angiogenic substances such as fibroblast growth factor (FGF) 1 and 2 and vascular endothelial growth factor-A (VEGF-A),[6–8] the field has rapidly progressed to phase-III double-blind

C. Seiler, *Collateral Circulation of the Heart*, DOI 10.1007/978-1-84882-342-6_5,
© Springer-Verlag London Limited 2009

Fig. 5.1 Cumulative number of publications found in Pubmed under the keywords 'angiogenesis OR arteriogenesis AND heart NOT cancer' (*vertical axis*) between the years 1967 and June 2008 (*horizontal axis*)

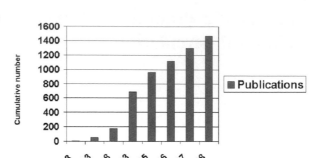

randomized trials. However, the initial enthusiasm seemingly justified by the results of the first non-randomized clinical studies was tempered by the subsequent disappointing outcome of controlled trials, which included the administration of single angiogenic agents either as the protein or as the gene encoding the protein.[9–17] Similarly, initial hype in the context of animal and small clinical studies for strategies using progenitor or adult stem cells for improving collateral function has also been moderated following the publication of larger randomized clinical trials reporting either negative results, or if positive, lacking biological relevance.[18–20] There are several factors that might explain the discordance between the positive results in animal studies and the rather disappointing observations made in randomized patient trials. First, collaterogenesis involves multifaceted processes leading to the balanced and coordinated expression of not just a single but many angiogenic and arteriogenic growth factors (see below).[21–23] Second, collateral remodelling or arteriogenesis involves physical forces in the form of

Fig. 5.2 Changes in exercise time (*left side*) and maximal double product (heart rate times systolic blood pressure; *right side*) before and after 20 treadmill exercise sessions with (closed symbol, *solid line*) and without (*open symbol, broken line*) heparin pre-treatment. *$p<0.001$ compared with values before exercise sessions

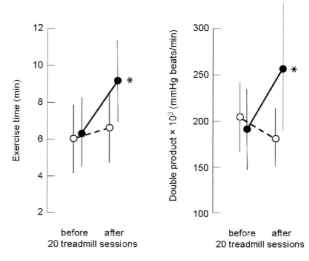

increased fluid shear stress as trigger along preformed coronary anastomoses, which has itself multiple effects, i.e. expression of various adhesion molecules and chemoattractant molecules contributing to homing of cellular elements on the vascular endothelial (VE) surface.[24]

In this context, the subsequent chapters on promotion of the human coronary collateral circulation are partitioned according to the current understanding of neovascularization with particular focus on angiogenic as opposed to arteriogenic and to progenitor or stem cell therapy; further chapters focus on physical strategies of coronary collateral promotion and on issues to be solved in neovascularization. The term neovascularization includes the processes of angiogenesis (capillary sprouting), arteriogenesis (remodelling of collateral conduits) and vasculogenesis (blood vessel formation from progenitor cells) (Fig. 5.3).[25]

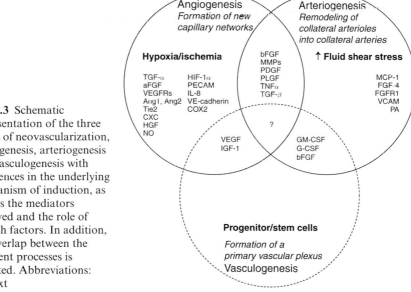

Fig. 5.3 Schematic representation of the three forms of neovascularization, angiogenesis, arteriogenesis and vasculogenesis with differences in the underlying mechanism of induction, as well as the mediators involved and the role of growth factors. In addition, the overlap between the different processes is depicted. Abbreviations: see text

5.2 Angiogenic Therapy

Angiogenesis refers to the sprouting of endothelial cells from post-capillary venules leading to capillary networks. It is initiated by tissue ischaemia with local hypoxia and overexpression of hypoxia-inducible genes. Stimulators of angiogenesis include over 50 growth factors, proteases and cytokines. The result of angiogenesis in ischaemic tissue is an increase in the capillary bed size, but this is ineffective in augmenting overall blood flow. VEGF and FGF are the most extensively studied families of angiogenic growth factors. The advance leading to the purification of endothelial cell mitogens in the early 1980s related to the observation that an endothelial cell growth factor had a marked affinity for heparin.

The FGFs are potent regulators of cell proliferation, differentiation, survival, adhesion, migration, motility and apoptosis. FGFs have been shown to stimulate angiogenesis in animal models of hindlimb ischaemia, in ischaemic porcine and canine hearts. The first uncontrolled clinical trials not only provided evidence of feasibility and safety of FGF treatment, but also suggested therapeutic efficacy. Subsequent, sizeable, randomized and placebo-controlled clinical studies using FGF protein and gene therapy have not supported the efficacy data of the previous smaller trials.

The VEGFs possess a secretory signal sequence, are secreted and bind with different affinities to one, two or all three VEGF receptor tyrosine kinases. VEGF-A with five different human isoforms was the first identified and is the most extensively studied VEGF family member. Knockout mice for VEGF have been shown to die of heart failure within 14 days after birth due to impaired postnatal myocardial angiogenesis. Evidence that VEGF can stimulate angiogenesis in vivo has been plentiful in animal models of coronary and peripheral ischaemia. In phase-I trials, protein therapy with human recombinant VEGF has been well tolerated, and has appeared efficacious with regard to myocardial perfusion. However, efficacy data could not be confirmed in a more sizeable, randomized, placebo-controlled trial of VEGF protein treatment. Clinical trials in peripheral and CAD using VEGF gene therapy have employed non-viral and viral methods. Though safe, direct intramyocardial injections of naked plasmid DNA encoding VEGF and of adenoviral VEGF have yielded inconsistent results with regard to efficacy.

In conclusion, angiogenic therapy using FGFs or VEGFs in patients with CAD has not hold promise of investigations in mostly young and healthy animals of different species.

5.2.1 Angiogenesis

Pioneering work in the field of angiogenesis, particularly with regard to the vascularization of tumours was performed by Folkman.[26] In fact, an angiogenic factor was first isolated by Folkman et al. in 1971 from the homogenate of a breast tumour of Sprague-Dawley rats.[27] This angiogenically active fraction was subsequently called tumour angiogenesis factor.[27] *Angiogenesis* refers to the sprouting of endothelial cells from post-capillary venules leading to capillary networks.[21] This involves dilation of existing vessels, activation of endothelial cell with increase in vascular permeability, degradation of extracellular matrix, proliferation of endothelial cell and migration to distant sites, and maturation and stabilization of the new blood vessel by recruitment of pericytes.[28] Stimulators of angiogenesis include over 50 growth factors, proteases and cytokines (Fig. 5.3), among them are the VEGF family (VEGF-A to -D; VEGF receptor 1–3), placental growth factor (PLGF), the angiopoietin family (ang1 and ang2) and their endothelial receptor Tie2, FGF, platelet-derived growth factor (PDGF), insulin-like growth factor-1 (IGF-1), hepatocyte growth factor (HGF), tumour necrosis factor α (TNFα), transforming growth factors (TGF), plasminogen activator (PA), over 20 matrix metalloproteinases (MMP), platelet endothelial cell adhesion molecule (PECAM), VE–cadherin, nitric oxide (NO), hypoxia-inducible factor-1α (HIF-1α), interleukin-8 (IL-8), erythropoietin, epidermal growth factor, etc.[29] Similarly, about as many natural inhibitors of angiogenesis have been uncovered.[29] The most widely known anti-angiogenic substance is thalidomide, a potent teratogen with not only sedative and hypnotic but also anti-myeloma qualities. From 1956 to 1962, approximately 10,000 children were born with severe malformities (Fig. 5.4), because their mothers had taken thalidomide during pregnancy.[30]

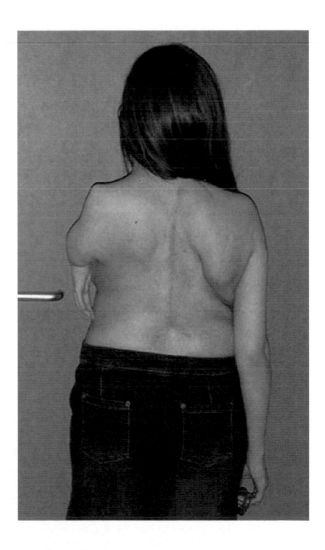

Fig. 5.4 A 20-year-old woman with left-sided phocomelia

Defective oxygenation of cells, as can be observed during pathological events like cancer, stroke and ischaemic vascular disease, leads to the expression and activation of the transcription factor HIF-1 (Fig. 5.3). HIF-1 is a heterodimer formed by a constitutive HIF-1β subunit and an oxygen-regulated HIF-1α subunit.[31] HIF-1α is known to control the expression of several angiogenic mediators, namely VEGF, the VEGF receptor Flt-1, nitric oxide synthase (NOS), PLGF, ang1, ang2 and ang4, PDGF, neuropilin-1 and others.[32] Also, HIF-1α can function as an activator or inhibitor of ang1 and ang2 gene expression, thus controlling endothelial cell proliferation and endothelial cell–smooth muscle cell interaction.[33] HIF-1α can also be activated by inflammatory cytokines, such as TNFα and IL-1. Endothelial cell proliferation and migration with capillary lumen formation are tightly controlled by proteinases of the PA/plasmin system, the MMP and heparanase, an enzyme that acts both at the cell surface and within the extracellular matrix to degrade polymeric heparan sulfate molecules into shorter chain length oligosaccharides. The PAs u-PA and tissue-type PA (tPA) convert the ubiquitous plasma protein plasminogen to plasmin, which itself activates certain MMP and degrades proteins such as fibronectin (FN), laminin and proteoglycans. This process is balanced by inhibitors including tissue inhibitors of MMP and by PA inhibitor-1. The maturation of the new capillaries probably involves PDGF, TGFβ and ang1-induced stabilization of the immature endothelial cell network by promoting pericyte growth and differentiation and by reprogramming endothelial cells. The result of angiogenesis in ischaemic tissue is a large increase in the capillary bed size, but it is ineffective in augmenting overall blood flow to the tissue, particularly in the presence of a flow-limiting atherosclerotic lesion in the upstream arterial conduit.

Theoretically, many of the above-mentioned substances involved in angiogenesis are candidates for therapeutic angiogenesis. Practically, only a few (VEGF, FGF, TGFβ) have been thoroughly evaluated, whereby VEGFs and FGFs are the most extensively studied families of angiogenic growth factors.[34] The ultimate goal of any therapeutic strategy to promote angiogenesis (also arteriogenesis and vasculogenesis) is to augment the level of angiogenic growth factors at the site of ischaemia (in the case of angiogenesis). This can be achieved most directly by local or systemic delivery of recombinant human or mammalian proteins.

5.2.2 Angiogenic Protein and Gene Delivery

The first angiogenic molecules were discovered in the 1980s.[35] A considerable advance in the purification of endothelial cell mitogens was achieved by the observation that an endothelial cell growth factor derived from rat chondrosarcoma had a marked affinity for heparin.[36] Subsequently, heparin affinity chromatography was employed to purify acidic and basic FGF (aFGF, bFGF)[36,37] as well as VEGF.[38,39] These factors have been shown to stimulate endothelial cell growth and migration in vitro as well as angiogenesis in vivo.

5.2.2.1 Fibroblast Growth Factors

The FGF family consists of 23 structurally related members, of which aFGF (FGF-1) and bFGF (FGF-2) are the most frequently described.[40] Both are stored in the extracellular matrix, but lack a signal sequence for secretion. FGFs bind to high-affinity receptors possessing tyrosine kinase activity as well as to syndecan-4, i.e. a transmembranase heparin sulphate carrying core protein.[41] FGFs are potent regulators of cell proliferation, differentiation, survival, adhesion, migration, motility and apoptosis. Additionally, effects of FGF administration include cardioprotection, angiogenesis, vascular remodelling and cardiac hypertrophy.[42] FGFs were shown to stimulate angiogenesis in animal models of hindlimb ischaemia,[43,44] in ischaemic porcine[45-47] and canine hearts.[48,49] Depending on the mode of FGF delivery (aFGF delivered epicardially by a sponge attached to an internal mammary artery pedicle), efficacy of angiogenic therapy could not be consistently documented.[50] Yanagisawa-Miwa et al. documented in a canine experimental myocardial infarct model that intracoronary injection of bFGF improved cardiac systolic function and reduced infarct size.[48] In that study, treatment with bFGF also increased the number of arterioles and capillaries in the infarct zone. The authors concluded that the angiogenic action of bFGF might lead to a reduction in infarct size and that the application of bFGF might bring about a therapeutic modality for the salvage of infarcted myocardium.[48] In this context, myocardial salvage by an angiogenic peptide in an acute myocardial infarction model is explainable only in an animal species with sufficiently preformed collateral arterioles, because infarct prevention can only occur if blood flow to the ischaemic region is restored immediately, i.e. in far less time than bFGF would require to induce angiogenesis. Harada et al. studied the effect of bFGF administration on regional myocardial function and blood flow in chronically ischaemic hearts of 26 pigs instrumented with proximal left circumflex coronary artery (LCX) ameroid constrictors.[47] In 13 animals, bFGF was administered extraluminally to the proximal left anterior descending (LAD) and LCX arteries with heparin–alginate beads, and 13 other animal served as controls. The bFGF-treated pigs showed a relevant reduction in left ventricular (LV) infarct size compared to untreated controls (Fig. 5.5).[47] In a study by Lazarous et al., dogs were subjected to progressive ameroid-induced occlusion of the LCX artery.[51] The animals were randomized to receive bFGF 1.74 mg/d (n = 10) or saline (n = 9) as a left atrial injection for 4 weeks. Relative collateral blood flow was assessed serially with radiolabelled microspheres in the conscious state during maximal coronary vasodilatation. Initiation of bFGF treatment was temporally associated with a marked acceleration of collateral development. However, collateral flow in control dogs improved toward the end of the study, approaching that of bFGF-treated dogs at the 38-day endpoint (Fig. 5.6).[51]

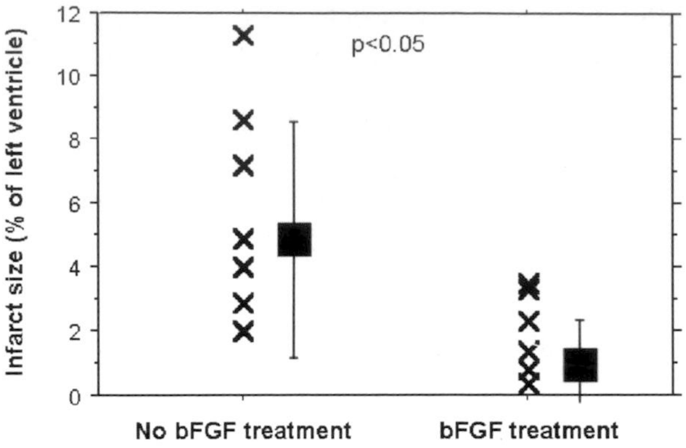

Fig. 5.5 Left ventricular infarct size (*vertical axis*) in pigs that underwent left circumflex coronary artery ameroid constriction as a function of absence or presence of treatment with basic fibroblast growth factor (bFGF; *horizontal axis*). The squared symbols and error bars indicate mean ± values standard deviation. Diagram according to Harada et al.[47]

Fig. 5.6 Line plot of maximal collateral flow over time for dogs as the ratio of ischaemic zone and normal zone blood flow. A marked increase in collateral flow occurred in treated dogs during the 10- to 17-day interval after ameroid placement. The difference was maintained regardless of whether basic fibroblast growth factor (bFGF) treatment was continued for 9 weeks (bFGF 9 weeks) or suspended after 5 weeks (bFGF 5 weeks). However, the level of ischaemic zone blood flow under bFGF treatment finally reached only about half that in the normal region

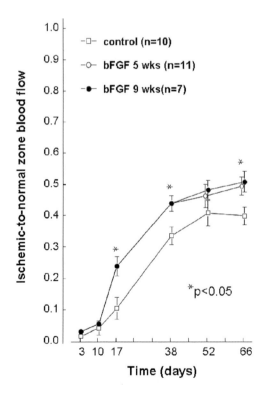

These early experimental studies provided proof of principle that the coronary and peripheral collateral circulation can be promoted. However, as the study by Lazarous et al. implicated,[51] the support could be just temporary in the sense of accelerating the restitution of perfusion (Fig. 5.6). Also, the recompensation of ischaemic-to-normal zone blood flow might not be complete, i.e. the collateral blood flow to the ischaemic zone in response to bFGF would reach 50% and not 100% of normal level. In addition, a subsequent investigation by

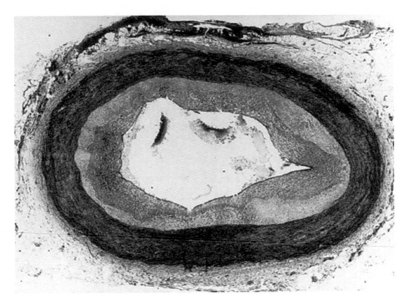

Fig. 5.7 Neointimal formation in response to injury in the iliac artery of a dog treated with vascular endothelial growth factor. Magnification ×40

the same group using the same model suggested that angiogenic therapy might be pro-atherogenic (Fig. 5.7).[52]

The first uncontrolled clinical trials not only provided evidence of feasibility and safety of FGF treatment, but also suggested therapeutic efficacy, and thus, supported the results from the above-described animal experiments (Table 5.1). In an early clinical investigation, Schumacher et al. injected FGF-I (0.01 mg/kg body weight; control group: heat-denatured FGF) close to the LAD after the completion of internal mammary artery anastomosis in 20 patients with three-vessel CAD.[6] All patients had additional peripheral LAD stenoses or diagonal branch obstructions. Twelve weeks later, the internal mammary bypasses were selectively imaged by digital subtraction angiography and quantitatively evaluated, whereby it was claimed that a capillary network sprouting from the proximal part of the coronary artery had formed and bypassed the stenoses and rejoined the distal parts of the vessel (Fig. 5.8).[6] The latter statement was entirely speculative, because there was no baseline internal mammary artery angiography to ascertain similar myocardial blush grades obtained at the onset of the study.[53] During conventional coronary artery bypass grafting, Sellke et al. included eight patients in an uncontrolled trial, whereby 10 heparin–alginate devices with 1 or 10 μg of bFGF were implanted in the epicardial fat at multiple sites of the unrevascularizable territory and also in the distal territory of a grafted or patent artery.[7] Three months after the operation, all patients remained free of angina pectoris. Seven patients were examined with stress perfusion scans. Three patients revealed enhancement of perfusion to the non-revascularized myocardium, one

Table 5.1 Angiogenic growth factor-based therapy: Clinical trials

Growth factor	Patient number	Delivery	Study phase and design	Results	Reference
FGF	20	Human recombinant aFGF	I, open label, uncontrolled	Safe, efficacious	{Schumacher, 1998 552}[6]
	8	FGF-2 (heparin–alginate)	I, open label, uncontrolled	Safe	{Sellke, 1998 553}[7]
	25	FGF-2 (intracoronary bolus)	I, open label, dose-ranging	Tolerated, hypotension	{Unger, 2000 594}[14]
	59	FGF-2 (intracoronary or i.v.)	II, open label, uncontrolled	↑ perfusion	{Udelson, 2000 593}[15]
	24	FGF-2 (heparin–alginate)	II, randomized, placebo-controlled	Safe, ↑ perfusion	{Laham, 2000 592}[54]
	337	Human recombinant bFGF (i.c.)	II, randomized, placebo-controlled	No↑ in ETT, perfusion	{Simons, 2002 598}[10]
	79	Adenovirus FGF-4 (i.c.)	I, randomized, placebo-controlled	Safe	{Grines, 2002 603}[56]
	52	Adenovirus FGF-4 (i.c.)	I, randomized, placebo-controlled	Trends to ↑ ETT, to ↑ perf.	{Grines, 2003 604}[57]
	532	Adenovirus FGF-4 (i.c.)	II, randomized, placebo-controlled	No↑ in ETT	{Henry, 2007 599}[58]
VEGF	14	I.c. human recombinant VEGF	I, open label, uncontrolled	Dose-dependent ↑ perfusion	{Hendel, 2000 608}[68]
	15	I.c. human recombinant VEGF	I, open label, uncontrolled	Tolerated	{Henry, 2001 607}[11]
	178	I.c. human recombinant VEGF	III, randomized, placebo-controlled	Tolerated, not improved	{Henry, 2003 602}[69]
	5	Plasmid (VEGF165) (i.m.)	I, open label, uncontrolled	Safe, ↑ perfusion	{Losordo, 1998 555}[8]
	20	Plasmid (VEGF165) (i.m.)	I, open label, uncontrolled	Safe, ↑ collateral score	{Symes, 1999 620}[72]
	13	Plasmid (VEGF165) (i.m.)	I, open label, uncontrolled	Safe, ↑ perfusion	{Vale, 2000 621}[73]
	6	Plasmid (VEGF-2) (i.m.)	I, open label, uncontrolled	Safe, feasible	{Vale, 2001 623}[17]
	29	Plasmid (VEGF-2) (i.m.)	I/II, randomized, placebo-controlled	Safe, reduced angina	{Losordo, 2002 617}[12]
	21	Adenovirus (VEGF121) (i.m.)	I, open label, uncontrolled	Tolerated	{Rosengart, 1999 625}[16]
	103	Adenovirus (VEGF165) (i.c.)	II, randomized, placebo-controlled	Safe, ↑ perfusion	{Hedman, 2003 626}[77]

ETT = exercise treadmill time; FGF = fibroblast growth factor; i.c. = intracoronary; i.m. = intramyocardial; perf. = myocardial perfusion; VEGF = vascular endothelial growth factor; ↑ = increase.

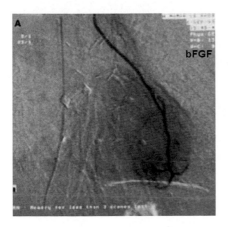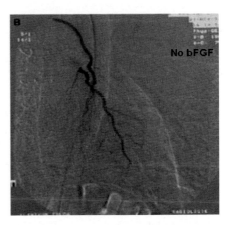

Fig. 5.8 Panel A: Angiography of the internal mammary artery graft to the left anterior descending coronary artery in a patient after treatment with intramyocardial basic fibroblast growth factor (bFGF). **Panel B:** Angiography of the internal mammary artery graft to the left anterior descending coronary artery in a patient without bFGF treatment. Radiographic contrast accumulation in the myocardium (myocardial blushing) is more pronounced in the treated than the untreated patient. However, it is unclear whether this is due to varying contrast injection dynamics, to different imaging technique or whether it represents a treatment effect

patient had a new fixed defect and three had minimal overall change but had evidence of new small, fixed perfusion defects. In three open-labelled phase-I trials, single intracoronary bFGF injections were well tolerated and associated with improved symptoms, exercise tolerance and augmented myocardial perfusion and LV systolic function (Table 5.1).[14,15,54]

In a placebo-controlled, randomized, double-blind study among 24 patients who underwent coronary artery bypass surgery, Laham et al. investigated the safety and efficacy of bFGF (bFGF; 10 or 100 µg versus placebo) delivered via sustained-release heparin–alginate microcapsules implanted in ischaemic and viable but ungraftable myocardial territories (n = 8 in each group; Table 5.1).[13] Clinical follow-up was available for all patients. Three control patients had recurrent angina, two of whom required repeat revascularization. One patient in the 10 µg bFGF group had angina, whereas all patients in the 100 µg bFGF group remained angina-free. Stress nuclear perfusion imaging at baseline and 3 months after bypass grafting showed a trend toward worsening of the defect size in the placebo group, no significant change in the 10 µg bFGF group and significant improvement in the 100 µg bFGF group (Fig. 5.9).[13] The symptomatic benefits of heparin–alginate-based bFGF therapy in the patients of the study just described were sustained 3 years later.[55] Also, late nuclear perfusion scans revealed a persistent reversible or a new, fixed perfusion defect in the ungraftable territory of four of five patients who received placebo versus only one of nine patients treated with bFGF (p = 0.02).[55]

The same application regimen of an intracoronary bFGF injection as in the above cited non-controlled trials[14,15,54] was then tested in a sizeable multicentre

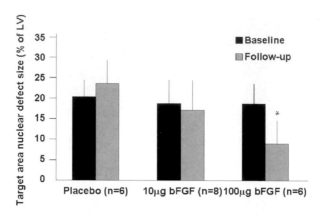

Fig. 5.9 Nuclear perfusion defect size of target left ventricular (LV) area (*vertical axis*) in three treatment groups of patients at baseline and 3 months after coronary artery bypass grafting. A significant (*) decrease in the perfusion defect is shown in the group of patients with 100 µg basic fibroblast growth factor delivered via epicardial, sustained-release heparin–alginate microcapsules

study (Table 5.1).[10] The FGF Initiating RevaScularization Trial (FIRST) was a randomized, double-blind, placebo-controlled study in 337 patients of a single intracoronary infusion of recombinant bFGF at 0, 0.3, 3 or 30 µg/kg. Efficacy was evaluated at 90 and 180 days by exercise tolerance test, myocardial nuclear perfusion imaging, angina assessment by questionnaire and Short-Form 36 questionnaire. Exercise tolerance was increased at 90 days in all groups and was not different between placebo and FGF-treated groups. Recombinant bFGF reduced angina symptoms as measured by the angina frequency score of the Seattle Angina Questionnaire (overall p = 0.035) and the physical component summary scale of the Short-Form 36 (pairwise p = 0.033, all FGF groups versus placebo).[10] These differences were more pronounced in highly symptomatic patients than in those with few symptoms. None of the differences were significant at 180 days because of continued improvement in the placebo group. Adverse events were similar across all groups, except for hypotension, which occurred with higher frequency in the 30 µg/kg bFGF group.

A similar picture of unfulfilled promise has emerged from FGF gene transfer studies. Two phase-I trials (Angiogenic GENe Therapy, AGENT) evaluated the safety and efficacy of escalating doses of adenovirus encoding FGF-4 from 3.3×10^8 to 10^{11} viral particles. The objectives of the first clinical angiogenic gene trial (AGENT-1) were to evaluate the safety and anti-ischaemic effects of five doses of a replication defective adenovirus (Ad) containing FGF-4 in patients with angina and to select potentially safe and effective doses for subsequent study.[56] Seventy-nine patients with chronic stable angina underwent double-blind randomization (1:3) to placebo (n = 19) or Ad-FGF-4 (n = 60). Safety evaluations were performed at each visit and exercise treadmill testing at baseline and at 4 and 12 weeks. Single intracoronary administration of Ad-FGF-4 seemed to be safe and well tolerated with no immediate adverse events. Overall, patients who received Ad-FGF-4 tended

Fig. 5.10 Change in total exercise treadmill time (*vertical axis*; mean ± standard error of mean) during follow-up (*horizontal axis*) for patients receiving an intracoronary infusion of adenoviral fibroblast growth factor-4 (Ad5 FGF-4; *solid line*) or placebo (*broken line*)

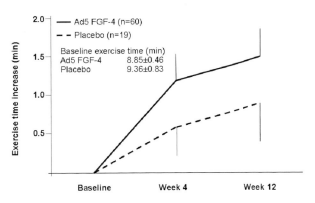

to have greater improvements in exercise time at 4 weeks (1.3 versus 0.7 minutes; Fig. 5.10).[56] The primary objective of the second clinical angiogenic gene therapy study (AGENT-2) was to determine whether intracoronary administration of Ad-FGF-4 can improve myocardial perfusion compared with placebo.[57] Grines et al. performed a randomized, double-blind, placebo-controlled trial of intracoronary injection of 10^{10} adenoviral particles containing a gene encoding FGF-4 to determine the effect on myocardial perfusion. Fifty-two patients with stable angina and reversible ischaemia comprising >9% of the LV on adenosine single-photon emission computed tomography (SPECT) imaging were randomized to gene therapy (n = 35) or placebo (n = 17). Clinical follow-up was performed, and 51 (98%) patients underwent a second adenosine SPECT scan after 8 weeks. Overall, the mean total perfusion defect size at baseline was 32% of the LV, with 20% reversible ischaemia and 12% scar. At 8 weeks, Ad-FGF-4 injection resulted in a significant reduction of ischaemic defect size (4.2% absolute, 21% relative; $p < 0.001$), but placebo-treated patients had no improvement.[57] However, the change in *reversible* perfusion defect size between Ad-FGF-4 and placebo was not significant. The authors concluded that intracoronary injection of Ad-FGF-4 showed a trend for improved myocardial perfusion.[57] The much larger AGENT-3 and -4 trials of a low and high dose of Ad-FGF-4 for chronic angina enrolled 532 patients in a randomized, double-blind, placebo-controlled fashion.[58] Both studies were stopped when an interim analysis of the AGENT-3 trial indicated that the primary endpoint change from baseline in total exercise treadmill time at 12 weeks would not reach significance. Henry et al. performed a pooled data analysis from the two nearly identical trials to investigate possible treatment effects on primary and secondary endpoints in prespecified subgroups.[58] The effect of placebo was large and not different from active treatment in men, but the placebo effect in the subgroup of women was negligible and the treatment effect was significantly greater than placebo (Fig. 5.11).[58] However, in the valid case population of both men and women, the change from baseline in the primary endpoint, exercise treadmill time (ETT) and most of the secondary endpoints revealed no difference between placebo and either dose group of Ad-FGF-4. This is in contrast to the results of the above-described AGENT-2 trial showing improvement in myocardial perfusion by SPECT imaging.

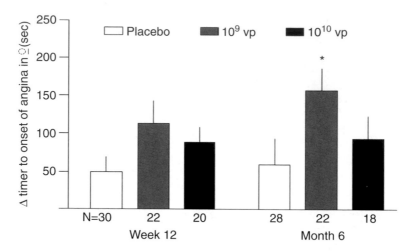

Fig. 5.11 Change from baseline in time to onset of angina pectoris during exercise (*vertical axis*) in female patients receiving placebo or different doses of intracoronary infusion of adenoviral fibroblast growth factor-4. Data are mean ± standard error. Vp: viral particles. *p<0.02

5.2.2.2 Vascular Endothelial Growth Factors

The VEGF family is composed of VEGF-A (VEGF-1), VEGF-B (VEGF-3), VEGF-C (VEGF-2), VEGF-D, VEGF-E and PLGF.[40] All forms posses a secretory signal sequence, are secreted and bind with different affinities to one, two or all three VEGF receptor tyrosine kinases: VEGFR-1 (Flt-1), VEGFR-2 (KDR/Flk-1) and VEGFR-3 (Flt-4). VEGF-A with five different human isoforms (121, 145, 165, 189, 206) (mouse isoforms: 115, 120, 164, 188) was the first identified and is the most extensively studied VEGF family member. VEGF 189 and 206 isoforms have strong heparin-binding ability and consequently are matrix bound. Conversely, VEGF 165 and 121 have no such heparin-binding properties and are present in the circulation. However, unlike VEGF 121, VEGF 165 binds another cell surface receptor, neuropilin-1, and as a result, is more active than VEGF 121 which has no neuropilin-binding region.[59] Knockout mice for VEGF 164 and VEGF 188 isoforms have been shown to develop ischaemic cardiomyopathy and to die of heart failure within 14 days after birth due to impaired postnatal myocardial angiogenesis.[60] VEGF 145 and 120 isoforms cannot rescue the lethal phenotype induced by VEGF 164 and 188 deficiencies.

Disruption of any of the VEGF receptor genes leads to embryonic lethality at the stage of not only vasculogeneis, but also angionesis and arteriogenesis, and thus, it appears that coordinated expression of all VEGF receptors is essential in early vascular development. A dramatic phenotype is demonstrated by VEGFR-2 deletion, which results in a complete failure of vasculogenesis.[61] Shalaby et al. reported the generation of mice deficient for VEGFR-2 by disruption of the respective gene using homologous recombination in embryonic stem cells.[61] Embryos homozygous for this mutation died in utero between 8.5 and 9.5 days post-coitum, as a result of an early defect in the development of haematopoietic and endothelial cells. Yolk-sac blood islands were absent at 7.5 days, organized blood vessels could not be observed in the embryo or yolk sac at any stage and haematopoietic progenitors were severely reduced. Fong et al. documented in VEGFR-1 knockout mice that it is an increase in the *number* of endothelial progenitors that leads to the vascular disorganization.[62] At the early primitive streak stage, i.e. prior to the formation of blood islands, haemangioblasts were formed much more abundantly in VEGFR-1 knockout embryos. This increase was primarily related to an alteration in cell fate determination among mesenchymal cells, rather than to increased proliferation, migration or reduced apoptosis of VEGFR-1 knockout haemangioblasts. It was shown in this study that the increased population density of haemangioblasts was responsible for the observed vascular disorganization, based on the following observations: (a) both VEGFR-1 knockout and VEGFR-1 wild-type endothelial cells formed normal vascular channels in chimaeric embryos; (b) wild-type endothelial cells formed abnormal vascular channels when their population density was significantly increased; and (c) in the absence of wild-type endothelial cells, VEGFR-1 knockout endothelial cells alone could form normal vascular channels when sufficiently diluted in a developing embryo.[62] Disruption of VEGFR-3 has been shown to lead to a defective remodelling of the primary vascular plexus and cardiovascular failure after embryonic day 9.5.[63] Dumont et al. demonstrated that targeted inactivation of the gene encoding VEGFR-3 resulted in defective blood vessel development in early mouse embryos. Hence, vasculogenesis and angiogenesis occurred, but large vessels became abnormally organized with defective lumens, leading to fluid accumulation in the pericardial cavity and cardiovascular failure at embryonic day 9.5.[63]

Evidence that VEGF can stimulate angiogenesis in vivo is plentiful in animal models of coronary and peripheral ischaemia.[44,64–67] Takeshita et al. administered the soluble isoform of VEGF 165 as a single intra-arterial bolus to the internal iliac artery of rabbits in which the ipsilateral femoral artery was excised to induce severe, unilateral hindlimb ischaemia.[64] Doses of 500–1,000 μg of VEGF produced statistically relevant augmentation of collateral vessel development by angiography as well as the number of capillaries by histology (Fig. 5.12). Consequently, improvement in the haemodynamic deficit in the ischaemic limb was larger in animals receiving VEGF than in untreated controls (collateralized-to-normal calf blood pressure ratio, 0.75 ± 0.14 vs. 0.48 ± 0.19, $p < 0.05$).[64] Banai et al. studied for the first time the effect of VEGF on *coronary* collateral blood flow in dogs subjected to gradual occlusion of the LCX artery.[65] Beginning 10 days after placement of an LCX artery-constricting device, 45 μg of VEGF (n = 9) or saline (n = 12) was administered daily via an indwelling catheter in the distal arterial stump. Treatment was maintained for 28 days. Collateral blood flow was determined with microspheres 7 days before treatment, immediately before treatment (day 0), and 7, 14, 21 and 28 days of the treatment period. Collateral blood flow was quantified during

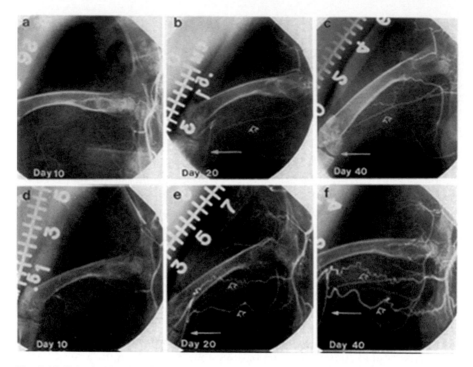

Fig. 5.12 Selective internal iliac artery angiography of rabbits with femoral artery excision before baseline (day 10). At baseline, at day 20 and at day 40, saline with 0.1% albumin (control group; **Panels a, b, c**) or vascular endothelial growth factor (VEGF; **Panels d, e, f**) was injected as a bolus into the internal iliac artery. Collateral arteries with their typical corkscrew-appearance are more extensively developed in the rabbit that underwent VEGF-treatment than in the rabbit receiving saline injections. Visibility of the distal vessel connection is better in the VEGF-treated animal (*closed arrow*) than in the control animal

chromonar-induced maximal vasodilation and expressed as a collateral zone/normal zone ratio. Treatment with VEGF was associated with a 40% increase in collateral blood flow (final collateral zone/normal zone blood flow of 0.49±0.06 and 0.35±0.02 in the VEGF-treated and control groups, respectively, p = 0.0037; Fig. 5.13).[65] Tsurumi et al. employed direct intramuscular gene transfer of naked DNA encoding VEGF, and observed augmentation of collateral development and tissue perfusion.[66] Ten days after ischaemia was induced in one rabbit hindlimb, 500 μg of naked plasmid DNA encoding VEGF165, or the reporter gene LacZ, was injected into the ischaemic hindlimb muscles. Thirty days later, angiographically recognizable collateral vessels and histologically identifiable capillaries were increased in VEGF transfectants compared with controls. In the study by Mack et al.,[67] Yorkshire swine that underwent ameroid constriction of the LCX artery were employed as the experimental model for testing the hypothesis that direct administration of adenovirus vector expressing the VEGF121 complementary DNA into regions

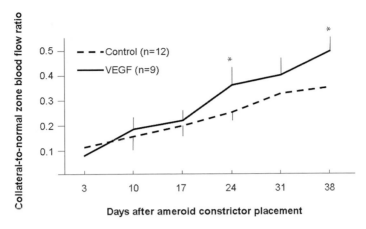

Fig. 5.13 Plot of transmural collateral-to-normal zone blood flow (*vertical axis*) as a function of time (*horizontal axis*); vascular endothelial growth factor (VEGF)-treated dogs versus controls. Collateral-to-normal zone blood flow was obtained during maximal vasodilation (mean ± standard error). Treatment with VEGF or placebo was started 10 days after collateral blood flow measurement. Collateral flow in VEGF-treated dogs increased more than in placebo-treated dogs. * p<0.05

of ischaemic myocardium would enhance collateral vessel formation and improve regional perfusion and function. SPECT, 4 weeks after vector administration, demonstrated a smaller ischaemic area at stress in VEGF-treated animals compared with control animals (p = 0.005).[67] Stress echocardiography at the same time demonstrated improved segmental wall thickening in animals that underwent VEGF gene therapy compared with control animals, with VEGF-treated animals showing nearly normalized function in the LCX territory.

In patients with CAD and limited options for revascularization, the safety and efficacy of recombinant human VEGF was tested by intracoronary and intravenous routes. In phase-I trials protein therapy with human recombinant VEGF appeared well tolerated, and augmented myocardial perfusion as expected from the above-cited experimental work.[11,68] Hendel et al. were the first to investigate in humans the effect of intracoronary recombinant human VEGF on myocardial perfusion (Table 5.1).[68] Fourteen patients underwent qualitative myocardial perfusion SPECT at rest and during hyperaemia before and 30 and 60 days, respectively, after VEGF administration. Stress and rest perfusion improved in >2 segments infrequently in patients treated with low-dose VEGF, but five of six patients showed improvement in >2 segments at rest and stress with the higher VEGF doses (Table 5.1).[68] In a dose escalation trial designed to determine the safety and tolerability of intracoronary recombinant human VEGF infusions, Henry et al. treated 15 patients with chronic stable CAD who were not candidates for conventional revascularization therapy with two sequential intracoronary infusions of VEGF, each for 10 minutes, at rates of 0.005 (n = 4), 0.017 (n = 4), 0.050 (n = 4) and 0.167 mg/kg/min (n = 3).[11] The maximally tolerated dose of VEGF was 0.050 mg/kg/min. Minimal haemodynamic changes were seen at 0.0050 mg/kg/min (2±7% mean decrease in systolic blood pressure from baseline to nadir systolic blood pressure), whereas at 0.167 mg/kg/min there was a 28±7% systolic blood pressure decrease from baseline to nadir (136 to 95 mmHg). Myocardial perfusion imaging was improved in 7 of 14 patients at 60 days (Table 5.1). All the seven patients with follow-up angiograms had improvements in the collateral density score (Fig. 5.14).[11] However, a more sizeable, randomized, placebo-controlled trial using the same application protocol of human recombinant VEGF could not confirm the initial efficacy data on VEGF protein therapy.[69] The Vascular endothelial growth factor in Ischemia for Vascular Angiogenesis, VIVA, trial was a phase II/III study with randomization of 178 CAD patients to placebo, low-dose VEGF (17 ng/kg/min), or high-dose VEGF (50 ng/kg/min) by intra-coronary infusion on day 0, followed by intravenous infusions on days 3, 6 and 9 (Table 5.1).[69] At day 60 following study inclusion, the change in ETT from baseline was not different between groups (placebo +48 seconds; low dose +30 seconds; high dose +30 seconds; Fig. 5.15). Angina class and quality of life were significantly improved within each group, with no difference between groups. By day 120, placebo-treated patients demonstrated reduced benefit in all three measures, with no significant difference compared with low-dose VEGF. High-dose VEGF resulted in significant improvement in angina class and non-significant trends in ETT time (p = 0.15) and angina frequency (p = 0.09) as compared with placebo.[69]

Gene therapy as an alternative to protein treatment potentially offers more sustained presence of the angiogenic growth factor in target tissues. Clinical trials in peripheral and CAD using VEGF gene therapy have employed non-viral (delivery of naked plasmid encoding VEGF or of DNA material in liposomal vehicle) and viral (adenoviral or retroviral vectors) methods.

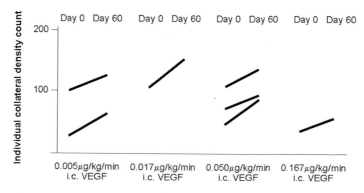

Fig. 5.14 Mean angiographic collateral density count at baseline and at day 60 for each patient of four groups receiving different dosages of intracoronary vascular endothelial growth factor

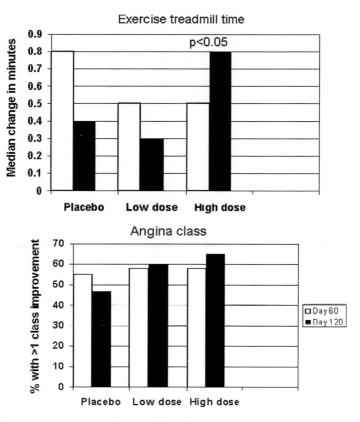

Fig. 5.15 Comparison from day 60 to day 120 of the change from baseline in exercise treadmill time and in the Canadian class of angina pectoris for three study groups that received intracoronary and intravenous infusions of placebo, low-dose vascular endothelial growth factor (17 ng/kg/min) or high-dose vascular endothelial growth factor (50 ng/kg/min)

In peripheral artery disease, Isner et al. pioneered the field by providing first clinical evidence of angiogenesis after arterial gene transfer of VEGF165 in a 71-year-old patient with limb ischaemia.[70] Two milligrams of human plasmid VEGF165 was administered that was applied to the hydrogel polymer coating of an angioplasty balloon. By inflating the balloon, plasmid DNA was thought to be transferred to the distal popliteal artery. Digital subtraction angiography 4 weeks after gene therapy showed an increase in collateral vessels at the knee, mid-tibial and ankle levels, which persisted at a 12-week view (Fig. 5.16).[70] In addition, three spider angiomas developed on the right foot/ankle of this female patient about a week after gene transfer; one lesion was excised and revealed proliferative endothelium, the other two regressed. The patient developed oedema in her right leg, which was treated successfully.[70] The objectives of a subsequent phase-I clinical trial by the same group were to document the safety and feasibility of intramuscular VEGF gene transfer by use of naked plasmid

Fig. 5.16 Digital subtraction angiography below the knee before and 4 weeks after gene therapy with vascular endothelial growth factor plasmid delivered via the angioplasty balloon in a 71-year-old patient with an ischaemic right leg. There is an increase in the number of collateral vessels at the knee, mid-tibial and ankle levels

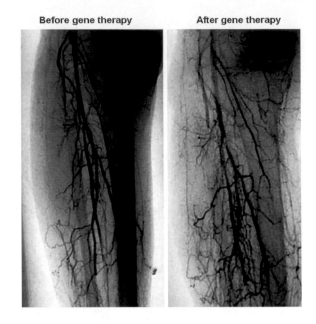

Before gene therapy   After gene therapy

DNA encoding, and to analyse the potential therapeutic benefits in patients with critical limb ischaemia.[71] Baumgartner et al. performed gene transfer in 10 limbs of 9 patients with non-healing ischaemic ulcers and/or rest pain due to peripheral arterial disease. A total dose of 4 mg of naked plasmid DNA encoding the 165 amino acid isoform of human VEGF was injected directly into the muscles of the ischaemic limb. The ankle–brachial index improved significantly (0.33 ± 0.05 to 0.48 ± 0.03, $p = 0.02$), and newly visible collateral blood vessels were directly documented by contrast angiography in seven limbs. Ischaemic ulcers healed or markedly improved in four of seven limbs, including successful limb salvage in three patients.[71]

The VEGF gene therapy for *myocardial* angiogenesis was first performed in a phase-I clinical trial among five male patients who had failed conventional CAD herapy (Table 5.1).[8] Naked plasmid DNA encoding VEGF (phVEGF165) was injected directly into the ischaemic myocardium via a mini left anterior thoracotomy. Injections caused no changes in heart rate, systolic or diastolic blood pressure, and ventricular arrhythmias were limited to single unifocal premature beats at the moment of injection. Serial ECG showed no evidence of new myocardial infarction in any patient. All patients had significant reduction in angina pectoris following gene therapy. Post-operative LV ejection fraction was unchanged (n = 3) or improved, and evidence of reduced ischaemia was documented using dobutamine SPECT in all patients (Table 5.1). Coronary angiography showed improved collateral score (0–3) in five of five patients.[8] This and a second uncontrolled study using the same protocol showed that the selected approach was generally safe and resulted in symptomatic as well as angiographic improvement of collateral filling (Table 5.1).[72] Additional positive results have been obtained using LV electromechanical mapping to monitor infarcted, ischaemic and normal myocardium before and after direct intramyocardial administration of naked plasmid DNA encoding VEGF 165 in patients with chronic stable CAD.[73] Similar results were found following catheter-based, transmyocardial injection of VEGF plasmid (Table 5.1),[12,17,74] whereby these findings have not been confirmed in a well-powered study using the same protocol.[75] In the Euroinject One phase-II randomized double-blind trial, therapeutic angiogenesis of percutaneous intramyocardial plasmid gene transfer of VEGF 165 on myocardial perfusion, LV function and clinical symptoms was assessed.[75] Eighty patients with severe stable CAD were randomly assigned to receive, via transmyocardial injection, either 0.5 mg of EVGF 165 (n = 40) or placebo plasmid (n = 40). After 3 months, myocardial stress perfusion defects did not differ significantly between the VEGF gene transfer and placebo groups.[75] Similarly, semiquantitative analysis of the change in perfusion in the treated region of interest did not differ significantly between the two groups. Compared with placebo, VEGF gene transfer improved the local wall motion disturbances, assessed by contrast ventriculography (p = 0.03). Canadian Cardiovascular Society functional class classification of angina pectoris improved significantly in both groups but without difference between the groups. A subanalysis of the study by Kastrup et al.[75] revealed that projection of the electromechanically guided injection area onto SPECT polar maps permitted quantitative evaluation of myocardial perfusion in regions treated with angiogenic substances, and that injections of VEGF 165 plasmid improved, but did not normalize, the stress-induced perfusion abnormalities.[76]

The utility of adenoviral VEGF gene therapy was assessed in a phase-I clinical trial of adenoviral VEGF 121 given by direct intramyocardial injection into a region with reversible ischaemia and as an adjunct to conventional coronary artery bypass or as sole therapy via minithoracotomy.[16] The patients received 100 μl-injections at 10 sites per patient with one of five dose groups. The study was documented to be safe related to the adenovirus injections and possibly efficacious with regard to myocardial perfusion, angina pectoris and treadmill exercise performance (Table 5.1).[16] Hedman et al. performed the Kuopio Angiogenesis trial (KAT),[77] which evaluated the safety and feasibility of adenoviral VEGF gene transfer via catheter-based intracoronary adminis-tration in 103 patients with CAD (Canadian Cardiovascular Society class II to III; mean age 58±6 years; randomized, placebo-controlled, double-blind phase-II study; Table 5.1). PCI was performed followed by gene transfer with a perfusion–infusion catheter. Thirty-seven patients received VEGF adenovirus [2x10^{10} particle units,[28] patients received VEGF plasmid liposome (2 mg of DNA] and 38 control patients received Ringer's lactate. Follow-up time was 6 months. Gene transfer to coronary arteries was feasible and well tolerated. The overall clinical coronary restenosis rate was 6%. Using quantitative coronary angiography, the minimal lumen diameter and percent diameter stenosis did not significantly differ between the study groups. Myocardial perfusion showed a significant improvement in the VEGF-adenovirus-treated

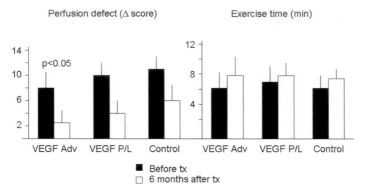

Fig. 5.17 Myocardial perfusion defect Δ score (perfusion score at rest minus perfusion score during adenosine infusion; *vertical axis; left side panel*) before and 6 months after therapy (tx) with adenoviral vascular endothelial growth factor (VEGF Adv), VEGF plasmid liposome (VEGF P/L) or Ringer lactate. *Right side panel*: exercise time (*vertical axis*) before and 6 months after therapy (tx) with VEGF Adv, VEGF P/L or Ringer lactate

patients after the 6-month follow-up (Fig. 5.17).[77] In the REVASC study, cardiac gene transfer was performed by direct intramyocardial delivery of a replication-deficient adenovirus-containing VEGF (4×10^{10} particle units). Sixty-seven patients with severe angina due to CAD and no conventional options for revascularization were randomized to VEGF121 gene transfer via minithoracotomy or continuation of maximal medical treatment.[78] Exercise time to 1 mm ECG ST-segment depression, the predefined primary end-point analysis, was increased in the VEGF121 group compared to control at 26 weeks (p = 0.026), but not at 12 weeks. Total exercise duration and time to moderate angina at weeks 12 and 26, and angina symptoms as measured by the Canadian Cardiovascular Society Angina Class and Seattle Angina Questionnaire were improved by VEGF gene transfer (all p-values at 12 and 26 weeks < or = 0.001). However, the results of nuclear perfusion imaging favoured the control group, although the VEGF121 group achieved higher workloads.[78]

As some of the above-cited trials have suggested potential benefits of VEGF therapy, none demonstrated so unequivocally in a controlled, well-powered investigation. The experience with FGF therapy demonstrates (see above) that positive efficacy results from open label phase-I trials do not easily translate into large, double-blind phase II/III study outcomes. Also, in the absence of convincing pharmacokinetic data after either protein or plasmid administration, it is unlikely that such delivery methods result in effective angiogenesis. However, one intriguing effect of VEGF 165 gene transfer is an increase in plasma levels of circulating endothelial progenitor cells (EPC), thus providing a potential link of this angiogenic substance to other concepts of neovascularization (see below).[79] An alternative concept to the use of single growth factors for collateral promotion could be the delivery of a *combination* of angiogenic and arteriogenic factors to the ischaemic myocardium in order to establish stable collateral networks. Lu et al. recently demonstrated in pigs that a combination of bFGF with PDGF-BB, two factors primarily targeting endothelial cells and vascular smooth muscle cells, promoted myocardial collateral growth and stabilized the newly formed collateral networks, which restored myocardial perfusion and function.[80] Using various members of the PDGF family together with bFGF in an angiogenesis assay, it was documented that PDGFR-α was mainly involved in angiogenic synergism, whereas PDGFR-β mediated vessel stability signals.

5.2.3 Other Pharmacological Substances with Potential Angiogenic Activity

5.2.3.1 Heparin

The above-cited work by Fujita et al.[5] reporting the results of the first clinical study on 'angiogenic' therapy opened the spectrum to angiogenic candidates other than the intensely studied factors FGF and VEGF. Although Fujita et al. concluded that heparin accelerated exercise-induced coronary collateral development by promoting angiogenesis,[5] they did not declare heparin to be an angiogenic factor. In a subsequent study, Unger et al. developed a canine model for the in vivo utilization of angiogenesis factors to promote revascularization of a collateral-dependent area of the heart and assessed the potential of heparin in this preparation.[81] Ameroid constrictors were placed on the proximal LAD coronary artery of 29 dogs, and the left internal mammary artery was implanted in an intramyocardial tunnel close to the LAD. A tube positioned in the distal internal mammary artery provided a continuous retrograde infusion directly into the vessel from an implanted pump. Heparin (15 or 150 U/h) or saline vehicle was infused. After 8 weeks, regional myocardial blood flow was assessed in the anaesthetized state during adenosine-induced vasodilatation, before and during occlusion of the internal mammary artery. The latter yielded a greater proportion of maximal collateral flow in heparin-treated dogs ($22\pm5\%$, n = 17) than in saline-treated dogs ($9\pm2\%$, n = 12, $p < 0.05$).[81] Apart from those two investigations, several others have supported the observation that heparin plays an important role in angiogenesis.[82–86] However, it is acknowledged that heparin itself is not angiogenic but interacts with FGF. FGF have a high-binding affinity for heparin,[36] and it is actually this property that facilitates their purification.[87] Additionally, heparin protects FGF from heat and acid inactivation, prolongs the half-life of aFGF and potentiates its mitogenic activity.[88] The role of heparin in collateral promotion may also be related to the interaction of FGF with glycosaminoglycans (such as heparin) in the extracellular matrix.[89] More recently, Masuda et al. evaluated whether external counterpulsation therapy combined with intravenous heparin injection is effective for augmenting exercise capacity and oxygen metabolism of ischaemic myocardium in stable angina.[90] Eleven patients with stable angina were treated with external counterpulsation therapy. Seven patients with stable angina were treated with external counterpulsation therapy with 5000 IU heparin pretreatment. At baseline and after completion of treatment with heparin, seven patients underwent [(11)C] acetate positron emission tomography to examine the change in regional myocardial oxygen metabolism. Although the total treadmill exercise time was prolonged after treatment in both groups, the extent of the improvements was significantly greater in the heparin-treated group compared with the control group.[90]

5.2.3.2 Dipyridamole

There has been evidence that oral dipyridamole, a nucleoside uptake blocker that increases myocardial adenosine levels, lessens myocardial ischaemia by inducing coronary collateral growth in animal models of ischaemic heart disease.[91,92] In this context, Belardinelli et al. studied 30 male patients with CAD and LV systolic dysfunction (ejection fraction >40%).[93] Patients were randomized to three matched groups. Ten patients received dipyridamole alone at a dose of 75 mg/d orally for 8 weeks; 10 patients underwent exercise training at 60% of peak oxygen uptake three times a week for 8 weeks and received dipyridamole, and 10 patients had neither exercise testing nor dipyridamole. On study entry and after 8 weeks, all patients underwent an exercise test with gas exchange analysis, dobutamine stress echocardiography, 201-thallium myocardial scintigraphy and coronary angiography. Maximum oxygen uptake increased significantly only in trained patients. Thallium uptake of the collateral-dependent myocardium, coronary collateral score and wall-thickening score increased significantly only in groups receiving dipyridamole, the greatest improvement being in patients with exercise training plus dipyrdiamole.[93] The effect of dipyrdiamole has been attributed to the elevation of the endogenous adenosine concentration.[94] Adenosine induces vascular relaxation through the activation of A2 adenosine receptors present in vascular smooth muscle and presumably in endothelial cells.[95] Adenosine has also been implicated in a variety of processes related to angiogenesis. In particular, adenosine can increase the number of endothelial cells,[96] augment DNA synthesis and vascular density.[97–99]

On the other hand, it is methodologically difficult to ascribe the myocardial salvaging effect of adenosine to its vasodilating action, to an eventual pro-angiogenic effect or both. In principle, adenosine could elicit its infarct-reducing effect as a vasodilator of preformed collateral arterioles before actual remodelling of collateral arteries takes place (arteriogenesis). Clinically, adenosine has been shown to reduce the occurrence of the no-reflow phenomenon in the context of rotational atherectomy during PCI.[100] The half-life of adenosine amounts only to seconds, and thus, it is questionable whether the action of this drug would last long enough to serve merely as a 'bridge' to structural collateral development. A further, complicating aspect with regard to adenosine's function to lessen myocardial ischaemia relates to its action in ischaemic myocardial preconditioning during the early and delayed phase.[101] The fact that adenosine preconditions ischaemic myocardium during artificial coronary occlusion has also been suggested in humans.[102] However, such an effect of adenosine could not be reproduced using an identical study protocol by other groups, i.e. ECG signs of myocardial ischaemia diminished similarly and collateral flow was recruited identically in response to repetitive artificial coronary occlusions among patients treated with adenosine or saline infusion (Fig. 5.18).[103] Since both myocardial

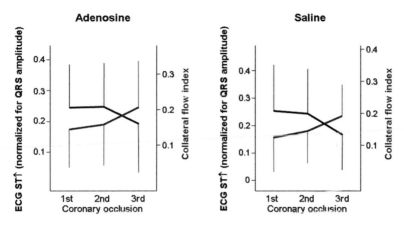

Fig. 5.18 Combined mean values (± standard deviation; *vertical axes*) of the normalized intracoronary ECG ST elevation (*black line; vertical axis, left side*) and the collateral flow index (CFI; *red line; vertical axis, right side*) during three subsequent 2-minutes coronary balloon occlusions (*horizontal axis*) for patients pre-treated with adenosine (*left panel*) and saline (*right panel*)

ischaemic preconditioning and coronary collateral recruitment are mechanisms of tolerance development against ischaemia, the contribution of each of these factors to lessening ischaemia can only be sorted out by a study design with simultaneous assessment of both.[103,104] Thus, it is not entirely certain whether the cardioprotective effect of adenosine is due to microvascular resistance reduction (including collateral dilation), to initiating a cascade of signal transduction events leading to opening of K_{ATP} channels with myocardial protection[105] or to collateral growth. In order to elucidate some of these questions, Zhao et al. determined the role of selected mediators of adenosine-induced late cardioprotection using pharmacological inhibitors.[106] Adult mice were treated with saline or an adenosine A1 receptor agonist, 2-chloro-N(6)-cyclopentyladenosine.[106] Twenty-four hours later, the hearts were perfused in Langendorff mode and subjected to 30 minutes of global ischaemia followed by 30 minutes of reperfusion. 8-Cyclopentyl-1,3-dipropylxanthine (DPCPX; 0.1 mg/kg IP) and S-methylisothiourea (3 mg/kg IP) were used to block adenosine receptors and inducible NOS (iNOS), respectively. Myocardial infarct size was reduced from 24.0±3.2% in the saline group to 12.2±2.5% in the adenosine-agonist-treated mice. The infarct-reducing effect of this substance was eliminated by DPCPX and by the iNOS blocker, and it was absent in mice with targeted ablation of iNOS.[106] Increased iNOS protein expression observed in adenosine-agonist-treated hearts was diminished by DPCPX. Thus, these data indicate that the factor crucial for cardioprotection, be it in the context of delayed preconditioning, angiogenesis or both, is NO rather than adenosine, in particular, inducible nitric oxide.

5.2.3.3 Nitric Oxide

There is substantial evidence that angiogenesis requires NO. A number of angiogenic factors upregulate endothelial expression of NOS and stimulate the release of endothelium-derived nitric oxide (eNOS).[107] VEGF enhances the endothelial expression of NOS and stimulates the synthesis of NO from cultured umbilical venous endothelial cells.[108] In segments of rabbit aorta, VEGF stimulates the production of NO, and pre-incubation of the model with L-arginine increases both basal and VEGF-stimulated NO release by 100%.[109] In case of TGFβ or bFGF being the angiogenic stimuli, endothelial cells also augment NO production.[110,111] The release of NO by angiogenic factors seems to play an important role in their effects. Capillary tube formation induced by bFGF and VEGF is abolished by the NO antagonist N^w-nitro-L-arginine methylester (L-NAME).[112] Similarly, NOS inhibition interrupts the angiogenic effects of TGFβ in vitro.[113] In a rabbit cornea model of angiogenesis, VEGF-induced angiogenesis is blocked by L-NAME.[113] The numerous effects of NO as a mediator of angiogenesis include inhibition of apoptosis,[114] proliferation of endothelial cell,[115] migration of endothelial cell migration[113] and enhancement of matrix-endothelial cell interaction.[115] Furthermore, the vasodilator effects of NO may play a role in its angiogenic effects, whereby increased microcirculatory flow has been observed to enhance endothelial cell proliferation.[116] Conversely and in the sense of a positive feedback mechanism, NO can induce the synthesis and release of VEGF from vascular cells.[117]

It is particularly the *endothelial* isoform of NO which has been demonstrated to be involved in the above-described actions. The eNOS knockout mice display a decreased neovascularization in response to ischaemia.[118] However, it has not been specified until recently that which form of neovascularization, i.e. angiogenesis, arteriogenesis, vasculogenesis or all three, is impaired most severely in the mentioned animal model. Mees et al. showed in a model of murine distal femoral artery ligation that endothelial NO activity is crucial for vasodilation of peripheral collateral vessels after arterial occlusion, but not for collateral artery growth in the sense of arteriogenesis.[119] The above-described function of iNOS as a mediator of delayed myocardial protection against ischaemia induced by adenosine suggests this isoform to be relevant as an angiogenic factor.[106] Along the same line, Fukuda et al. identified resveratrol (polyphenol) as a stimulus for the induction of new vessel growth, among others (VEGF and its tyrosine kinase receptor Flk-1) via increased endothelial as well as iNOS levels.[120]

Clinical studies on the therapeutic effect of NO donors on coronary collateral structure or function have been sparse and have focused rather on the vasodilating than the pro-angiogenic or arteriogenic effect of NO.[121,122] This has to do with the fact that, nowadays, it would be ethically unsuitable to withhold NO donors to patients randomly assigned to a treatment arm without nitrates. An observational study in 15 patients by Marfella et al. described the expression of angiogenic factors during acute coronary syndromes in human type 2 diabetes,[123] whereby HIF-1α and VEGF in specimens of human heart tissue were determined to elucidate the molecular responses to myocardial ischaemia in diabetic patients during unstable angina. Moreover, accumulation of a marker of protein nitration, nitrotyrosine, as well as the superoxide anion levels and iNOS were evaluated. Nondiabetic patients (n = 14) had higher HIF-1α and VEGF expressions compared with diabetic patients. As compared with non-diabetic specimens, diabetic specimens showed higher levels of both inducible NO mRNA and protein levels (p < 0.001) associated with the highest tissue levels of nitrotyrosine and superoxide anion (p < 0.001).[123] Accordingly, the relevance of, specifically, inducible NO with regard to the human coronary collateral circulation remains uncertain and appears to have both a pro-angiogenic and anti-angiogenic potential.

5.2.3.4 Sildenafil

In the context of the above-described putative role of inducible NO in cardioprotection, Salloum et al. found that sildenafil induces delayed preconditioning through an iNOS-dependent pathway in the mouse heart.[124] Adult male mice were treated with saline or sildenafil 24 hours before global ischaemia-reperfusion in the Langendorff mode. Infarct size was reduced from 27.6±3.3% in saline-treated control mice to 6.9±1.2% in sildenafil-treated mice.[124] Reverse transcription-polymerase chain reaction revealed a transient increase in eNOS and iNOS mRNA in sildenafil-treated mice. The magnitude of mRNA increase was less pronounced for eNOS than for iNOS (Fig. 5.19).[124] This study does, of course, not provide evidence in favour of sildenafil's angiogenic but just of its cardioprotective potential. It was a subsequent investigation by Vidavalur et al. which examined the angiogenic response of sildenafil in human coronary arteriolar endothelial cells.[125] The cells exposed to sildenafil (1–20 μM) demonstrated accelerated tubular morphogenesis with the induction of thioredoxin-1, haemeoxygenase-1 and VEGF. Sildenafil induced VEGF and angiopoietin-specific receptors such as KDR, Tie-1 and Tie-2. This angiogenic response was suppressed by tinprotoporphyrin IX, an inhibitor of HO-1 enzyme activity.[125] In a mouse model of peripheral artery disease with chronic hindlimb ischaemia, sildenafil has recently been demonstrated to exert angiogenic potential independent of NO production or NOS activity.[126] So far, there have been no clinical studies in the context of sildenafil as an angiogenic substance.

Fig. 5.19 Time course of inducible nitric oxide synthase (iNOS; *red line*) and endothelial NOS (eNOS; *black line*) mRNA expression determined with real-time polymerase chain reaction after sildenafil treatment (n = 3). * p<0.05 at corresponding time points

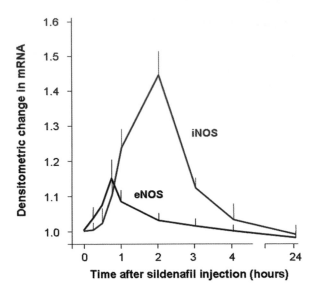

5.3 Arteriogenic Therapy

Arteriogenesis refers to an increase in the diameter of existing arterial vessels, and in the context of the coronary collateral circulation, to the outward remodelling of pre-existing collateral arterioles. It is arteriogenesis and not angiogenesis that accounts for sufficient bulk flow to myocardium at risk for infarction. Arteriogenesis is a process occurring independent of ischaemia. It is triggered mechanically by augmented tangential fluid shear forces. Monocyte–endothelial interaction is essential in the initiation of collateral artery formation, whereby shear stress-mediated upregulation of (ICAM-1) and vascular adhesion molecule-1 (VCAM-1) allows the binding of circulating monocytes.

Well-investigated substances with arteriogenic potency are monocyte chemoattractant protein-1 (MCP-1), colony stimulating factors (e.g. granulocyte–monocyte colony-stimulating factor, GM-CSF), TGFβ1, FGF, TNFα and MMP. Although being a strong arteriogenic factor, MCP-1 is not suitable for clinical use because of its atherogenic side effects. In patients with chronic stable CAD, GM-CSF has been shown to be efficacious in small randomized, placebo-controlled trials. However, safety issues have been raised in the context of the occurrence of acute coronary syndromes during GM-CSF treatment. Granulocyte-colony stimulating factor (G-CSF) appears to elicit a significant arteriogenic effect in patients with chronic stable CAD without exhibiting pro-atherogenic side effects. So far, TGFβ1 has been tested only in the experimental animal model. It seems to be efficacious and not to act pro-atherogenic. There has been evidence of impaired arteriogenic action of monocytes under conditions of hypercholesterolaemia that can be potentially reversed by statin therapy. VEGF-A-induced monocyte chemotaxis has been found to be impaired in hypercholesterolaemic CAD patients when compared with age-matched healthy controls. However, results from clinical work on the arteriogenic effect of statins have been controversial. In a sufficiently powered study including 500 CAD patients with quantitative collateral function measurements, statin treatment was not associated with extensively developed collaterals.

5.3.1 Arteriogenesis

In PubMed, the term arteriogenesis appears for the first time in the context of bridging defects in large arteries.[127] A total of three articles between 1955 and 1956 was dedicated to that topic, and from 1984 to 1991, Weiner et al. published five reports under the keyword arteriogenesis focusing on endocrinological tumours.[128] Another 367 articles on 'arteriogenesis' were published subsequently until June 2008 over the course of 10 years, whereby the term arteriogenesis in the currently used sense of collateral growth or, more precisely, remodelling of preformed collateral arterioles was coined by Schaper et al.[129] The results of that study in rabbits that underwent femoral artery occlusion indicated that monocytes play a major role in collateral artery growth, i.e. arteriogenesis.[129] However, functional collateral arteries were described already in 1669 by the English anatomist Richard Lower[130]: 'Coronary vessels describe a circular course to ensure a better distribution, and encircle and surround the base of the heart. From such an origin they are able to go off, respectively, to the opposite regions of the heart, yet around the extremities they come together again and here and there communicate by anastomoses. As a result fluid injected into one of them spreads at one and the same time through both. There is everywhere an equally great need of vital heat and nourishment, so deficiency of these is very fully guarded against by such anastomoses'. Since this initial observation of functional collateral arteries, numerous studies have confirmed Lower's description, and Fulton demonstrated that in the human heart, such anastomoses between different coronary vascular regions were already preformed in the absence of CAD, but increased in size to above 1 mm in the presence of CAD.[131] In the clinical setting, the described historical findings can be confirmed regularly (Fig. 5.20), and it can also be observed that the presence of sizeable collateral arteries to an occluded coronary artery may be associated with absence of systolic ventricular dysfunction (Fig. 5.21). On the other hand, collateral arteries may develop only after sudden coronary occlusion, i.e. in approximately 75–80% they are not preformed sufficiently to prevent myocardial infarction.[132] The coronary collateral artery between a marginal branch of the left circumflex and the occluded right coronary (RCA) artery shown in Figs. 5.20 and 5.22 illustrates that the calibre of such an anastomosis can be large, and that its appearance is distinctly different from the other epicardial coronary arteries, i.e. it has a corkscrew structure. The latter is the macroscopic hallmark of the foregoing remodelling process, and it is

Fig. 5.20 Coronary angiography of the left coronary artery in a cranial LAO projection depicting a collateral branch artery ($\rightarrow$). The collateral artery is originating from a marginal branch of the left circumflex coronary artery, and it is supplying the right coronary artery (RCA; orifice at the posterolateral branch of the RCA). LAD: left anterior descending coronary artery

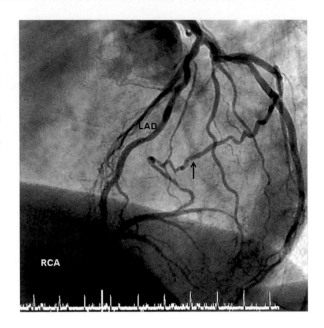

related to the non-directional growth of the preformed collateral arteriole not only in the radial but also in the longitudinal plane. Longitudinal arterial growth results in a meandering vascular path as long as the ventricular shape does not change accordingly (as in excentric ventricular hypertrophy or ventricular remodelling following myocardial infarction). Physically, the winding path of collateral arteries consumes part of the vascular conductance won during the cross-sectional vascular growth. However and according to Hagen-Poiseuille's law relating the perfusion pressure drop along a vessel to the volume flow in it, to its length and to the inverse of its radius raised to the fourth power, the energy dissipation for the transport of blood by vascular length increase is

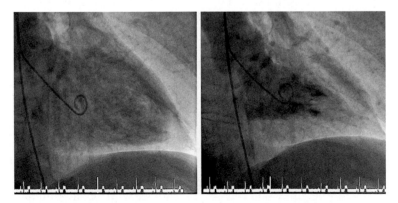

Fig. 5.21 Normal left ventricular angiography in RAO projection at end-diastole (*left side*) and systole (*right side*) of the same patient as depicted in Fig. 5.20

Fig. 5.22 Coronary
angiography of the left
coronary artery in a cranial
LAO projection of a patient
different from that of the
previous two illustrations.
Identical origin and orifice
of the collateral branch
artery ($\rightarrow$) as the path shown
in the previous figures.
However, in this case,
collateral growth occurred
only after occlusion of the
long stent in the proximal
right coronary artery (RCA)

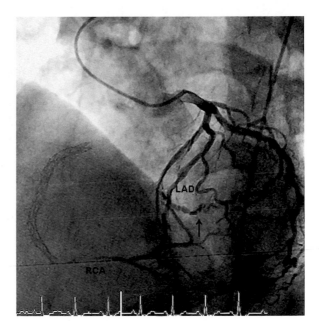

much less pronounced than that spared by the concurrently occurring calibre
growth. In the same physical context, it is the collateral artery growth (arteriogenesis) and not collateral capillary sprouting (angiogenesis) that accounts
for sufficient bulk flow to a myocardial region at risk for infarction.

5.3.1.1 Mechanisms of Arteriogenesis

Arteriogenesis has been known to be a process independent of ischaemia,
because clinical observations had demonstrated development of collateral
arteries distant from regions of ischaemia. For example (Fig. 5.23), in the
presence of an occlusion of the abdominal aorta, signs of ischaemia may
manifest in the muscles of the lower extremities as intermittent claudication,
but collateral arteries are located adjacent to the aortic occlusion. Also, ligation
of the femoral artery in rabbits is followed by a marked arteriogenic response in
the absence of a raise in ischaemia markers such as adenosine diphosphate,
adenosine monophosphate or lactate.[133] Deindl et al. studied the expression of
VEGF and its receptors in a rabbit model of collateral artery growth after
femoral artery occlusion.[134] The expression level of distinct hypoxia-inducible
genes and metabolic intermediates indicative for ischaemia (adenosine triphosphate, creatine phosphate and their catabolites) were also investigated. Arteriogenesis was not associated with an increased expression of VEGF or the
hypoxia-inducible genes. Furthermore, the high-energy phosphates and their
catabolites were entirely within normal limits. In this context, a backward
biochemical signalling mechanism has been postulated acting via products of

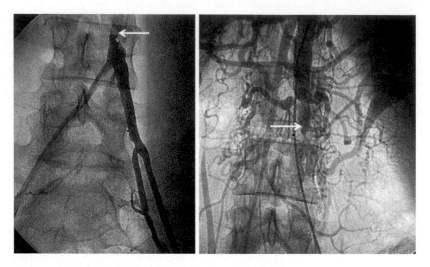

Fig. 5.23 Chronic occlusion of the abdominal aorta immediately proximal to the iliac artery bifurcation (*arrows*). *Left panel*: Contrast injection from the left superficial femoral artery. *Right panel*: Contrast injection from the thoracic aorta descendens: imaging of multiple corkscrew-like collateral arteries bypassing the occlusion

anaerobic metabolism and inducing collateral artery development, but its existence has not been proven yet. Rather than a biochemical mechanism, a biophysical one for initiating collateral artery growth was postulated early on by Schaper et al.[135] Meanwhile, there is compelling evidence that a chronic change of vascular fluid shear stress is the most important stimulus for arterial enlargement (Fig. 5.24; see also Chapter 3). Shear stress is caused by the flow of the viscous blood along the inner vascular surface, and is sensed by the

Fig. 5.24 Lower limb angiography in a rat with bilateral femoral artery ligation performed 14 days (d) earlier. The left femoral artery was ligated without any additional procedure; only a few corkscrew-shaped collateral arteries are visible (*). In addition to the right femoral artery ligation, an arterio-venous shunt was created between the distal stump of the femoral artery and the adjacent vein. On this side ('shunt 14d'), numerous collateral arteries are visible

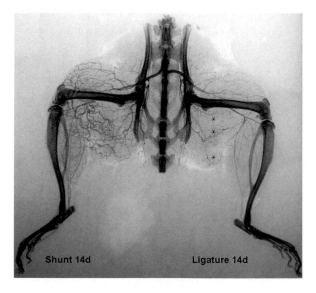

endothelial cell layer. It acts as a force tangential to the vascular wall, and in the arterial circulation it ranges between 10 and 70 dyn/cm^2. Following the gradual or abrupt occlusion of a main epicardial coronary artery, an increased perfusion pressure gradient between the pre- and post-stenotic myocardial perfusion territories augments blood flow through the small, preformed coronary anastomoses, thus bypassing the obstruction or occlusion and increasing shear stress on the collateral endothelium. In a pig model of femoral artery ligation, Eitenmüller et al. induced a constant increase in shear stress by means of an arterio-venous shunt, and they observed a very strong stimulation of arteriogenesis.[136] Also, they found three signalling pathways converging to allow the growth of collateral arteries beyond conductance values of the healthy femoral artery by a factor of two: (a) the RAS-ERK pathway, typically activated by the binding of growth factors to their cell surface receptors and regulating, e.g. cell migration; (b) the Rho pathway, influencing vascular proliferation and (c) the NO pathway, partially controlling endothelial function and leucocyte adhesion.[136] While the role of vascular shear stress as a trigger of arteriogenesis is evident, the endothelial mechanism to sense it is not. Tzima et al. recently described a mechanosensory complex that mediates the endothelial cell response to fluid shear stress.[137] Whereas earlier it was demonstrated that the conversion of integrins to a high-affinity state mediates a subset of shear responses, including cell alignment and gene expression, Tzima et al. investigated the pathway upstream of integrin activation. Together, the receptors PECAM-1 (which directly transmits mechanical force), vascular endothelial cell cadherin (which functions as an adaptor) and VEGFR2 (which activates phosphatidylinositol-3-OH kinase) were shown to be sufficient to confer responsiveness to flow in heterologous cells[137] (see also Chapter 3). Several transcription factors have been identified that are differentially expressed in growing collateral arteries. However, a specific functional relevance for arteriogenesis is documented only for a few of them, such as cardiac ankyrin repeat protein[138] and the transcription factors early growth response-1.[139]

Particularly important in the mediation of arteriogenesis appears to be a group of genes which is related to the chemoattraction and infiltration of circulating cells.[140] Schaper et al. first described the adhesion of monocytes to the activated endothelium of growing collateral vessels (Fig. 5.25), and they noted the accumulation of macrophages in the perivascular space.[135] A number of chemokines and growth factors contribute to endothelial leucocyte infiltration, such as MCP-1,[141] TNFα[142,143] and GM-CSF.[144] Monoctye–endothelial interaction is essential in the initiation of collateral artery formation, whereby shear stress-mediated upregulation of ICAM-1 and VCAM-1 allows the binding of circulating monocytes via the leucocyte-integrin Mac-1. Blood monocyte concentration is critical for collateral artery formation as an attenuation of arteriogenesis by leucocyte depletion can be mitigated by transfusion of monocytes.[145] The function of perivascular macrophages in arteriogenesis is currently under investigation. Several macrophage-derived factors have been identified to be essential for arterial remodelling.[146]

Other arteriogenic mediators of monocyte and macrophage origin are the FGF, and enzymes related to extracellular matrix turnover such as MMP and

Fig. 5.25 Collateral vessel
in the scanning electron
microscope: The endothelial
cell layer is activated and
oedematous

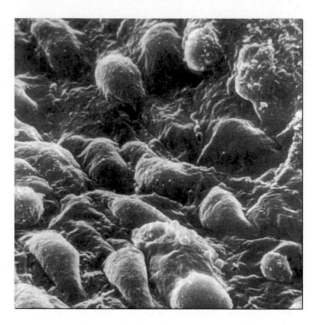

arginase-1. The fact that total mRNA levels of FGF remain constant in a model
of rabbit femoral artery ligation, whereas the FGF-1 receptor is upregulated,[147]
indicates that arteriogenesis is affected by receptor expression rather than
ligand availability. However, this pathogenetic aspect may differ between
species, since in patients with CAD, plasma levels of bFGF and VEGF have
been observed to be elevated among individuals with well-developed versus
those with poorly developed collaterals.[148] Remodelling of the adventitia is
indispensable to create the necessary space for collateral artery enlargement
(Figs. 5.26 and 5.27),[149] and proteolytic MMP as well as anti-proteolytic proteins

Fig. 5.26 Localization of
growing collateral vessels
on the surface of the left
ventricle of a dog heart.
The coronary circulation
was perfused with gelatine
and bismuth sulfate through
a branch of the left
circumflex coronary artery
(LCX; *injection site).
Several collateral arteries are
depicted (→) originating
from the left anterior
descending artery (LAD)
and supplying the occluded
(C, ameroid constrictor)
LCX territory

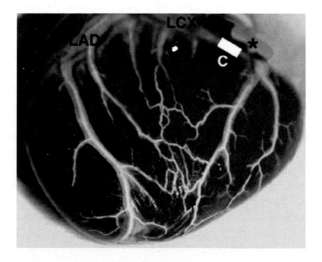

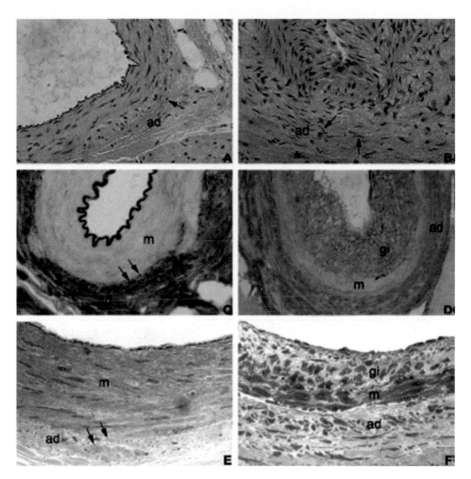

Fig. 5.27 Histology of the adventitia (ad) in normal vessels (*left column of panels*) and growing collateral vessels (*right column of panels*). **Panels A and B**: haematoxylin–eosin staining. Only a few fibroblasts are seen in the adventitia in normal vessels (**Panel A**), but many are visible in the adventitia of collateral vessels (**Panel B**; →). * Cardiomyocyte. **Panels C and D**: elastica van Gieson staining; m: media; gi: growing intima. Many elastic fibres are present in the adventitia of normal vessels (**Panel C**; →), but not in the adventitia of collateral vessels (**Panel D**). **Panels E and F**: semithin section. Many elastic fibres are present in the adventitia of normal vessels (**Panel E**; →), but not in the adventitia of collateral vessels (**Panel F**). A large number of fibroblasts can be seen in the adventitia of collateral vessels. Magnification: ×40 in **Panels A, B, C, and D** and ×63 in **Panels E and F**

(PA inhibitor-1, tissue inhibitor of MMP-1) reveal a specific temporal-expression pattern in growing collateral arteries of the dog heart.[150] In that context, Cai et al. studied the role of the adventitia in adaptive arteriogenesis during the phase of active growth of coronary collateral vessels induced by chronic occlusion of the LCX coronary artery in canine hearts (Fig. 5.26).[149] Electron microscopy and immunoconfocal labelling was used for bFGF, MMP-2, MMP-9, tPA, its inhibitor (PAI-1), FN and Ki-67. Proliferation of smooth muscle cells and adventitial fibroblasts was evident (Fig. 5.27). Immunoconfocal labelling showed that adventitial MMP-2, MMP-9 and FN were 9.2-, 7.5- and 8.6-fold, bFGF 5.1-fold and PAI-1 was 3.4-fold higher in collateral than in normal vessels.[149] The number of fibroblasts was fivefold elevated in collateral arteries, but the elastic fibre content was 25-fold greater in normal than in collateral vessels. Perivascular myocyte damage and induction of eNOS in pericollateral vessel capillaries indicated expansion of collateral arteries.[149] Leucocytes other than monocytes have also been shown to be relevant during arteriogenesis.[151,152] The contribution of pluripotent progenitor cells to vascular proliferation and repair will be discussed below in Section 5.4. In summary, the localization of bone marrow-derived cells (BMC) to the vascular wall is well documented,[153] although it is uncertain in how far they differentiate into endothelial or smooth muscle cells.[154]

5.3.2 Arteriogenic Substances

With the accumulating knowledge of the basic mechanisms of arteriogenesis, several factors have been identified, which are candidates for stimulation of arteriogenesis. While some of them reached clinical testing in pilot studies, others had to be abandoned preclinically because of significant side effects.

5.3.2.1 Monocyte Chemoattractant Protein-1

One of the most potent arteriogenic substances is MCP-1 (Fig. 5.28). In order to investigate whether MCP-1 enhances collateral growth after femoral artery occlusion, Ito et al. investigated 12 rabbits randomly assigned to receive either MCP-1, saline, or no local infusion via osmotic minipump. Both collateral and peripheral conductances were significantly elevated in animals with MCP-1 treatment compared with the control group, reaching values of non-occluded hindlimbs after only 1 week of occlusion (Fig. 5.29).[155] Because the efficacy of MCP-1 with regard to arteriogenesis was shown to depend on monocyte attraction, an aggravation of atherosclerosis was and is an obvious concern. In the acute coronary syndrome, monocyte activation is believed to play an important pathogenetic role. Among more than 4,200 patients with that condition, Lemos et al. observed that the rates of death and the composite endpoints of death or myocardial infarction and other major adverse cardio-vascular events increased across baseline quartiles of MCP-1.[156] The objective of a study by van Royen et al. was to quantify the arteriogenic potency of MCP-1 under hyperlipidaemic conditions and to determine the effects of locally applied MCP-1 on systemic serum lipid levels as well as on atherosclerosis.[157] Sixty-four Watanabe rabbits were treated with either low-dose MCP-1 (1 μg/kg/week), high-dose MCP-1 (3.3 μg/kg/week) or saline. Substances were applied directly into the collateral circulation via an osmotic minipump with the catheter placed in the proximal stump of the ligated femoral artery. MCP-1 accelerated arteriogenesis upon femoral artery ligation under hyperlipidaemic

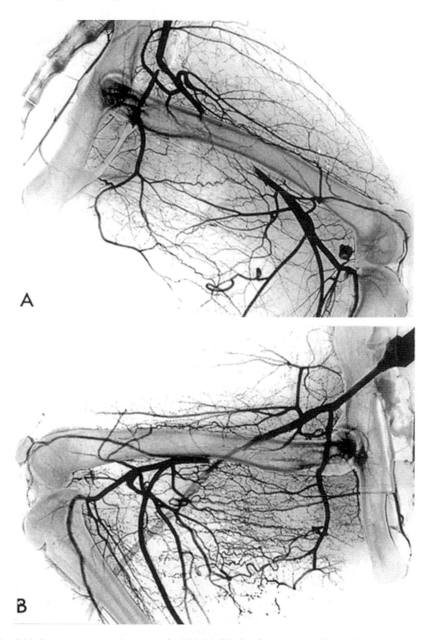

Fig. 5.28 Post-mortem angiograms of rabbit hindlimbs after 1 week of femoral artery occlusion. **Panel A**: without monocyte chemoattractant protein-1 (MCP-1) treatment. **Panel B**: after 1 week of local MCP-1 infusion. The density of collateral vessels with typical corkscrew appearance is markedly increased in hindlimbs of animals treated with MCP-1

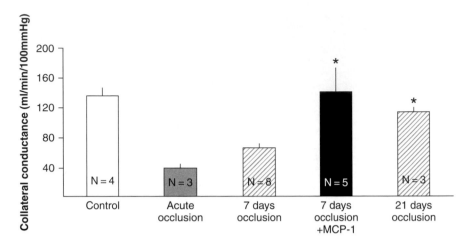

Fig. 5.29 Coronary collateral conductance of rabbit hindlimbs after 1 week of femoral artery occlusion with local monocyte chemoattractant protein-1 (MCP-1) infusion compared with control hindlimbs after acute, 1-week, 3-week, or no occlusion. The conductance in animals treated with MCP-1 was significantly higher than in control animals after the same time of femoral artery occlusion and reached values of non-occluded legs. *p<0.05 compared with acute occlusion

conditions, but 6 months after treatment, these arteriogenic effects of MCP-1 could no longer be observed. This study in Watanabe rabbits did not show an effect of local MCP-1 treatment on serum lipids or on atherosclerosis.[157] In Apo-E-deficient mice (n = 78) treated similarly as described above with local infusion of MCP-1 in two doses or saline after unilateral ligation of the femoral artery, increases in collateral flow could be observed for up to 2 months after the treatment.[158] However, the local treatment did not preclude systemic effects on atherogenesis, leading to increased atherosclerotic plaque formation and changes in cellular content of plaques (Fig. 5.30).[158] The cited clinical and experimental findings render MCP-1 unsuitable for future clinical use.

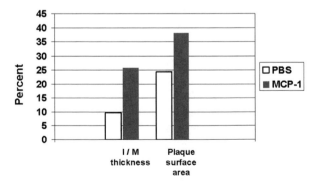

Fig. 5.30 Treatment with high-dose MCP-1 versus saline (PBS) is associated with an increased percentage of aortic intima-to-media thickness (I/M; *left side*), and with more atherosclerotic plaque surface area in total aortas 2 months after initiation of the treatment (*right side*; 24.3±5.2% for PBS versus 38.2±9.5% for MCP-1; p<0.01)

5.3.2.2 Colony-Stimulating Factors

Another group of cytokines exerting a positive effect on arteriogenesis via circulating cells are the GM-CSF and the G-CSF. Although the mechanisms by which GM-CSF induces arteriogenesis are partially unclear, a modulatory effect on monocyte survival with reduced apoptosis has been shown to play a role.[159] Human GM-CSF is a glycoprotein hormone that stimulates the growth of haematopoietic progenitor cells and enhances the functional activity of mature myeloid effector cells. Nimer et al. documented also a serum cholesterol-lowering activity of GM-CSF.[160] In that study, GM-CSF was administered to eight patients with severe aplastic anaemia in an attempt to restore adequate haematopoiesis. Relevant decreases in serum cholesterol concentrations were observed during GM-CSF therapy that were not dependent on changes in the patients' peripheral blood cell counts. Serum cholesterol concentrations returned to baseline in all patients after discontinuation of GM-CSF therapy.[160] Similarly, the goal of a study by Shindo et al. in Watanabe heritable hyperlipidaemic rabbits was not to promote collateral growth but to prevent the progression of atherosclerosis using GM-CSF via changes in the cellular and extracellular composition of atherosclerotic lesions (Fig. 5.31).[159] GM-CSF (10 μg/kg/d) was administered to 4-month-old rabbits (n = 9) 5 days a week for 7.5 months, whereas an equal dose of human serum albumin was administered to controls (n = 9). Of notice, the cholesterol levels were not changed by the treatment. Age-matched 4-month-old rabbits (n = 7) had extensive atheromatous plaques on the inner surface area of the aortic arch. After treatment, the percentages of surface atheromatous plaques to total aortic arch area were 45.0±12.6% in the GM-CSF group and 74.3±11.0% in controls (Fig. 5.32).

Even before the availability of respective experimental data, the mentioned evidence of an anti-atherosclerotic effect of GM-CSF together with the knowledge of monocytes acting at the forefront of arteriogenesis prompted a pilot study in 21 patients with severe CAD in order to investigate safety and

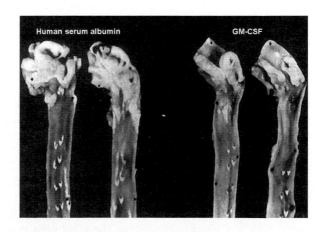

Fig. 5.31 Photographs of inner surface of two aortas in Watanabe heritable hyperlipidaemic rabbits treated with granulocyte–macrophage colony-stimulating factor (GM-CSF; *right 2 aortas*) or human serum albumin (*left 2 aortas*)

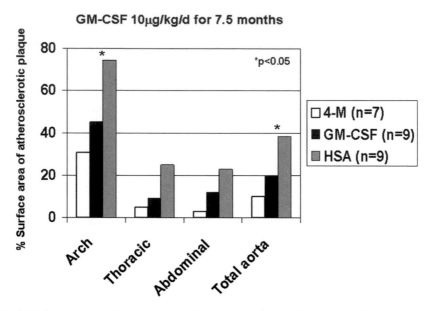

Fig. 5.32 Percentages of inner aortic surface area involving atheromatous plaques (*vertical axis*; same study as in Fig. 5.32). Extent of inner surface area of aorta involving atheromatous plaques was estimated in age-matched 4-month-old Watanabe heritable hyperlipidaemic rabbits (4-M) and GM-CSF-treated or human-serum-albumin (HAS) -treated 11.5-month-old rabbits. A significant reduction in the extent of atheromatous plaques is shown in the aortic arch (p<0.0001) and total aorta (p<0.05) in rabbits treated with GM-CSF (n = 9) compared with control animals (n = 9). The control group of untreated young rabbits has the least extensive atherosclerosis

pro-arteriogenic efficacy of GM-CSF.[144] In this 2-week randomized, placebo-controlled study, the cholesterol-lowering effect of GM-CSF (10 µg/kg subcutaneously every second day) was confirmed (change from 5.3±0.8 mmol/l to 4.1±0.6 mm/l, p = 0.02). The study protocol consisted of an invasive collateral flow index (CFI; Fig. 5.33) measurement immediately before intracoronary injection of 40 µg of GM-CSF (n = 10) or placebo (n = 11) and after a 2-week period with subcutaneous GM-CSF or placebo, respectively. CFI was determined by simultaneous measurement of mean aortic pressure, distal coronary occlusive pressure using intracoronary sensor guidewires and central venous pressure (CVP) (Fig. 5.33). CFI, expressing collateral flow during coronary occlusion relative to normal antegrade flow during vessel patency, changed from 0.21±0.14 to 0.31±0.23 in the GM-CSF group and from 0.30±0.16 to 0.23±0.11 in the placebo group (Figs. 5.33 and 5.34). The treatment-induced difference in CFI was +0.11 ± 0.12 in the GM-CSF group and –0.07±0.12 in the placebo group (p = 0.01). ECG signs of myocardial ischaemia during coronary balloon occlusion occurred in 9 of 10 patients before and 5 of 10 patients after GM-CSF treatment (p = 0.04; Fig. 5.33), whereas they were observed in 5 of 11 patients before and 8 of 11 patients after placebo (p = NS).[144] CFI changes during the treatment period were associated with

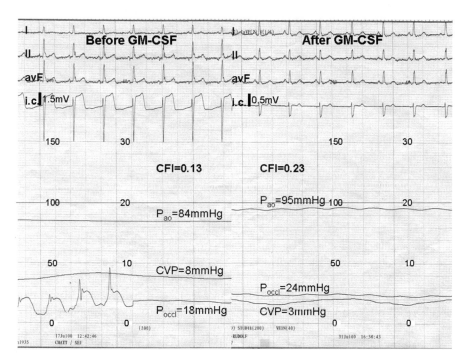

Fig. 5.33 Determination of collateral flow in a patient receiving granulocyte–macrophage colony-stimulating factor (GM-CSF) before (*left*) and after (*right*) therapy. Top, Surface (I, III, and avF) and intracoronary (i.c.) ECG lead recordings are shown. After 1 minute of vessel occlusion before GM-CSF treatment, there are marked ST-segment elevations on the i.c. ECG lead, indicating coronary collaterals insufficient to prevent myocardial ischaemia. After therapy, i.c. ECG signs of myocardial ischaemia have disappeared. CFI (no unit) is calculated by dividing distal coronary mean occlusive pressure (P_{occl}, mmHg) minus CVP (mmHg) by mean aortic pressure (P_{ao}, mmHg) minus CVP; before GM-CSF CFI amounts to $(18–8)/(84–8) = 0.13$. CFI increases to 0.23 after GM-CSF treatment (*right side*)

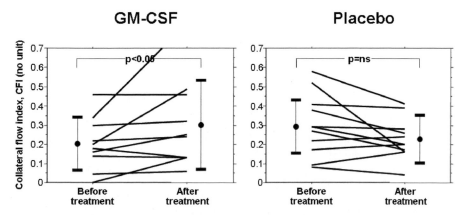

Fig. 5.34 Individual changes of CFI (no unit; *vertical axes*) before and after treatment (*horizontal axes*) in patients who received granulocyte–macrophage colony-stimulating factor (n = 10; left) and placebo (n = 11; right). Dots with error bars indicate mean ± standard deviation

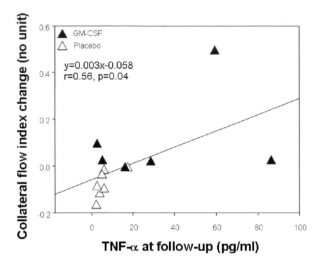

Fig. 5.35 Direct correlation between tumour necrosis factor-α plasma concentration (TNFα; *horizontal axis*) measured after 2 weeks of treatment with GM-CSF (*closed triangles*) or placebo (*open triangles*; same study as in Fig. 5.34) and collateral flow index (CFI) change from baseline to follow-up (*vertical axis*)

changes in TNFα serum concentrations (Fig. 5.35). Also, a direct relationship of the CFI response to GM-CSF and an increase in peripheral blood monocyte concentration were observed (Fig. 5.36).[161]

Experimental data on the arteriogenic effect of GM-CSF in the rabbit model of femoral artery occlusion were published subsequently by Buschmann et al.,[162] who claimed to have discovered a new function of the haemopoietic stem cell factor GM-CSF. GM-CSF was continuously infused for 7 days into the proximal stump of the acutely occluded femoral artery. This produced a marked arteriogenic response as demonstrated by a twofold increase in number and size of collateral arteries on post-mortem angiograms and by the increase in maximal blood flow during vasodilation measured in vivo (Fig. 5.37). When

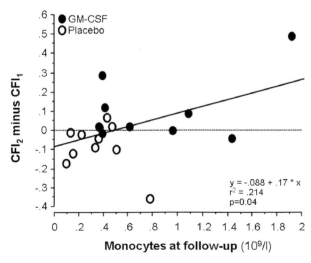

Fig. 5.36 Direct correlation between the number of monocytes per volume of whole blood (*horizontal axis*) measured after 2 weeks of treatment with GM-CSF (*closed symbols*) or placebo (*open symbols*; same study as in Fig. 5.34) and collateral flow index (CFI) change from baseline to follow-up (*vertical axis*)

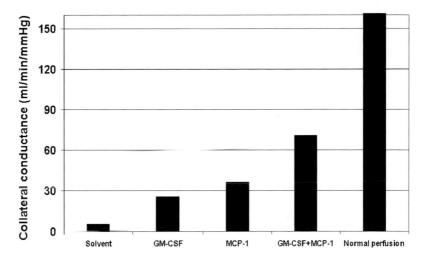

Fig. 5.37 Average values of collateral conductance (*vertical axis*) the first week after femoral artery occlusion in rabbits with continuous infusion of either monocyte chemoattractant protein-1 (MCP-1), granulocyte–macrophage colony-stimulating factor (GM-CSF), a combination of both or solvent over 7 days

GM-CSF and MCP-1 were simultaneously infused, the effects on arteriogenesis were additive on angiograms as well as on conductance (Fig. 5.37). GM-CSF was also able to extend the effect of MCP-1: MCP-1 treatment alone was ineffective when given after the third week following occlusion (Fig. 5.38). When administered together with GM-CSF, about 80% of normal maximal conductance of the artery replaced by collaterals was achieved (Fig. 5.38). In a

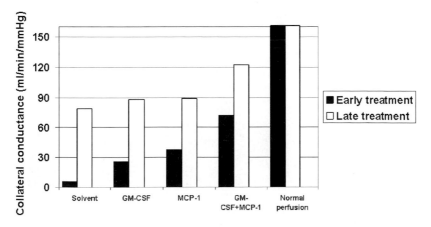

Fig. 5.38 Average values of collateral conductance (*vertical axis*) the first week and 3 weeks after femoral artery ligation and 1 week treatment with either MCP-1, GM-CSF, combination of both or solvent (conductance units in ml/min per mmHg; same study as in Fig. 5.37). Late treatment: treatment in the last week before conductance measurement

rat model of the ischaemic brain (bilateral occlusion of vertebral plus left carotid artery), Buschmann et al. later documented that the subcutaneous application of GM-CSF led to structural and functional improvement of cerebral arterial supply via collaterals (Fig. 5.39).[163] Schneeloch et al. using the same animal model,[164] observed that GM-CSF-induced arteriogenesis reduced energy failure in haemodynamic stroke.

While the above-described first study in patients with CAD has not provided evidence for adverse, pro-atherogenic side effects of GM-CSF,[53] a second, randomized, placebo-controlled safety/efficacy investigation using GM-CSF for the promotion of coronary collateral growth was prematurely stopped, because two patients in the GM-CSF group presented with an acute coronary syndrome on days 7 and 9, respectively, of the 14-day study protocol (Fig. 5.40).[165] Similarly as above,[144] the protocol consisted of an invasive CFI

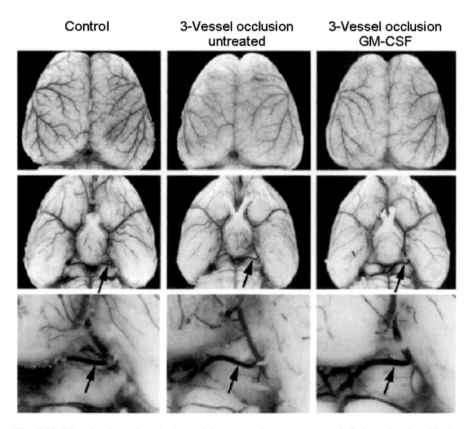

Fig. 5.39 Visualization of cerebral arterial structure by post-mortem infusion of carbon black-stained latex in rats. Comparison of control brain with untreated and granulocyte–macrophage colony-stimulating factor (GM-CSF)-treated brains at 1 week after three-vessel occlusion (bilateral occlusion of vertebral plus left carotid artery). Note the marked enlargement of ipsilateral posterior cerebral artery ($\rightarrow$) in GM-CSF-treated animals compared with the control group and untreated animals

Day 0   Day 9   Day 9

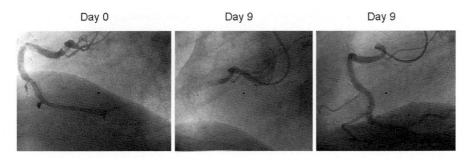

Fig. 5.40 Angiograms showing the right coronary artery of a patient who received granulocyte–macrophage colony-stimulating factor (GM-CSF). On the image taken before treatment (day 0), multiple proximal stenoses with hazy appearance are visible. At day 9 of the treatment protocol, the patient was admitted to the hospital with an acute coronary syndrome; the extensively calcified right coronary artery was proximally occluded (*middle panel*), and could be successfully recanalized (*right panel*)

measurement in a stenotic, but differently, also in a normal coronary artery before and after a 2-week period with subcutaneous-only GM-CSF (10 μg/kg; n – 7) or placebo (n = 7).[165] CFI in the placebo group remained unchanged, whereas it increased from 0.116±0.05 to 0.159±0.07 in the GM-CSF group (Figs. 5.41 and 5.42). Among 11 determined cytokines, chemokines and their monocytic receptor concentrations, the treatment-induced change in CFI was predicted by the respective change in TNFα concentration (Fig. 5.43).

The fact that none of the 40 atherosclerotic patients with peripheral artery disease, included in a 14-day randomized, placebo-controlled study[166] on the collateral-promoting effect of GM-CSF suffered a serious adverse event, may challenge the above-described interpretation of GM-CSF-induced atherosclerotic coronary plaque rupture by Zbinden et al. [165]. However, for ethical reasons, safety issues of a drug cannot be assessed by the same statistical rules as efficacy, i.e. already the suspicion of a safety risk is sufficient irrespective of statistical relevance. With regard to safety aspects of G-CSF, Hill et al. reported 2 of 16 refractory angina patients treated with this substance for over 5 days having had suffered an acute myocardial infarction including one with fatal outcome.[167] On the other hand, none of the larger clinical trials found an increased incidence of adverse events,[166] and also, no increase in in-stent neointima formation was observed.[168] Also, a recent meta-analysis on the clinical use of G-CSF in acute myocardial infarction (n = 445) did not observe an increased rate of major adverse cardiac events among patients treated with G-CSF in comparison to control patients.[169]

In the cited investigation by van Royen et al., patients with moderate or severe intermittent claudication were treated with placebo or subcutaneously applied GM-CSF (10 μg/kg) for a period of 14 days.[166] GM-CSF treatment led to a strong increase in total white blood cell count and C-reactive protein. Monocyte fraction initially increased, but decreased thereafter as compared

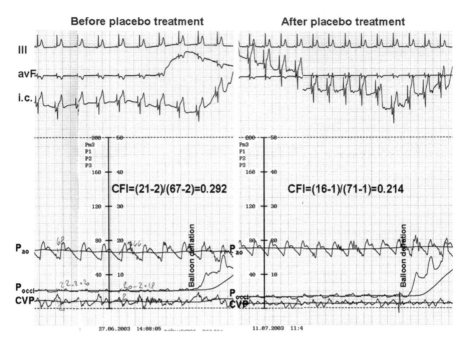

Fig. 5.41 Determination of collateral flow index (CFI) in a patient who received placebo before (*left panel*) and after treatment (*right panel*). Surface (III, avF) and intracoronary ECG lead recordings are shown in the upper part of the panels. After 1 minute of vessel occlusion before and after treatment, there are ST-segment elevations on the intracoronary ECG lead indicating coronary collaterals insufficient to prevent myocardial ischaemia. CFI is calculated by dividing distal mean coronary occlusive pressure (P_{occl}, mmHg) minus central venous pressure (CVP, mmHg) by mean aortic pressure (P_{ao}, mmHg) minus CVP. In comparison to Fig. 5.33, the constant value of CFI in the absence of arteriogenic treatment is illustrated here

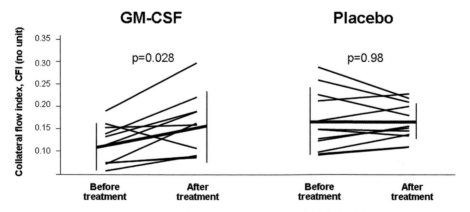

Fig. 5.42 Individual data of collateral flow index (CFI, *vertical axis; black lines*) obtained in stenotic as well as normal coronary arteries before and after treatment (*horizontal axis*) in patients of the granulocyte–macrophage colony-stimulating factor (GM-CSF, *left panel*) and the placebo group (*right panel*). The blue lines connect the mean (± standard deviation) CFI before and after treatment

Fig. 5.43 Correlation between treatment-induced change in collateral flow index (ΔCFI, *vertical axis*) and the respective change in tumour necrosis factor-α concentration (ΔTNFα, *horizontal axis*). Black symbols indicate values obtained in stenotic, blue symbols in normal vessels, respectively. *Value after minus value before treatment

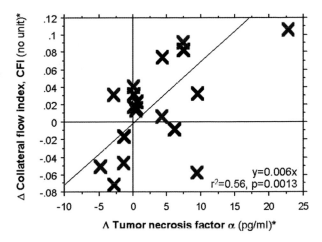

with baseline. Both the placebo group and the treatment group showed a significant increase in walking distance at day 14 (placebo: 127 ± 67 versus 184 ± 87 meters, p = 0.03, GM-CSF: 126 ± 66 versus 189 ± 141 meters, p = 0.04) and at day 90. Change in walking time, the primary endpoint of the study, was not different between groups. No change in ankle–brachial index was found in response to GM-CSF treatment at day 14 or at day 90. Since GM-CSF regularly induces flu-like symptoms as a side effect (more muscle pain, fever and loss of appetite in the GM-CSF group), the absence of efficacy in the cited study could have been due to a disadvantage in the GM-CSF group of a drug-induced impaired exercise tolerance.

In a pig model of peripheral artery disease, Grundmann et al., on the other hand, documented pro-arteriogenic properties of GM-CSF in this larger animal species, revealing comparable efficacy of continuous and intermittent intra-arterial infusion.[170] Twenty-four pigs underwent unilateral occlusion of the right femoral artery and received GM-CSF continuously, GM-CSF intermittently, or saline. After 1 week, collateral conductance was determined under maximal vasodilatation with adenosine and by using a pump-driven extracorporal shunt system. Collateral conductance in ml/min/mmHg showed a significant stimulatory effect of GM-CSF on arteriogenesis (saline 37.7 ± 5.4; GM-CSF continuous 69.2 ± 12.5; GM-CSF intermittent 71.5 ± 11.1; Fig. 5.44).[170]

The related G-CSF is another potent agent to mobilize bone marrow-derived stem cells (see below) and was found to reduce myocardial damage and ventricular dysfunction following myocardial infarction in the pig model.[171] Several mechanisms of action including the stimulation of arteriogenesis and angiogenesis have been hypothesized to contribute to this beneficial effect, since G-CSF receptors are expressed on cardiomyocytes and endothelial cells as well as circulating cells and their precursors. However, the arteriogenic effect of G-CSF has not been tested so far in patients with CAD. Preliminary data from our laboratory obtained in 52 patients with chronic stable CAD who underwent

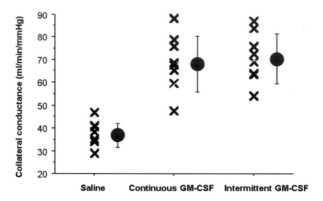

Fig. 5.44 Individual collateral conductance measurements (*black cross symbols; filled blue circles*: mean ± standard deviation) under maximal vasodilatation achieved by continuous adenosine infusion and extra-corporal circulation. Collateral conductance (mL/min/mmHg; *vertical axis*) as a parameter of flow-increase per increase in blood pressure gradient is higher in the granulocyte–macrophage colony-stimulating factor (GM-CSF)-treated groups, although there is no significant difference between continuous and intermittent drug application

invasive CFI measurements before and after 14 days of treatment randomized to G-CSF (10 μg/kg subcutaneously every second day) or placebo have revealed a statistically relevant benefit of G-CSF with an absolute change of CFI of $+0.05$ (Fig. 5.45). The arteriogenic effect of G-CSF appears to be associated with the respective change in peripheral blood CD34$^+$ mononuclear cells (Fig. 5.46).

The monocyte colony-stimulating factor (M-CSF) has not been investigated in clinical trials for cardiovascular disease so far. Exogenous application of M-CSF following experimental myocardial infarction in rats has had beneficial effects on myocardial repair and ventricular function.[172] However, further

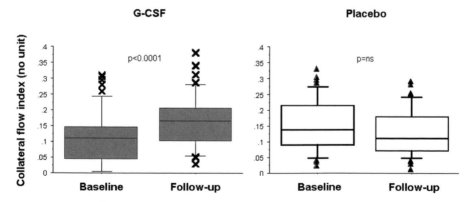

Fig. 5.45 Values of collateral flow index (CFI, vertical axis; mean, 75 and 95% confidence intervals) obtained in stenotic as well as normal coronary arteries of patients before and after treatment (*horizontal axis*) withgranulocyte colony-stimulating factor (G-CSF, *left panel*) or placebo (*right panel*)

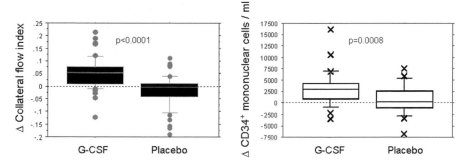

Fig. 5.46 Change (Δ) in collateral flow index and CD34⁺ progenitor cell count (*vertical axis*; value at follow-up minus value at baseline) during 2 weeks of treatment with granulocyte colony-stimulating factor (G-CSF) or placebo (*horizontal axis*). The box plots indicate mean, 75 and 95% (*error bars*) confidence interval

investigations on its arteriogenic potential in humans are discouraged by its documented promotion of tumour angiogenesis and atherosclerosis.[173,174]

5.3.2.3 Transforming Growth Factor β1

Another cytokine undergoing preclinical testing for arteriogenesis is TGFβ1. This pluripotent cytokine is overexpressed in regions of collateral artery growth. Aside from its effects on endothelial cells,[175] it is also a chemoattractant and activator of monocytes.[176] In a New Zealand White rabbit model of femoral artery ligation, van Royen et al. observed increased expression of active TGFβ1 around proliferating arteries, and the exogenous application of TGFβ1 led to an increase in both the number of visible collateral arteries as well as the conductance of the collateral circulation.[177] Fluorescence activated cell sorting analysis showed an increase in the expression of the MAC-1 receptor in both rabbit and human monocytes after treatment with TGFβ1.[177] The strong arteriogenic action is particularly interesting because TGFβ1 might also have a beneficial effect on the underlying atherosclerosis.[178,179] Grainger et al. showed that a population of patients with advanced atherosclerosis had less active TGFβ1 in their sera than patients with normal coronary arteries, with a fivefold difference in average concentration between the two groups.[179] This correlation with atherosclerosis was stronger than for other known major risk factors. The transition from stable to rupture-prone atherosclerotic plaques involves many processes, including an altered balance between inflammation and fibrosis. An important mediator of both appears to be TGFβ1, and an important role for TGFβ1 in atherogenesis has been postulated. Lutgens et al. determined the in vivo effects of TGFβ1 inhibition on plaque progression and phenotype in atherosclerosis, and found a crucial role for TGFβ1 in the maintenance of the balance between inflammation and fibrosis in atherosclerotic plaques.[178] Recently, Grundmann et al. tested a new intra-arterial, stent-based delivery platform for pro-arteriogenic compounds to induce arteriogenesis via TGFβ1 release.[180] For continuous delivery of a pro-arteriogenic substance, such a local platform could be essential. Different polymer stent coatings were tested regarding their suitability for cytokine release. Fifty-four rabbits underwent implantation of bare-metal stents, polymer-only coated stents and polymer-coated TGFβ1-eluting stents in the iliac artery, or bolus infusion of TGFβ1 and subsequent femoral artery ligation.[180] Perfusion measurements revealed an increase in collateral conductance after TGFβ1 stent implantation compared with the control groups (Fig. 5.47).[180]

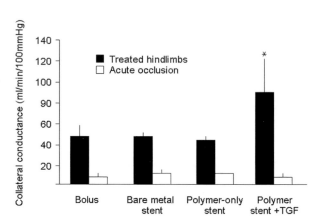

Fig. 5.47 Microsphere-based assessment of collateral conductance (*vertical axis*). Implantation of transforming growth factor (TGF)-β1-eluting stents results in an increase in collateral conductance compared with animals that received a bolus infusion of TGFβ1 (bolus), a bare-metal stent (BMS), or a stent coated with the polymer only

Conversely, new insights regarding the pathogenesis of Marfan syndrome have shown fibrillin-1 deficiency associated with excess signalling by TGFβ1.[181] TGFβ antagonists like the AT1 antagonist losartan have shown success in improving or preventing several manifestations of Marfan syndrome in these mice, including aortic aneurysm.[181] The link of these findings to arteriogenesis may be found in the upregulation of MMP-2 and -9 during progression of aortic aneurysm in Marfan syndrome, which has been shown to be accompanied by an overexpression of TGFβ with degenerated elastic fibres.[182] So far, it is unknown whether hypertensive patients undergoing a long-term therapy with an AT1 blocker exhibit more often a poorly functional collateral circulation than those with anti-hypertensive treatment not involving the renin–angiotensin system.

5.3.2.4   Fibroblast Growth Factors

During arteriogenesis, peri-vascular macrophages are an important source of bFGF, which stimulates the proliferation of smooth muscle cells via activation of the FGF-receptor 1.[147] Deindl et al. reported that collateral artery growth in its early phase is associated with an increased expression of FGF receptor 1 (FGFR-1) and syndecan-4 on mRNA and protein levels as well as with an increased kinase activity of FGFR-1 in a rabbit model of arteriogenesis.[183]

Notwithstanding this finding and that of an increased bFGF concentration in patients with chronic total occlusion and high coronary collateral resistance,[184] genetic knockout of the bFGF gene does not affect neovascularization following femoral artery ligation in mice.[185] However and in the experimental animal model, exogenous application of bFGF results in a stimulation of arteriogenesis.[49] In 190 patients with intermittent claudication caused by infra-inguinal atherosclerosis, Lederman et al. tested the efficacy of bFGF on 90-day change in peak walking time (random assignment to bilateral intra-arterial infusions of placebo on days 1 and 30, n = 63; to bFGF single dose 30 mg/kg, n = 68; or double dose n = 61).[186] Peak walking time at 90 days was increased by 0.60 min with placebo, by 1.77 min with single-dose and by 1.54 min with double-dose. The difference between groups was not statistically different (p = 0.075). However, the results were interpreted by the authors as evidence of clinical therapeutic angiogenesis by intra-arterial infusion of an angiogenic protein.[186] As described in the above chapter on angiogenesis, large randomized clinical trials on the effect of FGFs in CAD were similarly disappointing with regard to clinical outcome parameters.

5.3.2.5 Statins

Therapy with 3-hydroxy-3-mehtylglutaryl coenzyme A reductase inhibitors (statins) has been investigated as a possible means to improve the function of circulating monocytes and EPC. Experimental data have documented impairment of the pro-arteriogenic action of monocytes under conditions of hypercholesterolaemia that can be potentially reversed by statin therapy. In a study by Czepluch et al., [187] the migratory response of monocytes to the arteriogenic ligands VEGF-A and MCP-1 in hypercholesterolaemic CAD patients (n = 14), hypercholesterolaemic controls (n = 8) and age-matched healthy controls (n = 19) was analysed.[187] VEGF-A-induced monocyte chemotaxis was impaired in hypercholesterolaemic CAD patients when compared with age-matched healthy controls (p < 0.001). The same was true for the migratory response to MCP-1 (p < 0.001). VEGF-A- and MCP-1-induced monocyte chemotaxis of hypercholesterolaemic controls was also decreased in comparison with the healthy control group, but not as severe as that observed in the hypercholesterolaemic CAD patients.[187] Also, statins have been reported to enhance mobilization of EPC.[188] Since statins enhance endothelial NO availability by both increasing its production and reducing NO inactivation, Landmesser et al. studied the effect of statin treatment on endothelial NO availability after myocardial infarction and tested its role for EPC mobilization, myocardial neovascularization, LV dysfunction, remodelling and survival after myocardial infarction.[188] Atorvastatin improved mobilization of EPC and myocardial neovascularization of the infarct border zone in wild-type mice after myocardial infarction while having no effect in eNOS knockout mice. LV dysfunction and interstitial fibrosis were markedly attenuated by the statin in wild-type mice, whereas no effect was observed in the knockout mice.[188]

Neovascularization and capillary density, respectively, were assessed in that study by counting endothelial cells in high-power micropscopic fields focused on four areas within the infarct border zone.

Results from clinical work on the arteriogenic effect of statins have been controversial. In a retrospective analysis by Pourati et al.,[189] 51 patients were taking statins before admission and 43 were not. Their angiograms were reviewed and coronary collaterals angiographically graded from 0 to 3. The statin-treated group revealed a higher mean collateral score compared with the patients not taking statins (2.05 vs 1.52, p = 0.005). Another clinical study by Dincer et al., in 149 diabetic patients employing also angiographic collateral qualification, observed that statin therapy and the presence of stable angina pectoris were the only independent predictors of good collateral formation.[190] The methodological ambiguity of such low-powered clinical studies using post-hoc analysis of a very blunt instrument for collateral assessment, i.e. non-occlusive angiographic collateral scoring, is emphasized by the finding in Dincer et al.'s study that coronary artery stenosis severity was *not* one of the factors independently predicting collateral degree.[190] Coronary stenosis severity is *the* most consistently found variable across different species influencing the state of the collateral circulation. Contradictory to the mentioned study results, Zbinden et al. found that in a total of 500 CAD patients (186 with and 314 patients without statin treatment) who underwent quantitative CFI measurements long before data analysis for the respective study, the statin treatment was not associated with CFI.[191]

5.4 Cell-Based Promotion of the Collateral Circulation

Vasculogenesis is the process of in situ formation of blood vessels from EPC. The EPC were considered restricted to embryonic development, until their occurrence at sites of angiogenesis in the adult organism changed this view. There has been evidence in favour of endogenous EPC mobilization and incorporation into new blood vessels in response to tissue ischaemia. Flow cytometry revealed that circulating CD34$^+$ mononuclear cells significantly increased in patients with acute myocardial infarction. The functional impact of EPC-induced vasculogenesis on blood flow restoration has not been established yet. Estimates of the extent of BMC EPC incorporation into ischaemic tissue differ considerably between 0 and 50%. Another way than vasculogenesis for progenitor cells to contribute to neovascularization could be via a paracrine effect, i.e. via release of pro-angiogenic and pro-arteriogenic factors to the ischaemic myocardium.

All clinical trials have been performed in the setting of acute or chronic myocardial infarction, whereby coronary bone marrow cell therapy has been inconsistently found to improve LV ejection fraction. If one of the mechanisms for myocardial salvage is the putative action of stem cells on neovascularization, then no substantial effect on systolic function can be expected in myocardial infarction, because coronary collateral growth should have taken place before this event in order to be effective.

5.4.1 Introduction

Although cell-based strategies for improving myocardial or lower extremity ischaemia have been shown to be successful in animals, clinical trials to date have not revealed consistently beneficial results.[192] Even more so, the mechanism(s) by which a possible benefit is conferred remains obscure, i.e. it is uncertain whether it is angiogenesis, arteriogenesis, vasculogenesis or a combination of them, which leads to the uncertain effect of ischaemia reduction. Hence, the following paragraph on vasculogenesis does not imply the latter to be the principal mechanism involved in cell-based collateral promotion, but vasculogenesis was selected to be described here because of its intimate connection to EPC.

5.4.2 Vasculogenesis

Vasculogenesis is the process of in situ formation of blood vessels from EPC. Endothelial and haematopoietic cells share a common progenitor, the haemangioblast. In the yolk sac, haemangioblasts form cellular aggregates or blood islands, in which the inner cell population differentiates into haematopoiteic precursors, and the outer population into endothelial cells. In the past, EPC or angioblasts were considered restricted to embryonic development until their isolation from peripheral blood and indications of their occurrence at sites of angiogenesis in the adult organism changed this paradigm.[193,194] It is possible that in association with angiogenesis and arteriogenesis, vasculogenesis contributes to neovascularization in adult tissues, though the extent of this contribution has not been clarified yet.[195] EPC and haematopoietic progenitors share many surface markers such as CD34, CD133, Flk-1, Tie-2, c-Kit and Sca-1. Therefore, no straightforward definition of EPC exists. EPC have been shown to express vascular endothelial cadherin and an orphan receptor specifically expressed on EPC (AC133), which is lost once the EPC differentiates into a mature endothelial cell.[196] In addition to haematopoietic stem cells, EPC can originate from other bone marrow stem cells such as the highly enriched haematopoietic stem cells, the so-called side population cells (CD34$^-$, c-Kit$^+$ and Sca-1$^+$),[197] and multipotent adult progenitor cells (CD34$^-$, CD45$^-$, c-Kit$^-$ and GlyA$^-$,).[198] Factors that induce EPC mobilization from bone marrow to the peripheral circulation stimulate also their homing to an angiogenic, arteriogenic or vasculogenic site, but signals for tissue-specific differentiation have not been defined yet. There has been evidence in favour of endogenous EPC mobilization and incorporation into new blood vessels in response to tissue ischaemia.[199,200] Shintani et al. investigated whether EPC and their putative precursor, CD34$^+$ mononuclear cells, are mobilized into peripheral blood in acute ischaemic events in humans.[200] Flow cytometry revealed that circulating CD34$^+$ mononuclear cell counts significantly increased in patients with acute myocardial infarction (n = 16), peaking on day 7 after onset, whereas they were unchanged in control subjects (n = 8) who had no evidence of cardiac ischaemia. During culture, peripheral blood CD34$^+$ mononuclear cells formed multiple cell clusters, and EPC-like attaching cells with endothelial cell lineage markers sprouted from clusters. In patients with acute myocardial infarction, more cell clusters and EPC developed from cultured peripheral blood CD34$^+$ mononuclear cells obtained on day 7 than those on day 1.[200] However, the functional impact of EPC-induced vasculogenesis on blood flow restoration has not been established yet. Haematopoietic stimulators such as GM-CSF,[201] G-CSF,[202] Ang-1,[203] SDF-1[196] and VEGF[203] could contribute to EPC mobilization and homing. Human EPC expanded ex vivo and injected in athymic nude mice with an ischaemic hindlimb[204] or athymic nude rats with myocardial infarction[205] were incorporated in neovasculature, and improved blood flow and myocardial function. Freshly aspirated bone marrow delivered into ischaemic myocardium of pigs that underwent ameroid constriction of a coronary artery has been shown to augment coronary vascularity.[206] Estimates of the extent of BMC incorporation into ischaemic tissue differ considerably between 3% endothelial cells and 0.02% cardiomyocytes, respectively, originating from bone marrow and much higher rates.[197] Orlic et al. reported that newly formed murine myocardium occupied 68% of the infarcted portion of the ventricle, 9 days after transplanting autologous bone marrow cells.[207] The developing tissue comprised proliferating myocytes and vascular structures. The authors concluded that locally delivered bone marrow cells could generate de novo myocardium, ameliorating the outcome of CAD.[207]

The highly variable incorporation rates of trans-differentiation are difficult to explain. This is even more so in the context of studies such as that by Ziegelhoeffer et al.,[154] who found no incorporation of BMC into the adult growing vasculature of C57BL/6 wild-type mice. In that study, mouse models of hindlimb ischaemia (arteriogenesis and angiogenesis) and tumour growth were used.[154] The wild-type mice were lethally irradiated and transplanted with bone marrow cells from littermates expressing enhanced green fluorescent protein. Six weeks after bone marrow transplantation, the animals underwent unilateral femoral artery occlusions with or without pretreatment with VEGF or were subcutaneously implanted with fibrosarcoma cells. After 7 and 21 days of surgery, proximal hindlimb muscles with growing collateral arteries and ischaemic gastrocnemius muscles as well as grown tumours and various organs were excised for histological analysis. No green fluorescent protein signals could be colocalized with endothelial or smooth muscle cell markers. The use of high-power laser scanning confocal microscopy occasionally uncovered false-positive results because of overlap of different fluorescent signals from adjacent cells. Nevertheless, accumulations of green fluorescent protein-positive cells were observed around growing collateral arteries and in ischaemic distal hindlimbs. These cells were identified as fibroblasts, pericytes and primarily leucocytes that stained positive for several growth factors and chemokines (Fig. 5.48).[154] Another way than vasculogenesis for progenitor cells to contribute to neovascularization could be via a paracrine effect. The release of pro-angiogenic and pro-arteriogenic factors to the ischaemic myocardium by cells recruited from the bone marrow may lead to collateral growth and inhibition of apoptosis.[206,208,209]

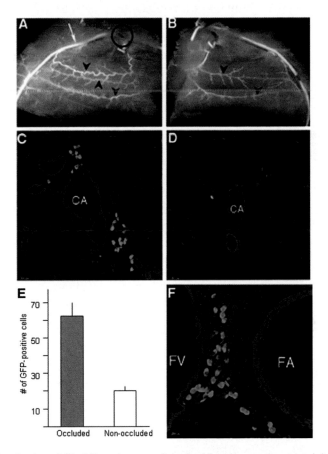

Fig. 5.48 Panels A and B: Microphotographs of adductor muscles containing collateral arteries filled with bismuth/gelatine contrast agent. **Panel A**: Corkscrew pattern of growing collateral arteries (*arrowheads*) connecting the deep femoral artery (*red arrow*) with the femoral artery (*white arrow*) 21 days after femoral artery ligation (*circle* ndicates ligation site). **Panel B**: Pre-existing collateral vessels (*arrowheads*) on the contralateral non-ligated side. **Panel C, D, and E**: Accumulation of bone marrow-derived cells around growing collateral arteries. Red indicates BS-1 lectin; blue, nuclei. **Panel C**: Numerous green fluorescent protein (GFP)-positive cells are clustered around growing collateral artery (CA) 3 weeks after femoral artery occlusion. **Panel D**: Only a few GFP-positive cells are found around quiescent collateral arteries. **Panel E**: Graph showing quantification of the number of GFP-positive cells around collateral arteries. A threefold, significant increase was found in growing (3 weeks after surgery) compared with quiescent collateral arteries. **Panel F**: GFP-positive cells were frequently found in the perivascular space between the femoral artery (FA) and femoral vein (FV). Red indicates αactin; blue, nuclei

5.4.3 Cell-Based Therapy of Myocardial Ischaemia in Humans

Aside from myocardial repair, the stimulation of collateral growth (angio-, arterio- and/or vasculogenesis) is one of the goals of the steadily increasing number of clinical trials using bone marrow or progenitor cell populations for the treatment of patients with CAD and peripheral artery disease. Whereas the clinical evaluation of isolated and expanded tissue resident stem cells is just beginning,[210] results of several more or less sizeable, randomized clinical trials infusing bone marrow mononuclear cells are available (Table 5.2). Chen et al. investigated 69 patients who underwent primary PCI within 12 hours after onset of acute myocardial infarction.[211] They were randomized to receive intracoronary injection of autologous bone marrow mesenchymal stem cells or standard saline. Several imagining techniques demonstrated that bone marrow-derived stem cells improved myocardial perfusion but also LV function (Table 5.2).[211] Wollert et al. observed, in 60 CAD patients with acute myocardial infarction and primary PCI, that 6 months after bone marrow cell or saline injection, mean global LV ejection fraction had increased by 0.7 percentage points in the control group and by 6.7 percentage points in the bone marrow cell group ($p = 0.0026$).[212] Transfer of bone marrow cells enhanced LV systolic function primarily in myocardial segments adjacent to the infarcted area. Cell transfer did not increase the risk of adverse clinical events, in-stent restenosis, or pro-arrhythmic effects. In a follow-up study of the same group, no long-term benefit on LV systolic function of a single intracoronary bone marrow cell injection could be observed.[213] The randomized Autologous Stem cell Transplantation in Acute Myocardial Infarction (ASTAMI) trial included 100 patients, and did not find an effect of intracoronary BMC injection on LV ejection fraction 6 months after primary PCI (Table 5.2).[18] A similar study in 67 patients with acute ST-elevation myocardial infarction was performed by Janssens et al.[214,] who, in addition to LV ejection fraction measurement, obtained myocardial perfusion and oxidative metabolism with serial positron emission tomography. Mean global LV ejection fraction 4 days after PCI was $47\pm8\%$ in controls and $49\pm7\%$ in BMC patients, and increased after 4 months to $49\pm11\%$ and $52\pm9\%$ (Table 5.2).[214] In patients with acute as well as chronic healed myocardial infarction who underwent PCI of the culprit coronary lesion, Schächinger et al.[20] and Assmus et al.[19] observed a beneficial effect of coronary bone marrow injection on LV ejection fraction (Table 5.2). Meluzin et al. studied the impact of the dose of transplanted cells on myocardial function and perfusion in patients with acute myocardial infarction.[215] At 3 months of follow-up, the baseline peak systolic velocities of longitudinal LV contraction of the infarcted wall of 5.2, 4.5 and 4.3 cm/s in the control, low-dose (10^7 cells) and high-dose (10^8 cells) BMC groups increased by 0.0, 0.5 ($p < 0.05$ vs control group) and 0.9 cm/s ($p < 0.05$ vs low dose group, $p < 0.01$ vs control group), respectively, as demonstrated by

Table 5.2 Bone marrow/stem cell trials: Randomized clinical trials

Study	Year	Cells	Disease	Patients	Perfusion assessment	Perfusion endpoint	Primary endpoint	Result	Reference
Chen et al.	2004	BMC	CAD, AMI	69	PET	Positive	LVEF	Positive	{Chen, 2004 768}[211]
BOOST	2004	BMC	CAD, AMI	60	No	–	LVEF	Positive	{Wollert, 2004 774}[212]
ASTAMI	2006	BMC	CAD, AMI	100	No	–	LVEF	Negative	{Lunde, 2006 558}[18]
Janssens et al.	2006	BMC	CAD, AMI	67	PET	Negative	LVEF	Negative	{Janssens, 2006 769}[214]
REPAIR-AMI	2006	BMC	CAD, AMI	204	No	–	LVEF	Positive	{Schächinger, 2006 561}[20]
TOPCARE-CHF	2006	BMC, Progenitors	CAD	92	No	–	LVEF	Positive	{Assmus, 2006 559}[19]
Meluzín et al.	2006	BMC	CAD, AMI	66	SPECT	Negative	LVEF	Positive	{Meluzín, 2006 770}[215]
MAGIC Cell-3-DES	2006	PBSC	CAD, AMI	96	No	–	LVEF	Positive*	{Kang, 2006 771}[216]
Ruan et al.	2005	BMC	CAD, AMI	20	No	–	LV TDI	Positive	{Ruan, 2005 773}[217]
TCT-STAMI	2006	BMC	CAD, AMI	20	SPECT	Positive	LVEF	Positive	{Ge, 2006 772}[218]
HEBE	2008	BMC	CAD, AMI	Enrolling					{Hirsch, 2008 765}[224]
Baxter		CD34$^+$	CAD	Enrolling					
BONAMI		BMC	CAD	Enrolling					

AMI = acute myocardial infarction; BMC = bone marrow-derived cells; CAD = coronary artery disease; LVEF = left ventricular ejection fraction; PBSC = peripheral blood stem cells; PET = positron emission tomography; SPECT = single photon emission computed tomography.
* Negative for old myocardial infarction.

Doppler tissue imaging.[215] Baseline LV ejection fractions of 42, 42 and 41% in control, low-dose and high-dose groups increased by 2, 3 and 5%, respectively (Table 5.2). Intracoronary infusion of mobilized peripheral blood stem cells with G-CSF was found to improve LV ejection fraction and remodelling in patients with acute myocardial infarction but this was less definite in patients with old myocardial infarction.[216] Two other small trials investigating the efficacy of coronary BMC injection in the setting of acute myocardial infarction were positive (Table 5.2).[217,218]

Considering the evidence from the described clinical trials on cell-based therapy of myocardial ischaemia, several conclusions can be drawn: The majority of trials has been performed in the setting of acute myocardial infarction, and in this situation, coronary bone marrow cell therapy has been inconsistently found to improve LV ejection fraction. If one of the mechanisms for myocardial salvage is the hypothesized action of BMC on neovascularization, then a substantial effect on LV ejection fraction can conceptually not be expected in acute myocardial infarction, because coronary collateral growth should have taken place already before this event in order to be effective. The presence of sufficiently preformed coronary collateral vessels is essential for rescuing myocardial tissue and reducing cardiac mortality in the event of an acute coronary occlusion.[219] Collateral growth in response to an angiogenic or arteriogenic stimulus requires several days to weeks to occur (Figs. 5.49 and 5.50),[133] and as a consequence, the newly developed collateral vessels are not able to prevent myocardial necrosis if they are not sufficiently functional before coronary occlusion. If neovascularization occurs only after infarction, it is just the border zone or penumbra of the infarct territory, which may benefit from improved myocardial perfusion. In the above-cited trials, actual myocardial perfusion has been obtained only in four of them, whereby just half have revealed augmented perfusion following BMC treatment. Thus, the hypothesis of a pro-angiogenic effect of cell-based therapy for myocardial ischaemia has hardly been tested nor has it been verified.

In this context, it is not surprising that G-CSF therapy with mobilization of bone marrow stem cells soon after acute myocardial infarction in the STEM cells in Myocardial Infarction (STEMMI) trial, did not improve LV systolic function when compared to placebo.[220] These results have been confirmed by the REVIVAL-2 trial and the G-CSF-STEMI trial.[221,222] G-CSF was hypothesized to be beneficial on the myocardium both indirectly by mobilizing bone marrow stem cells into the peripheral circulation and directly by inhibiting apoptosis of myocardial cells.[223] The efficacy – though inconsistently reported – of direct coronary bone marrow injection in acute myocardial infarction appears all the more puzzling in light of the mentioned negative clinical effect of G-CSF on systolic ventricular function, which has also been confirmed by a recent meta-analysis in 445 patients with acute myocardial infarction.[169] Why should pharmacological mobilization of bone

Fig. 5.49 Post-mortem angiograms of rabbit hindlimbs without (**a**) and after acute femoral artery ligation (**b**). One week after femoral artery ligation, several collateral arteries spanning the occlusion site can be detected (**c**). Continuous infusion of monocyte chemoattractant protein-1 (MCP-1) for the same time period significantly increases collateral vessel density (**d**). Animals treated for a 1-week period 3 weeks after femoral artery occlusion showed no significant difference between phosphate-buffered saline (PBS; **e**) and MCP-1 (**f**) infusion

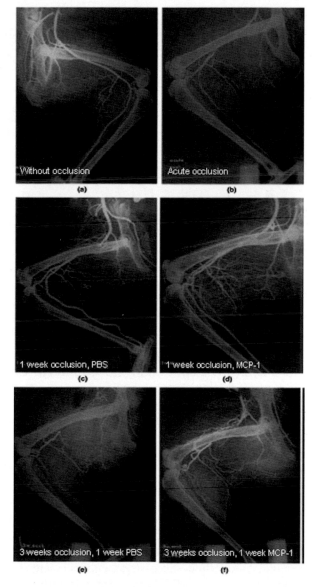

marrow be useless, but direct coronary infusion of bone marrow aspirated cells be efficacious?

Further trials in patients with acute myocardial infarction undergoing primary PCI and BMC injection are ongoing, and in part, more meaningful endpoints aside from LV ejection fraction are obtained, such as gadolinium-derived infarct size by magnetic resonance imaging (Table 5.2).[224]

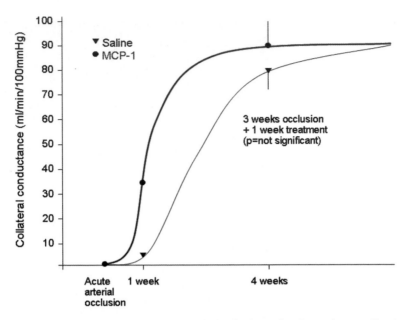

Fig. 5.50 Increase in collateral conductance index in time after femoral artery ligation for monocyte chemoattractant protein-1 (MCP-1) -treated and control animals

5.5 Physical Promotion of the Collateral Circulation

Any physical strategy for chronic augmentation of vascular fluid shear stress indirectly leads to monocyte activation, i.e. the pivotal element in the context of arteriogenesis. Aside from the beneficial process of arterial remodelling, increased shear stress and activated monocytes are also related to the harmful development of atherosclerosis. Thus, the risk of suffering an acute coronary syndrome in an untrained individual is elevated by a factor of 100 *during* an event of physical exercise. However, the absolute risk of such an event can be lowered to baseline at rest depending on the number and level of exercise training sessions. While recurring physical exercise is the most common way of repetitively increasing fluid shear stress, several other forms of global or regional blood fluid shear stress enhancement also exist: extension of the endothelial contact to fluid shear stress, by induction of bradycardia. Diastolic pressure augmentation with elevation of coronary flow and thus, fluid shear stress. An unevenly distributed coronary back pressure with elevation at the origin and lowering at the orifice of collaterals could have an arteriogenic effect.

It is primarily the repetitive increase in cardiac output during physical exercise sessions, which offers itself as the candidate physiological promoter of arteriogenesis. However, endurance exercise training has several effects, and variables alternative to augmented cardiac output may cause structural and functional changes of coronary arteries. It has been proved in the living healthy human without CAD that endurance exercise training augments coronary collateral function. In patients, a self-selection bias for or against exercise training may play an important role in the study outcome, i.e. the patient with a priori well-developed collaterals may choose to engage in exercise and this may be falsely interpreted as an arteriogenic effect of exercise. Such a selection bias is likely to be present even in *randomized* human investigations with an exercise and sedentary group. The first studies in humans on the arteriogenic effect of exercise training did not provide positive evidence; they were all statistically underpowered and employed coronary angiographic collateral grading as the study endpoint. A study in 178 patients with CAD who underwent allocation to a 1-year exercise programme or to a 'usual care' programme could not discern between the effect of CAD progression and exercise on angiographic collateral degree. Quantitatively obtained coronary collateral function in 40 patients who underwent initial removal of the most severe atherosclerotic lesion was positively influenced by an endurance exercise programme. Since one of the effects of exercise training is the development of bradycardia at rest, one element of the arteriogenic action of exercise could be the extension of diastole. In comparison, diastolic expansion by β-blockers cannot be expected to induce arteriogenesis, because the β-sympathomimetic collateral dilation as the first step in the cascade of collateral growth is prevented. Humans without CAD and no β-blockers have more preformed coronary collaterals as assessed invasively by measuring collateral relative to normal antegrade flow in the presence of low versus high heart rate. Preliminary data in patients with chronic stable CAD randomly assigned to low (80 mmHg) or high (300 mmHg) pressure external counterpulsation for a total of 30 hours have revealed no effect on collateral function in the 80 mmHg-pressure group and a significant increase in the 300-mmHg group.

5.5.1 Introduction

Aside from directly influencing the monocyte/macrophage contributions to arteriogenesis, there are several physical strategies, which can stimulate collateral growth. Based on the relevance of fluid shear stress as a molding force of vascular remodelling,[24] it is not just chronic physical exercise but several other ways of mechanically augmenting fluid shear stress, which may lead to vascular and thus, principally also collateral enlargement. There is a biophysical and a 'biochemical' aspect of vascular adaptation to altering fluid shear stress, whereby the latter provides the mechanism involved in the former aspect.

The biophysical side of fluid shear stress as a molding force relates to a general law in nature regarding the design of biological vascular trees, i.e. the law of minimum frictional energy dissipation during the transport of fluids.[225–228] The design of all vascular trees for which there exist morphometric data in the literature (coronary arteries, pulmonary airways and arteries, vessels of various skeletal muscles, mesenterial arteries, omentum and conjunctiva) obeys a set of scaling laws which are based on the hypothesis that the net cost spent for constructing the tree and operating the fluid conduction is minimized.[225] The laws consist of scaling relationships between (a) length and vascular volume of the tree, (b) lumen cross-sectional area and blood flow rate in each branch and (c) cross-sectional area and length of vessel branches. The exponent of the relationship between vascular cross-sectional area and flow rate is not necessarily 2/3 as suggested by Murray's law (see also Chapter 2), but depends on the ratio of metabolic to viscous power dissipation. Viscous or frictional energy loss during the transport of blood in a circulation is directly related to blood viscosity and to the flow velocity at the endothelial surface (shear rate), the latter of which is changing with volume flow rate for a given vascular calibre. It has been consistently demonstrated that chronic change of blood volume flow rate leads to a directly related vascular remodelling.[136,227,229–231]

The 'biochemical' mechanism behind flow-related vascular remodelling (as detailed in Chapter 3) is triggered by endothelial sensing of altered tangential fluid shear stress (the product of shear rate and viscosity of the fluid), which leads to a cascade of events, such as mechanotransduction by integrins on the endothelial surface, activation of tyrosine kinase receptors (transcription factor early growth response-1 switching on MCP-1 gene expression), stretching of sensitive sodium and chloride channels and activation of the actin cytoskeleton of the endothelial cell with transmission of the mechanical signal to the nucleus; furthermore, expression of eNOS is modulated by shear stress.[24] Endothelial cell activation in response to fluid shear stress is reflected by initial cell swelling, coinciding with a number of processes conditioning for the attraction of circulating cells, especially monocytes. Upregulated genes encode for chemoattractant or activating cytokines or for adhesion molecules, whereby MCP-1 plays a pivotal role in monocyte recruitment. Following adhesion, endothelial transmigration of monocytes into deeper parts of the vessel wall and surrounding tissue can be observed. Monocytes and macrophages with their function as 'power plants' of chemokines, proteases and growth factors play a pivotal role in the induction and proliferation of vascular wall cells as well as in outward arterial remodelling.

Thus, any strategy for chronically augmenting vascular fluid shear stress indirectly leads to monocyte activation, the pivotal element in the context of vascular remodelling. Aside from the beneficial process of arterial remodelling during arteriogenesis, increased fluid shear stress and activated monocytes are also related to the harmful development of atherosclerosis and rupture of atheromatous plaques. Epidemiologically, this is reflected in the observation that the risk of suffering an acute coronary syndrome in an untrained individual is elevated by a factor of 100 *during* an event of physical exercise.[232] However, the absolute risk of such an event can be lowered to the baseline risk at rest depending on the number and level of exercise training sessions (Fig. 5.51).[232] While recurring physical exercise is the most common way of repetitively increasing fluid shear stress in a general way by augmentation of cardiac output,

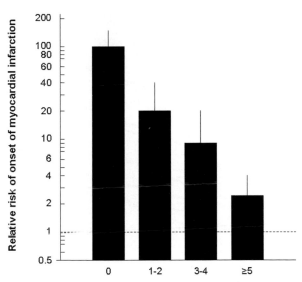

Fig. 5.51 Relative risk of myocardial infarction according to the usual frequency of heavy exertion defined as physical activity at a level of 6 MET or more. The relative risk is shown on a logarithmic scale. Sedentary persons have a high relative risk (107), whereas those with heavy exertion five or more times per week have a risk only 2.4 times higher than the base-line risk (p<0.001). The error bars indicate the 95% confidence limits. The dotted line indicates the base-line risk

several other forms of global or regional blood fluid shear stress enhancement are discussed subsequently. In principle and aside from (a) global increase in cardiac output, it is conceivable in the context of the diastolic predominance of coronary artery flow that (b) extension of the endothelial contact to fluid shear stress might be favourable for vascular remodelling. (c) Diastolic perfusion pressure augmentation with elevation of coronary flow and thus, fluid shear stress could lead to regional arterial remodelling and (d) an unevenly distributed coronary back pressure with elevation at the origin and lowering at the orifice of collaterals could have the same effect.

5.5.2 Recurrent Increase in Cardiac Output

5.5.2.1 Native Epicardial Coronary Artery Remodelling and Exercise

The results from a few human autopsy studies indicate that habitual physical activity is related to a larger cross-sectional area of the major epicardial arteries.[233–235] In healthy volunteers, it has been shown that invasively obtained epicardial coronary artery calibres adapt to physical endurance exercise by enlargement.[231,236] Haskell et al. recruited 11 men who had participated in ultradistance running during the past 2 years and 11 physically inactive male patients who had been referred for arteriography but had no visible CAD.[236] Before the administration of nitroglycerin, the sum of the cross-sectional areas for the proximal right, LAD and LCX arteries was insignificantly larger for the runners than the inactive men: 22.7±4.79 versus 21.0±7.97 mm^2, respectively.

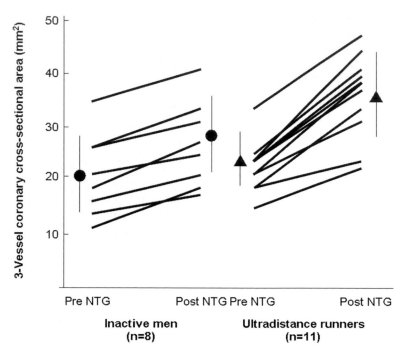

Fig. 5.52 Combined cross-sectional area (*vertical axis*) of the proximal right coronary artery, left anterior descending and left circumflex coronary artery before (pre-NTG) and after (post-NTG) nitroglycerin (NTG) for sedentary men (*circular symbols*) and ultra-distance runners (*triangular symbols*). Symbols with error bars indicate mean values ± standard error

However, the increase in the summed coronary artery cross-sectional area in response to nitroglycerin was greater for the runners (13.20±4.76 versus 6.00± 3.02 mm^2; p = 0.002; Fig. 5.52).[236] In a longitudinal study, Windecker et al. studied the effect of regular endurance exercise training on coronary artery structure and function in eight healthy physicians who underwent coronary invasive measurements before and immediately after a 5-months training phase.[231] The right, left main and LAD coronary artery cross-sectional area increased significantly in response to exercise (Fig. 5.53). Before versus at the end of the exercise programme, adenosine-induced LAD coronary artery cross-sectional area was 10.1±3.5 and 11.0±3.9 mm^2, respectively (p = 0.03), nitroglycerin-induced left coronary calibers increased significantly, and coronary flow velocity reserve changed from 3.8±0.8 to 4.5±0.7 (p = 0.001). Left coronary artery calibre correlated significantly with ventricular mass and maximum oxygen uptake, and coronary flow velocity reserve was significantly associated with maximum workload.[231]

Considering shear stress to be the trigger for vascular outward remodelling, it is primarily the repetitive increase in cardiac output during physical exercise sessions, which offers itself as the candidate physiological promoter of

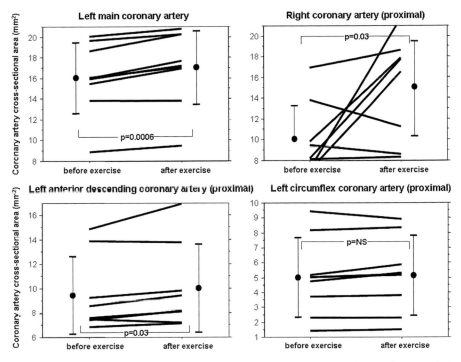

Fig. 5.53 Individual changes of coronary artery cross-sectional area before (before exercise) and at the end (after exercise) of the endurance exercise programme. Circular symbols with error bars denote means ± standard deviation. NS: not significant

arteriogenesis. However, endurance exercise training has several effects, and thus, variables alternative to augmented cardiac output may cause structural and functional changes of coronary arteries. The beneficial influence of exercise on cardiovascular risk factors likely improves coronary structure (anti-atherosclerosis) and endothelial function. Prolongation of diastole at rest as a training effect more effectively exposes the endothelium to fluid shear stress than a shortened diastolic phase (see below). In the living organism with manifestation of a net effect of exercise training on the vasculature, it is challenging to discern which component of the physiological response to repetitive bouts of exercise is responsible for a measured vascular effect.

5.5.2.2 Exercise and Functional Changes of Coronary Anastomoses Without CAD

Are repetitive increases in cardiac output related to physical exercise training able to affect preformed anastomoses between coronary arteries, i.e. does coronary flow augmentation reach anastomotic vessels in the absence of CAD? This question relates to the issue whether there is any flow in preformed collateral vessels in the normal epicardial coronary circulation. The general view on this subject is that a perfusion pressure gradient between two coronary territories linked by anastomoses is necessary as the driving force for collateral flow.[237] Based on this undisputed concept, the notion is derived that there is no collateral flow in the absence of epicardial coronary atherosclerotic lesions because of the absence of stenoses-related pressure gradients. This simplistic model of the epicardial coronary arterial circulation does not account for two facts potentially influencing the perfusion pressure balance between different vascular territories: there is a slight downstream perfusion pressure loss of 5–10 mmHg within the epicardial coronary tree,[238] and the proximity of the origin and orifice of epicardial coronary anastomoses is principally unequal and not identical as mutually assumed.[237] Figure 5.54 exemplifies the very proximal, aortic origin of the collateral artery from the RCA and the distal orifice in the chronically occluded LAD via the fourth septal branch. As a consequence, there is a potential vector of blood flow along preformed coronary collaterals even in the absence of CAD. Thus, increased cardiac output can principally affect preformed coronary collaterals in the absence of CAD. The direct verification of this hypothesis in the living organism is essentially unattainable, since detection of collateral function requires temporary occlusion of the collateral recipient artery (see also Section 5.3), and thus, the conditions described above for a perfusion pressure imbalance in the patent and non-obstructed epicardial coronary circulation are not met. However, the concept has been proved in living healthy human without CAD that repetitive increases of cardiac output

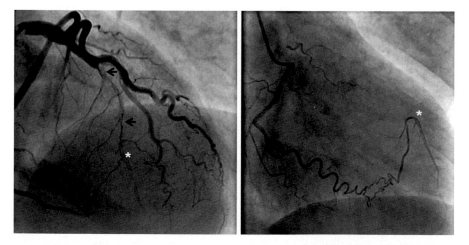

Fig. 5.54 Coronary angiogram of the left coronary artery (RAO cranial view; *left side*) showing a thrombotic chronic occlusion of the mid-left anterior descending (LAD) artery (→). Injection of contrast into the right coronary artery (antero-posterior cranial view; *right side*) depicts a large right ventricular branch collateral artery with filling of a septal branch and the distal LAD. *Orifice of the collateral artery to the distal LAD. This figure exemplifies the *proximal origin* of a collateral vessel with a *distal orifice*

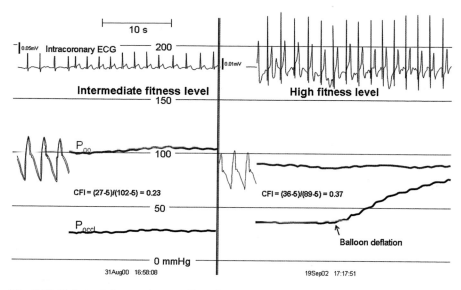

Fig. 5.55 Collateral flow at intermediate fitness (*left panel*) and at high fitness level (*right panel*). Intracoronary ECG lead recordings are shown in the upper part of the panels. On the left side of both panels, phasic aortic pressure tracings are shown; on the right side mean aortic (*upper curve*, P_{ao} = 102 and 89 mmHg respectively) and mean coronary occlusive (*lower curve*, P_{occl} = 27 and 36 mmHg respectively) pressure tracings at the end of a 1 minute coronary artery balloon occlusion. The calculation of CFI is shown for both examinations during intermediate and high fitness level (CVP = 5 mmHg; measured non-simultaneously)

in the context of endurance exercise training augment coronary collateral function (Fig. 5.55).[239]

5.5.2.3 Exercise and Functional Changes of Collaterals with Coronary Obstructions

In animal models, the effect of exercise on collaterals has not been tested in the absence of coronary obstruction to epicardial flow, but mostly in the presence of coronary occlusions in order to mimic severe human CAD, thus providing a situation with an entirely collateralized vascular area. At variance, Eckstein studied the effect of physical exercise and coronary artery narrowing, i.e. not complete occlusion, on the collateral circulation by applying different degrees of coronary narrowings.[240] Subsequently, one group of dogs underwent exercise training (15–20 minutes per session, four times a day, 5 days weekly for 6–8 weeks; n = 44) and a second group remained at rest in cages (n = 46). The data obtained in 90 of 117 dogs which had survived until after the training/sedentary period indicated that the degree of coronary artery narrowing determined the amount of collateral flow, which was even more pronounced in exercising as compared to sedentary animals (Fig. 5.56).[240] Eckstein also

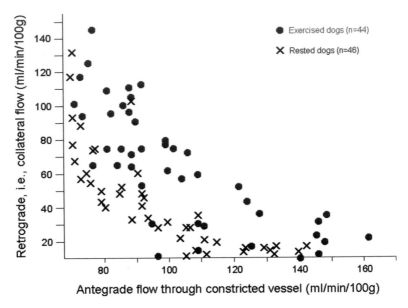

Fig. 5.56 Magnitude of retrograde collateral flow (*vertical axis*) with different degrees of left circumflex coronary artery narrowing (*horizontal axis*) in sedentary (*black crosses*) and exercised (*red circles*) dogs

observed that mild arterial narrowing failed to initiate retrograde, i.e. collateral flow as obtained during brief total coronary occlusion, but that the addition of exercise training effectively promoted the coronary collateral circulation (Fig. 5.56).[240] This is in agreement with the above-mentioned result in a healthy human individual, in whom improved coronary collateral function was measured in response to exercise training. However, later experiments in dogs carried out with more refined techniques and under nearly clinical conditions have produced conflicting results.[241–243] Scheel et al. found that exercise did not stimulate collateral growth in normal beagle dogs. However, exercise after coronary occlusion doubled collateral conductance to the impaired vascular bed compared to animals with only coronary occlusions.[243] In order to reconcile the conflicting observations, Schaper restudied the problem using a standardized canine model by obtaining regional myocardial blood flow with radioactive mircospheres during maximal vasodilation and under a wide range of coronary perfusion pressures.[244] In 45 German shepherd dogs, the LCX and the RCA were chronically occluded by implantation of ameroid constrictors. Before the operation, 27 dogs were trained on a treadmill until they could run 8 miles per hour on a 22% incline for 1 hour, 5 days per week. Two weeks after the operation, exercise was gradually resumed and continued for 4 weeks, until the preoperative fitness level had been regained. Preoperative exercise training lasted 1–3 months; post-operative training lasted 100±22 days. After the dogs had trained with two chronically occluded coronary arteries, collateral and coronary blood flows were measured with radioactive microspheres at maximal coronary vasodilation in an isolated, blood-perfused Langendorff preparation at perfusion pressures of 40, 60, 80, 100, 120 and 140 mmHg. Eighteen sedentary dogs that also had two-vessel coronary occlusion served as controls. Exercise of relatively high intensity at heart rates >200 beats/min before and after occlusion had no effect on coronary collaterals (Fig. 5.57).[244] In a further canine study (n = 13), Cohen et al. found that chronic exercise can stimulate coronary collateral development and the enhanced collateral vessels had a beneficial functional effect.[245] Thus, the majority of the cited experimental studies in dogs observed a positive effect of endurance exercise on functional collateral flow. However, the most rigorously performed investigation by Schaper did not confirm these results. The advantages of the latter study are that the intensity of exercise was by far the highest, the dogs were already well conditioned before the coronary operation and resumed training early after the procedure and the duration of post-operative training and the total distance covered were the longest of the mentioned studies; furthermore, collateral conductance measurements were based on pressure-flow curves using a wide range of coronary perfusion pressures and they were obtained under maximum vasodilation requiring the Langendorff preparation to keep perfusion pressures and heart rate constant. Considering that the dog model is one more similar to the human coronary collateral circulation than previously

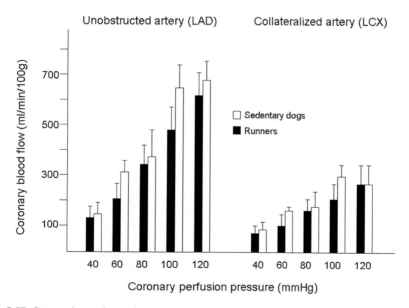

Fig. 5.57 Comparison of exercised and sedentary dogs for normal left anterior descending coronary artery (LAD) and collateral blood flow values (*vertical axis*) as a function of aortic or proximal coronary perfusion pressure during maximal vasodilation. *Error bars*: standard deviation

thought,[132] not only the results of the studies just discussed, but also the lack of evidence of exercise as arteriogenic factor are of considerable relevance with regard to human studies.

In the pig model of gradual coronary occlusion, endurance exercise appears to have a beneficial effect on collateral function. Roth et al. tested the effect of myocardial ischaemia, induced by long-term exercise, on regional myocardial function and coronary collateral development in pigs after gradual occlusion of the LCX with an ameroid occluder.[246] Thirty days after surgery, regional myocardial function and blood flow were assessed during exercise in 22 pigs separated into exercise (n = 12) and sedentary groups (n = 10). The exercise group trained on a treadmill for 25±1 days, 30–50 min/day, at heart rates of 210–220 beats/min. After 5 weeks, another exercise test was performed. Transmural and subendocardial myocardial blood flow in the LCX region expressed as a ratio of flow in the non-occluded region increased during severe exercise after 5 weeks (Fig. 5.58). The sedentary group showed no significant change in systolic wall thickening or myocardial blood flow ratios during severe exercise after 5 weeks.[246] The goal of a study by White et al. was to investigate the effects of training on capillary and arteriolar growth.[247] Minipigs were trained for 1, 3, 8 and 16 weeks and compared with sedentary controls. Capillary and arteriolar densities and diameters, and proliferation of vascular cells in these vessels, were determined in perfusion-fixed tissue. The total vascular bed cross-sectional area increased by 37% at 16 weeks of training, mainly because of an increase in the number of the small arterioles and in the diameter of the larger vessels. Capillary density increased at 3 weeks and then returned to control levels by 16 weeks; concomitantly, the number of arterioles increased at 16 weeks.[247] Since the surgical procedure used in the study by White et al. did not consist of gradual or abrupt coronary occlusion thus establishing a collateralized myocardial region, no direct inference from this study can be made on the efficacy of exercise regarding collateral growth, but only on its capacity to

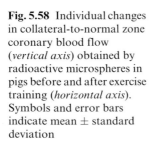
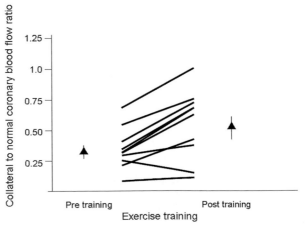

Fig. 5.58 Individual changes in collateral-to-normal zone coronary blood flow (*vertical axis*) obtained by radioactive microspheres in pigs before and after exercise training (*horizontal axis*). Symbols and error bars indicate mean ± standard deviation

induce vascular remodelling. Similarly as the cited work on exercise-induced vascular remodelling, a study by Indermuhle et al. in endurance athletes and hypertensive patients found that physiological and pathological LV hypertrophy could be differentiated non-invasively and accurately by obtaining relative myocardial blood volume, a measure of vascularization assessed by myocardial contrast echocardiography.[248] Hypertensive patients had lower relative myocardial blood volume (0.093 ± 0.013 ml m^{-1}, i.e. approximately 9%) than triathletes with the highest capillary and arteriolar density (0.141 ± 0.012 ml m^{-1}), football players (0.129 ± 0.014 ml m^{-1}), and sedentary individuals (0.126 ± 0.018 ml m^{-1}).

5.5.2.4 Exercise and Functional Changes of Collaterals in Human CAD

While it has been recognized for a long time that physical activity plays an important role in the relief of intermittent claudication among patients with peripheral artery disease, it has been controversial whether collateral growth importantly contributes to the beneficial effect of exercise.[249] Exercise studies in humans with peripheral artery disease have reported no or only a moderate increase in ankle–brachial index or calf blood flow and no correlation of blood flow with walking capacity.[249] Mechanisms alternative to arteriogenesis for the efficacy of physical exercise could be an optimized muscle metabolism and oxygen extraction, improved blood viscosity and red-cell aggregation, decreased inflammation, augmented walking biomechanics and beneficial influence on cardiovascular risk factors. In patients with CAD, the evidence favouring a benefit of exercise training for coronary arteriogenesis has been debated for a long time. The first time physical exercise was mentioned as a treatment option for angina pectoris was in 1785, when William Heberden reported the following observation[250]: ' know one who set himself a task of sawing wood for half an hour every day, and was nearly cured'. This reference has long been interpreted as a sign for coronary collateral recruitment. Alternatively, it could be taken as an indication for the effectiveness of exercise in the development of coronary collaterals. Conversely, a possible interpretation could be that the described patient engaged in daily physical exercise, because he had developed sufficient collateral function in the first place. Finally, a further reading would see ischaemic myocardial preconditioning as the mechanism of the development of tolerance to ischaemia. Basically, the quote can be used only methodologically in the sense that in human patients a self-selection bias for or against exercise training may play an important role, i.e. the patient with a priori well-developed collaterals may choose to engage in exercise and this may be falsely interpreted as an arteriogenic effect of exercise. In general, such a selection bias is likely to be present even in *randomized* human investigations with an exercise and sedentary group. In contrast, self-selection bias in exercise studies using animals is less likely to occur, because animals can be forced to adhere to the randomly selected protocol. From the statement cited from Eckstein's study,[240] it can be suspected that compelling an individual to a certain exercise protocol may be even difficult in animals: 'Of 117 operated dogs 12 died as a result of operation and 6 died of distemper'.

In humans, the effects of training on the collateral circulation have not been systematically studied until 1974, when Ferguson et al. performed an uncontrolled investigation in 14 CAD patients, who underwent coronary angiography before and after a 13-month physical exercise programme.[251] Treadmill exercise capacity increased in response to the training programme, but coronary angiographic follow-up data did not support the existence of a relationship between augmented physical fitness and the development of collateral vessels. Aside from the insufficient statistical power of this study, the principal methodological problem of investigations focusing on the effect of exercise programmes in humans is exemplified: how can it be distinguished between collateral growth in response to progression of CAD and to exercise? Kennedy et al. performed an open observational study in eight men with mild stable angina pectoris who participated in a 1-year exercise programme.[252] Coronary arteriography, left ventriculography, LV haemodynamics at rest and during supine leg exercise, treadmill testing with ECG monitoring and measurement of oxygen uptake were obtained before and 1 year after the exercise training programme. No change was noted in the arteriographic appearance of coronary artery lesions or of the collateral circulation. Considering the number of eight patients included in this study and the cursory way of coronary angiographic analysis, the absence of CAD progression and unchanged collateral appearance cannot be taken as hard evidence against an effect of exercise on arteriogenesis. Conner et al. tested the effects of exercise on coronary collateralization using baseline and repeat angiography in six post-infarction patients, who underwent a supervised exercise programme for 10–12 months.[253] All patients demonstrated the expected physical, physiological, metabolic and psychological benefits, and two of them showed an increased collateralization; however, in both of these the changes were possibly related to extension of the occlusive CAD and not to the exercise effect. The first controlled clinical investigation on the effect of exercise on the development of intercoronary collaterals was performed by Nolewajka et al.[254] They examined 20 men who had suffered an acute myocardial infarction and who were randomly allocated to an exercise group (10 patients) and a control group (10 patients). Both groups underwent coronary angiography, LV systolic function studies and myocardial perfusion studies with labelled microspheres, before and after the 7-month study period. Both groups had similar extent of CAD as visually estimated by angiography and both had mild progression of disease. Neither group showed changes in the extent of collateralization, myocardial perfusion or LV function. In fact and despite a history of myocardial infarction in all 20 patients (i.e. the majority of them with total coronary occlusions), angiographic collateral degree (range 0–3) remained unchanged during follow-up in all 20 patients. Even in the control group, some increase in collateralization to the acutely occluded vascular area would have been expected during follow-up, because the degree of a coronary artery stenosis (which had abruptly increased at the onset of the study) is the strongest determining factor of coronary collateralization.

Thus, the first four studies in humans did not provide evidence of a coronary arteriogenic effect of exercise; they were all statistically underpowered and employed a crude method as the study endpoint for collateral assessment (coronary angiography) and three of four studies were exploratory investigations without a sedentary control group.

Almost 20 years later, Niebauer et al. examined in a randomized fashion and in a sizeable population the effects of >3 hours of physical exercise per week and low-fat diet on collateral formation in patients with CAD (intervention group, n = 56), and compared the results with those of patients in a control group (n = 57), who received usual care by their private physicians.[255] Coronary lesions were assessed by quantitative coronary angiography at the beginning and after 1 year of study. After 1 year, there was a slowdown of progression of CAD in the intervention group as compared with the control group. In this study, angiographic evaluation of collateral formation revealed no difference between both groups, and changes in haemodynamic and metabolic variables or leisure-time physical activity were not related to changes in collateral formation. Although progression of the disease was significantly related to an increase in collateral formation, regression was significantly related to a decrease in collateral formation. In contrast, Belardinelli et al. observed, in 46 patients randomly assigned to an exercise group (n = 26; exercise training at 60% of maximum oxygen uptake for 8 weeks) or to a sedentary control group (n = 20), that angiographic coronary collateral degree had increased by at least one score point in all but one patient of the exercise group (Fig. 5.59; coronary angiography at baseline and follow-up in only 23 patients).[256]

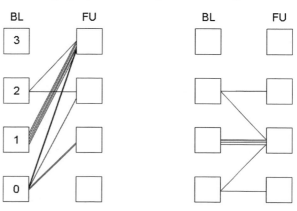

Exercise group   **Control group**

Angiographic coronary collateral degree

Fig. 5.59 Angiographic collateral score at baseline (BL) and after 8 weeks of follow-up (FU) in the exercise and control patients. Of 12 trained patients, all but 1 showed an improved collateral score after exercise training. Of 11 control patients, 9 had no changes, 1 a reduced score and 1 a greater score after 8 weeks

Employing as the principal study endpoint a more refined measure of collateral function than angiographic scoring, Senti et al. performed a prospective, cross-sectional study in order to evaluate an association between the level of long-term physical activity as well as other clinical and angiographic variables and an index of collateral flow to the vascular region undergoing PCI.[257] In 79 patients with CAD who underwent PCI, an intracoronary Doppler-derived coronary CFI was determined as the ratio between the distal flow velocity time integral during and after PCI of the treated stenosis. CFI was measured by Doppler guidewire. The level of long-term physical activity was determined by a structured interview (score from 1 to 4). Long-term physical activity during leisure time, but not during work hours', and the severity of the stenosis that underwent PCI were found to be independently and directly associated with CFI (Fig. 5.60).[257] The basic methodological problem of this study was its cross-sectional observational design, which did not allow to determine the cause and effect of the results obtained, i.e. it remained obscure whether patients had engaged more in exercise activities because of their better developed collateral function in comparison to the less-active patients, or whether more exercise had improved collateral function. A longitudinal, uncontrolled observation among 21 of the above-mentioned 78 patients revealed a direct association between change in leisure-time physical activity over time and change in CFI (Fig. 5.61).

Belardinelli et al. studied 30 male patients with CAD who were randomized into a group that received only dipyridamole at a dose of 75 mg/d orally for 8 weeks (n = 10), a group that underwent exercise training three times a week for 8 weeks plus dipyridamole (n = 10) and a control group (n = 10).[93] On study entry and after 8 weeks, all patients underwent an exercise test with gas

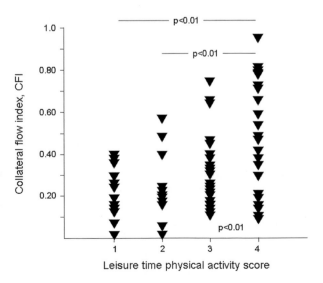

Fig. 5.60 Linear regression trend between individual collateral flow index data (CFI; *vertical axis*) and leisure-time physical activity score (*horizontal axis*). There is a trend between CFI and leisure-time physical activity score; p values between different activity scores obtained by analysis of variance

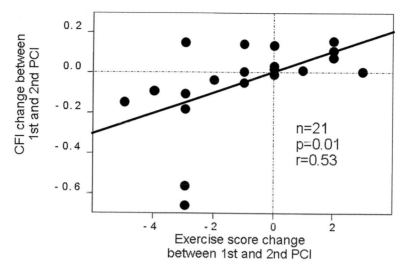

Fig. 5.61 Correlation between change of collateral flow index between two percutaneous coronary interventions (CFI; *vertical axis*) and change of physical activity score during the same follow-up period (*horizontal axis*)

exchange analysis, dobutamine stress echocardiography, 201-thallium planar myocardial scintigraphy and coronary angiography. Peak oxygen uptake increased significantly only in trained patients. Thallium uptake in the collateral-dependent myocardium, coronary collateral score and wall thickening score increased significantly only in groups receiving dipyridamole, the greatest improvement occurring in exercising patients.[93]

In the context of the close relationship between coronary stenosis change and alteration of collateral function, a study performed at our laboratory on the arteriogenic effect of exercise training tried to circumvent the issue by removing the most severe atherosclerotic lesion prior to the onset of the exercise programme.[258] In the study by Zbinden et al., the following hypotheses were tested[258]: The expected collateral flow reduction after PCI of a stenotic lesion is prevented by endurance exercise training; collateral flow supplied to an angiographically normal coronary artery improves in response to exercise training; there is a direct relationship between the change of fitness after training and the coronary collateral flow change. Forty patients underwent a 3-month endurance exercise training programme with baseline and follow-up assessments of invasively obtained, coronary pressure-derived CFI (collateral relative to normal flow). Patients were divided into an exercise training group (n = 24) and a sedentary group (n = 16) according to the fact whether they adhered or not to the prescribed exercise programme, and whether or not they showed increased endurance (maximum oxygen uptake) and performance (Watt/kg) during follow-up versus baseline bicycle spiroergometry. In the vessel that initially underwent PCI, there was an increase in CFI among exercising

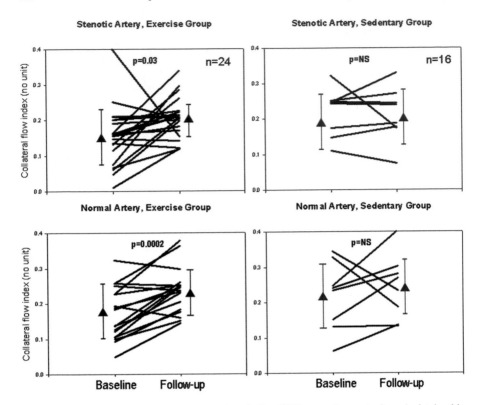

Fig. 5.62 Individual changes of collateral flow index (CFI, no unit; *vertical axes*) obtained in the previously stenotic (*upper panels*), and in the normal arteries (*lower panels*) before and after treatment (*horizontal axes*) among patients who underwent exercise training (*black lines*) or who belonged to the sedentary group (*blue lines*). The triangles with error bars indicate mean values ± standard deviation

but not sedentary patients from 0.155±0.081 to 0.204±0.056 and from 0.189±0.084 to 0.212±0.077, respectively (Fig. 5.62). In the normal vessel, CFI changes were from 0.176±0.075 to 0.227±0.070 in the exercise group, and from 0.219±0.103 to 0.238±0.086 in the sedentary group (Fig. 5.62). A direct correlation existed between the change in CFI from baseline to follow-up and the respective alteration of peak oxygen uptake (Fig. 5.63) and Watt (p = 0.03).[258]

It can be argued that the above study is limited by not meeting *the* major study design criterion employed to ascertain causality of a relationship being investigated: randomised allocation of the individuals to the treatment groups. Conversely and as already outlined above, there is a severe limitation inherent in randomising motivated or unmotivated individuals to make intense, long-term lifestyle changes.[259] In principle, highly motivated patients do not accept randomised assignment to a sedentary control group, and less-motivated patients do not adhere to the demands of an exercise training group. Therefore,

Fig. 5.63 Correlation between the change during follow-up in maximal oxygen uptake (VO$_2$max, *horizontal axis*) and the respective change in collateral flow index (CFI, *vertical axis*)

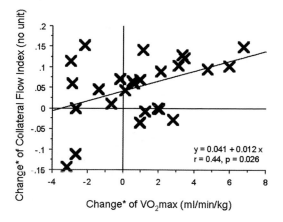

*: value after minus that before exercise

a randomised design to study the effect of exercise on coronary collateral flow likely introduces bias from motivated patients assigned to the control group and from poorly motivated subjects assigned to the exercise group with consequent little difference between groups and negative results.

5.5.3 Prolongation of Diastole

In the context of the arteriogenic function of vascular shear stress, *prolongation* of the endothelial contact to fluid shear stress might be favourable for vascular remodelling. The relative contribution of diastole to the cardiac cycle is enhanced during bradycardia. Since one of the effects of physical endurance exercise training is the development of bradycardia at rest, one element of the arteriogenic action of exercise could be the extension of diastole. In comparison, diastolic expansion by β-blockers cannot be expected to induce arteriogenesis, because the β-sympathomimetic collateral dilation as the first step in the cascade of collateral growth is prevented. There has been evidence from animal experiments that bradycardia has a pro-angiogenic effect. More importantly regarding the focus of this book, humans without CAD (no β-blockers) do have more preformed coronary collaterals as assessed invasively by measuring collateral relative to normal antegrade flow in the presence of low versus high heart rate (Fig. 5.64). The inverse relationship between resting heart rate and CFI is no longer present in patients with CAD irrespective of treatment with β-blockers. In a retrospective study, Patel et al. analysed ECG and rhythm tracings obtained during angiography of patients presenting to the cardiac catheterization laboratory.[260] Coronary angiograms of patients with heart rates ≤50 beats/min were reviewed. An equivalent number of consecutive

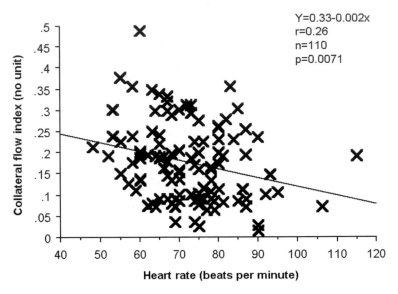

Fig. 5.64 Correlation between collateral flow index (CFI; *vertical axis*) obtained in patients with normal coronary arteries and their resting heart rate (*horizontal axis*)

patients with heart rates ≥60 beats/min served as controls. Patients with acute myocardial infarction, with rhythms other than sinus and without high-grade obstructive CAD were excluded from the study. The study population consisted of 61 patients, 30 having heart rates ≤50 beats/min and 31 controls with heart rates ≥60 beats/min. A significantly greater proportion of patients with bradycardia in comparison to the control group was demonstrated to have well-developed collaterals (97 versus 55% in p < 0.005).[260] The fact that the use of β-blocking agents (similar rate of around 75% in both groups) did not have an influence on the results of the latter, small study is puzzling.

Wright and Hudlicka determined in a rabbit model of chronic right atrial pacing to half the normal heart rate whether this procedure affected myocardial capillary density.[261] Following were the principal findings of this study:chronic bradycardic pacing produced a decreased heart rate even when pacing was turned off, pacing was not associated with development of ventricular hypertrophy, an increased stroke work was observed in response to norepinephrine and there was an increased capillary density in hearts paced for at least 10 days (Fig. 5.65).[261] By the same research group but in a larger animal species, the pig, bradycardia (approximately 30% decrease in heart rate) was induced by electrical pacing for 4–5 weeks.[262] There was no evidence of ventricular hypertrophy and capillary density was found to be significantly increased in the left, but not right, ventricle.[262] Zheng et al. hypothesized that VEGF is upregulated in response to low heart rate and, as a consequence, increased stroke volume. Bradycardia was induced in rats by administering the bradycardic drug alinidine twice daily.[263] Heart rate decreased by 32% for 20–40 minutes after

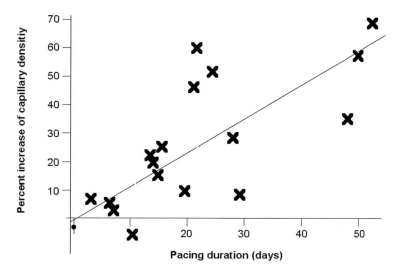

Fig. 5.65 Correlation between percent of capillary density increase (*vertical axis*) and atrial pacing duration (*horizontal axis*) in chronically paced rabbits. The circular symbol with error bars represents the mean value of eight sham-operated control animals (± standard deviation)

injection and was chronically reduced by 10, 14 and 18.5% after 1, 2 and 3 weeks of treatment, respectively. Arterial pressure and cardiac output were unchanged. LV capillary length density increased gradually with alinidine administration; a 15% increase after 2 weeks and a 40% increase after 3 weeks of alinidine treatment were documented. After 1 week of treatment and before an increase in capillary density, VEGF mRNA increased >2-fold and then declined to control levels after 3 weeks of treatment. VEGF protein was higher in alinidine-treated rats than in control animals after 2 weeks and increased further after 3 weeks of treatment. Using a similar rat model of alinidine-induced bradycardia but in addition, with coronary artery ligation, Lei et al. found that early on, VEGF, VEGF receptor 1 and bFGF proteins were higher in the bradycardia group, whereas VEGF receptor 2, ang-1 and ang-2 were not affected by the treatment.[264] After 3 weeks, VEGF protein remained elevated, and bradycardia was associated with a higher capillary length density in the border and remote regions and a higher arteriolar length density in the septum, despite a greater increase in LV mass. Although arteriolar length density increased in all size classes, the greatest increase occurred in the smallest arterioles.

Except for the last experimental work, the others provide no evidence for a pro-arteriogenic effect of bradycardia, because they just estimated capillary density, which does not provide bulk coronary flow to a vascular region in need. However, the recent investigation by Lei et al. offered evidence in favour of bradycardia-induced arteriogenesis of the heart together with a possible mechanism of induction of angiogenic (though not arteriogenic) pathways.[264]

5.5.4 Diastolic Perfusion Pressure Augmentation

It is intuitively evident that diastolic perfusion pressure augmentation leads to improved coronary perfusion. According to Ohm's law ($\Delta P = Q \times R$) coronary flow increase occurs in the context of flow-induced vascular resistance reduction. In comparison, systolic pressure augmentation does not have such an effect, because the coronary flow-inhibiting effect of myocardial contraction resulting in a predominant tissue compressive force on the circulation would even lead to an amplification of this effect because of elevated ventricular afterload.[265] Focusing on coronary collateral flow, Brown et al. investigated the effect of intraaortic balloon pumping on retrograde coronary flow collected from the cannulated distal bed of the ligated LAD in 10 dogs.[266] Mean systolic and mean diastolic aortic root pressures were varied, and it was observed that retrograde coronary flow remained practically constant with altering systolic pressure, but increased significantly in response to rising diastolic pressure (Fig. 5.66).[266] In a similar experimental study and in order to determine the influence of intraaortic balloon pumping on infarct size and collateral blood flow, Müller et al. occluded two small branches of the left coronary artery in each of 12 mongrel dogs.[267] The perfusion areas of both branches were similar in size. Intraaortic balloon pumping was started immediately before ligation of the first branch for a 90-minute period followed by reperfusion during 90 minutes. Subsequently the second vessel was occluded for 90 minutes as a control without intraaortic balloon pumping while myocardial oxygen consumption remained constant and was then reperfused. Infarct size was expressed as a percentage of the perfusion area. There was no difference in infarct size with and without intraaortic balloon pumping (18±17 and 18±10%, respectively). However, a significant increase in collateral blood flow due to intraaortic

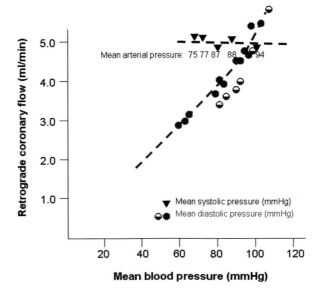

Fig. 5.66 Plot from a single dog of retrograde coronary collateral flow (*vertical axis*) in relation to altering values of mean systolic pressure at constant diastolic pressure (Ψ; *horizontal axis*) and to varying mean diastolic pressure at constant systolic pressure (red TΩ; *horizontal axis*) induced by intra-aortic counterpulsation. The *circular, half open symbols* (T) correspond to progressive *left ventricular* failure which occurred with prolonged ischaemia in the *left anterior* descending bed

balloon pumping in the subendocardial layer from 8.9±4.8 to 14.9±4.6 ml/min/ 100 g (p < 0.05) was observed. In the subepicardial layer, the augmentation from 23.7±19.9 to 26.9±15.2 was not significant.[267]

For similar conceptual reasons as those described for the setting of acute myocardial infarction with injection of BMC, it cannot be expected that diastolic pressure augmentation applied *after* the event is effective to salvage myocardium.[267] The myocardium at risk for infarction *before* acute coronary occlusion cannot be prevented from becoming necrotic, if the rescuing neovascularization is initiated only after the necrotizing event. In humans, direct translation of the mentioned experimental investigations using intraaortic balloon pumping is not feasible, if the focus is on the collateral circulation in chronic CAD. This is because it would be technically demanding and thus, ethically questionable to insert an intraaortic balloon pump in a stable patient with simultaneous coronary balloon-occlusive measurements in order to obtain quantitative collateral function on and off the assist device. More reasonably, application of *external* counterpulsation (Fig. 5.67) over a cumulative duration

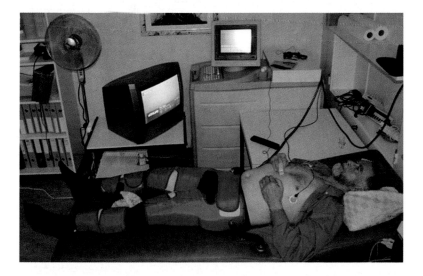

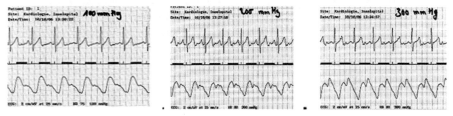

Fig. 5.67 External counterpulsation in a patient with coronary artery disease (*upper panel*) showing the blue lower leg cuffs which are sequentially inflated from distal to proximal as triggered by the ECG QRS complex (*lower panels*). The plethysmographic pressure tracings simultaneously recorded with the ECG register the increasing diastolic pressure augmentation at increasing cuff inflation pressures between 100 and 300 mmHg

of, e.g. 30–40 hours can be tested with regard to its effect on coronary collateral function. A radial artery Doppler flow velocity signal obtained without, during low (100 mmHg) and high-pressure (300 mmHg) external counterpulsation illustrates the effect on diastolic blood flow, and thus, on coronary perfusion (Fig. 5.68). Preliminary data from our laboratory, in 12 patients with chronic stable CAD randomly assigned to low (80 mmHg) or high (300 mmHg) pressure external counterpulsation for a total of 30 hours, have revealed no effect on CFI in the 80-mmHg pressure group and a significant increase in the 300-mmHg group (Fig. 5.69).

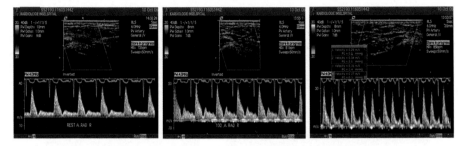

Fig. 5.68 Radial artery Doppler ultrasound recordings before (*left side*) and during external counterpulsation at cuff inflation pressures of 100 mmHg (*middle panel*) and 300 mmHg (*right side*). Note the progressively increased diastolic flow velocities in response to diastolic pressure augmentation. *Vertical axis*: flow velocity; *horizontal axis*: time (200 ms calibration)

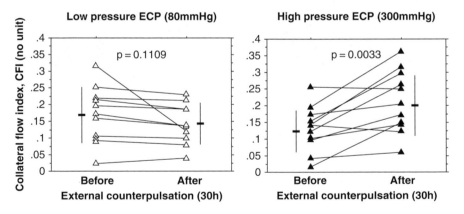

Fig. 5.69 Individual values of collateral flow index (CFI; *vertical axis*) before and after 30 hours of external counterpulsation in patients randomized to low- or high-inflation pressure

5.5.5 *Coronary Back Pressure Augmentation*

Considering the formula to calculate invasively obtained, pressure-derived CFI, it is counterintuitive that augmentation of coronary back pressure (CVP) should improve rather than impair collateral flow: CFI $= [P_{occl}-CVP]/[P_{ao}-CVP]$, where P_{occl} is coronary occlusive pressure, P_{ao} mean aortic pressure, and CVP central venous pressure or right atrial or coronary sinus pressure. However, the regional effect of a global increase in coronary sinus pressure is unlikely to be as uniform as the above formula implies, i.e. in certain vascular areas, the response is probably more pronounced than in other territories. Theoretically, it is conceivable that there is systematically more transmission of augmented coronary sinus pressure to a non-ischaemic than to an ischaemic coronary artery territory. Still in theory, this could be related to uneven ventricular wall stress distribution with lower wall stress in the non-ischaemic area, which is due to higher wall thickness with more pronounced systolic thickening than in the ischaemic region. As a consequence, it can be imagined that at the origin of preformed collateral channels in the non-ischaemic area, blood is diverged away from the downstream microcirculation due to regionally augmented back pressure. At the orifice of the preformed collaterals, perfusion pressure as well as back pressure is low resulting in a low driving pressure, i.e. the necessary condition to receive blood from the collateral-supplying region. Naturally, this scenario is limited by an exceedingly high ventricular wall stress in the collateral-receiving area, respectively by an extravascular tissue pressure beyond the so-called waterfall pressure which is equal to approximately 27 mmHg.[265]

In support of this theoretically derived mechanism, Sato et al. performed regional myocardial blood flow measurements with and without coronary sinus pressure elevation to 30 mmHg in dog hearts.[268] Coloured microspheres for myocardial perfusion measurements were injected into the left artery and RCA, after coronary perfusion of the left anterior descending coronary artery was stopped in seven isolated canine hearts with induced atrioventricular block paced at 120 beats/min. Regional myocardial blood flow in the collateralized LAD area of the beating heart with coronary sinus pressure augmentation to 30 mmHg was significantly greater than without coronary sinus pressure elevation, and than in the non-beating heart with coronary sinus pressure augmentation. The augmentative effect of the LAD area regional myocardial blood flow was observed only in the periphery of the ischaemic region but not in its centre.[268] Similarly, Ido et al. investigated 38 anaesthetized dogs that underwent occlusion of the left anterior descending coronary artery with or without coronary sinus occlusion and intact vasomotor tone.[269] Regional myocardial blood flow was obtained. With intact vasomotor tone, coronary sinus occlusion during ischaemia significantly increased regional myocardial blood flow in the collateralized region (Fig. 5.70). These effects of coronary sinus occlusion were partially abolished by adenosine.[269] In fact during adenosine-induced hyperaemia with coronary sinus occlusion, regional myocardial blood flow was increased in the non-ischaemic region at the cost of a decrease in the ischaemic territory, i.e. coronary steal via collateral vessels could be observed.

Despite the existence of only meagre explanations on the exact physical mechanism of collateral flow enhancement in response to coronary sinus occlusion provided by the mentioned experimental studies, Banai et al. performed a first open-labelled clinical study testing a coronary sinus reducer

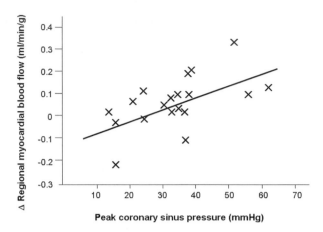

Fig. 5.70 Correlation between the change in regional myocardial blood flow to the occluded left anterior descending coronary artery of 19 dogs (*vertical axis*; change in response to coronary sinus occlusion) and the peak coronary sinus pressure obtained during coronary sinus occlusion (*horizontal axis*)

stent for the treatment of chronic refractory angina pectoris.[270] Fifteen CAD patients with severe angina pectoris and reversible myocardial ischaemia were electively treated by permanent implantation of a coronary sinus reducer stent. Clinical evaluation, dobutamine echocardiography, thallium SPECT and administration of an angina pectoris questionnaire were performed before and 6 months after implantation. Stent implantation was completed success-fully in all patients. No procedure-related adverse events occurred during the periprocedural and the follow-up periods. Angina score improved in 12 of 14 patients. Stress-induced ECG ST-segment depression was reduced in six of nine patients and was eliminated in two of those six. The extent and severity of myocardial ischaemia by dobutamine echocardiography and by thallium SPECT were reduced.[270] The authors considered the treatment with a coronary sinus reducer stent to be feasible and safe. Despite concluding it to be even efficacious, they did not provide any mechanistic insight into regional physical changes induced by coronary sinus obstruction, which could explain the results obtained.[270]

5.6 Issues of Neovascularization to be Resolved

The discrepancies between positive outcome of neovascularization trials in the experimental animal model and small clinical trials as compared to disap-pointing results in sizeable clinical trials may be related to issues such as poor conversion of animal to human data, influence of systemic atherosclerosis on the ability of promoting collateral growth and mode of growth factor delivery.

The majority of data on collateral promotion comes from non-atherosclerotic animal models. Conversely, the population addressed consists exclusively of diseased people, the most important conditions being systemic atherosclerosis and the presence of one or more risk factors for cardiovascular disease. The processes of angiogenesis and arteriogenesis have been shown to be less potent under atherosclerotic than under healthy conditions, and they appear also less susceptible to therapeutic promotion. Apart from the influence of atherosclerosis on the organism's responsiveness to angiogenic and arteriogenic treatment, there is potentially the accelerating effect of arteriogenic therapy on the course of atherosclerosis. However, arteriogenic factors, such as G-CSF or TGFβ1, without the adverse effect on atherosclerosis appear to exist.

Another obvious concern of collateral growth promotion is the potential stimulation of tumour angiogenesis. Despite evidence of the relevance of neovascularization in the growth of tumours and metastases, no increase in neoplastic diseases has been observed so far in clinical trials aiming to promote angiogenesis or arteriogenesis in patients with coronary or peripheral artery diseases. Nevertheless, the concern of stimulating tumour neovascularization requires careful patient selection and close surveillance during follow-up to detect side effects.

It is acknowledged that systemic delivery of factors for collateral promotion is less efficient than local application. There is consensus that extended exposure of the circulation to the collateral-promoting drug is important. With regard to the latter requirement, the following modes of delivery are well suited: intracoronary infusion instead of bolus injection, intramyocardial injection (transendo- or transepicardial), intrapericardial injection and retroperfusion from the coronary sinus. The evolving technology of biodegradable stents could offer a mode of slowly releasing arteriogenic substances into the coronary artery. A further possibility of local drug delivery potentially suitable for arteriogenic proteins and genes as well as cells is the ultrasound-mediated destruction of echocontrast microbubbles.

5.6.1 Introduction

Despite advances of the past years in promoting neavascularization, a discrepancy exists between successful promotion of neovascularization in experimental animal models as well as small clinical trials and the disappointing outcome in recent large clinical trials. Aside from the general problem that animal data are not directly translatable for the human situation (small size and young age of animal species, genetic background in favour or contra-preformed collaterals, absence versus presence of disease in animals versus humans), other issues of neovascularization remain to be addressed, such as potential pro-atherogenic and pro-neoplastic side effects and selection of the optimal delivery mode for collaterogenic promoters.

5.6.2 Arteriogenesis Versus Atherogenesis

The majority of data on neovacularization comes from non-atherosclerotic animal models. Conversely, the human population addressed consists exclusively of diseased people, the most important conditions being systemic atherosclerosis and the presence of one or more risk factors for cardiovascular disease. The processes of angiogenesis and arteriogenesis have been shown to be less potent under atherosclerotic than under healthy conditions, and they appear also less susceptible to therapeutic promotion.[271] In this context, van Weel et al. demonstrated in mice with femoral artery occlusion that hypercholesterolaemia reduces collateral artery growth more dominantly than hyperglycaemia or insulin resistance.[272] In addition, even the intrinsic ability to develop preformed collateral vessels may be affected in a young individual by cardiovascular risk factors.[271] Risk factor-induced impaired collateral growth and reduced response to collaterogenic therapy can involve any of the numerous steps involved in collateral development, such as the mobilization of bone marrow-derived progenitor cells, the efficacy of mononuclear effector cells and the responsiveness of developing collaterals to angiogenic or arteriogenic stimuli.

Apart from the influence of atherosclerosis on the organism's responsiveness to angiogenic and arteriogenic treatment, there is potentially the opposite effect, i.e. that of arteriogenic therapy on the course of atherosclerosis. The stimulation of neovascularization with growth factors is prone to harmful side effects, such as rupture of atherosclerotic plaques, because arteriogenesis shares common mechanisms with inflammatory diseases like atherosclerosis. Both arteriogenesis and atherogenesis undergo endothelial activation with upregulation of adhesion molecules on endothelial cells and monocytes and the infiltration of circulating cells into the vascular wall. Since most compounds evaluated for collateral growth promotion influence one of the mentioned parameters, an aggravation of plaque progression is frequently observed in experimental studies, so that the term 'Janus phenomenon' has been coined to describe the trade-off between arteriogenesis and atherogenesis.[273] However, though vascular infiltration of inflammatory cells is an important characteristic of both processes, they are not identical and arteriogenic factors, such as G-CSF or TGFβ1, without the adverse effect on atherosclerosis appear to exist. Differences in the transcriptional profile of macrophages with regard to arteriogenesis and atherogenesis may provide clues for identifying factors that specifically promote one without affecting the other process.[140,274] In the context of the consistent observation that patients with poor collateral function do often elicit an upregulation of anti-angiogenic or anti-arteriogenic genes, a novel strategy of collateral promotion could consist of inhibiting anti-angiogenic gene signalling,[140,274] thereby circumventing the atherogenic side effects of collateral promoting growth factors.

5.6.3 Neovascularization and Tumour Growth

Another obvious concern is the potential stimulation of tumour angiogenesis by pro-arteriogenic therapies. As in neovascularization, tumour-associated leucocytes are sources of angiogenic factors, which substantially influence tumour vascularization. Infiltrating T-lymphocytes express VEGF and macrophages release a variety of cytokines in neoplastic tissue, some of them, like TNFα, are also relevant in promoting collateral growth. In this context, Luo et al. recently targeted tumour-associated macrophages as a novel strategy against breast cancer.[275] Legumain, a member of the asparaginyl endopeptidase family functioning as a stress protein, overexpressed by tumour-associated macrophages, provided a target molecule. A legumain-based DNA vaccine served as a tool to prove this point, as it induced a robust CD8[+] T-cell response against tumour-associated macrophages, which dramatically reduced their density in tumour tissues and resulted in a marked decrease in proangiogenic factors released by macrophages such as TGFβ, TNFα, MMP-9 and VEGF. This, in turn, led to a suppression of both tumour angiogenesis and tumour growth and metastasis.[275] This strategy was demonstrated in murine models of metastatic breast, colon and non-small cell lung cancers, where 75% of vaccinated mice survived tumour cell challenges and 62% were completely free of metastases. Lewis and Pollard reviewed recently that macrophages are prominent in the stromal compartment of virtually all types of malignancy, and these cells respond to the presence of stimuli in different parts of tumours with the release of a repertoire of growth factors, cytokines, chemokines and enzymes that regulate tumour growth, angiogenesis, invasion and/or metastasis.[276] EPC also contribute to tumour angiogenesis.[277]

Despite the compelling evidence of the relevance of neovascularization in tumour growth and development of metastases, no increase in neoplastic diseases has been observed so far in clinical trials aiming to promote angiogenesis or arteriogenesis in patients with coronary or peripheral artery diseases. Nevertheless, the concern of stimulating tumour neovascularization requires careful patient selection and close surveillance during follow-up to detect side effects. Since tumour angiogenesis is predominantly driven by hypoxia, and fluid shear stress-induced vascular remodelling is less prominent in this form of neovascularization, therapies aiming at arteriogenesis instead of angiogenesis may be less at risk for the side effect of tumour growth.

5.6.4 Growth Factor Delivery Mode

A critical issue of studies aiming to stimulate collateral growth is the route of administration of the compound(s). Principally, growth factors, cytokines, proteases, growth factor genes and mononuclear cells can be delivered systemically or locally. It is generally acknowledged that systemic delivery is less efficient than local application. Even for systematically active growth factors such as GM-CSF, a high local concentration in collateral arteries appears to be important to achieve optimal effects.[166] Conversely, the efficacy results of two small randomized trials of GM-CSF for coronary collateral growth promotion can be interpreted differently[144,165]: systemic-only delivery of GM-CSF[165] was more consistently efficient than a combination of systemic and local intracoronary bolus delivery.[144] The cumulated dose of GM-CSF was likely higher in the subcutaneous-only GM-CSF than in the systemic/local protocol, because the first intracoronary bolus was probably washed out instantaneously. Accordingly, there is consensus that extended exposure of the collateral vasculature to the collateral-promoting drug is important. With regard to the latter requirement, the following modes of delivery are well suited: intracoronary infusion instead of bolus injection, intramyocardial injection (transendo- or transepicardial), intrapericardial injection and retroperfusion from the coronary sinus. Baklanov et al. recently compared two routes for myocardial delivery of arteriogenic therapeutics, transendocardial delivery with an intramyocardial injection catheter and retrograde coronary venous delivery with a balloon occlusion catheter in the interventricular vein. Transendocardial delivery and retrograde venous injection of neutron-activatable microspheres were compared in three healthy pigs, four pigs with a 1-week-old myocardial infarction and in four pigs with a 2-weeks-old myocardial infarction.[278] Myocardial infarction was induced by a 1-hour balloon occlusion in the LAD. Both methods were compared in the same animal using different microspheres. The retrograde injection catheter allowed for measurement of distal coronary pressure and microspheres were injected in 10 ml at 300 mmHg above balloon occlusion pressure. The transendocardial injections were targeted to the infarct zone and the same amount of microspheres were distributed over 10 injections. Retention of microspheres decreased with increase in infarct age, but was similar between devices within the groups.[278] In experimental studies, best results in the sense of achieving the highest efficacy of a treatment have been demonstrated by delivery of the neovascularizing agent directly into the donor artery of the developing collateral vessel.[133] In the clinical situation of CAD, this is difficult to realize, because the collateral-supplying artery cannot be identified with certainty or because injection of the agent into both coronary arteries is technically more demanding than single vessel injection.

The genetic transfection of the vascular wall is a possibility to circumvent the delivery problem encountered with protein-based treatments. In particular, trials employing adenoviral vectors for delivery of FGF or VEGF have shown promising results of neovascularization in both CAD and peripheral artery disease.[9,57,77] However, transfection of the vascular wall remains difficult and is at risk for safety concerns associated with gene therapy and because of the use of viral vectors.

With recent advances in drug-eluting stent technology, endovascular devices are emerging as a promising new platform for extended intracoronary drug delivery. New generation drug-eluting stents possess an enhanced drug delivery capacity, which can be used for other purposes than for coronary restenosis prevention. Specifically, the evolving technology of biodegradable stents could offer a mode of slowly releasing arteriogenic substances into the coronary artery. In this context, safety is, however, an important issue and any negative effect on thrombogenicity or enhanced in-stent restenosis must be excluded.

A further possibility of local drug delivery potentially suitable for arteriogenic proteins and genes as well as cells is the ultrasound-mediated destruction of echocontrast microbubbles. Imada et al. investigated the targeted delivery of bone marrow mononuclear cells by ultrasound destruction of microbubbles with regard to the angiogenic and arteriogenic response.[279] Ultrasound-mediated destruction of phospholipid-coated microbubbles was applied to the ischaemic hindlimb muscle of rats, and subsequently, BMC were transfused. A larger enhancement in blood flow recovery after microbubble destruction plus cell infusion was observed as compared with microbubble destruction alone.[279] Alternatively, microbubbles of only a few microns in size can be loaded with proteins, non-protein compounds or genetic constructs, and following intravenous injection, the circulation of the microbubbles can be traced by ultrasound. Upon arrival of the loaded echo contrast in the myocardium, the bubbles can be destroyed in the region of interest using a burst of increased ultrasonic mechanical energy.[280] By incorporating antibodies or other agents with specific affinity, microbubbles can be targeted to specific tissues or cells. Recently, Leong-Poi et al. detected endogenous and therapeutic arteriogenesis in rats with hindlimb ischaemia by contrast ultrasound molecular imaging of integrin expression.[281] Targeted contrast ultrasound imaging of alpha(v)- and $\alpha5\beta1$-integrin expression was performed with microbubbles bearing the disintegrin echistatin. A similar approach could be employed in order to deliver an arteriogenic substance selectively to a region of growing collateral vessels. In principle, developing collaterals can be detected on the basis of differential expression of endothelial surface markers.[282] Mazur et al. generated antibodies that specifically target collateral arteries, but not quiescent control arteries or tumour vessels.[282] Incorporating collateral antibodies in ultrasonic microbubbles could be employed for the targeted delivery of arteriogenic factors with a minimized risk for tumour neovascularization.

Abbreviations

Ang1/2	angiopoietin 1 / 2
aFGF	acidic fibroblast growth factor
bFGF	basic fibroblast growth factor
BMC	bone marrow-derived cell
CAD	coronary artery disease
CFI	collateral flow index (no unit)
CVP	central venous pressure (mmHg)
EPC	endothelial progenitor cell
ETT	exercise treadmill time
FGF	fibroblast growth factor

G-CSF	granulocyte colony-stimulating factor
GM-CSF	granulocyte-macrophage colony-stimulating factor
HGF	hepatic growth factor
HIF-1α	hypoxia-inducible factor 1 alpha
IGF-1	insulin-like growth factor-1
IL-8	interleukin-8
eNOS	endothelial nitric oxide synthase
iNOS	inducible nitric oxide synthase
IS	infarct size
LAD	left anterior descending artery
LCX	left circumflex coronary artery
LV	left ventricle, left ventricular
MCP-1	monocyte chemoattractant protein-1
MMP	matrix metallo proteinase
NO	nitric oxide
P_{ao}	mean aortic pressure (mmHg)
PCI	percutaneous coronary intervention
PDGF	platelet-derived growth factor
PECAM	platelet endothelial cell adhesion molecule
P_{occl}	mean coronary occlusive or wedge pressure (mmHg)
PLGF	placenta growth factor
RCA	right coronary artery
TGFβ	transforming growth factor beta
TNFα	tumour necrosis factor alpha
VEGF	vascular endothelial growth factor
VEGFR	vascular endothelial growth factor receptor

References

1. Boersma H, Doornbos G, Bloemberg B, Wood D, Kromhout D, Simoons M. Cardiovascular diseases in Europe. In: Cardiology ESo, ed. *European Registries of Cardiovascular Diseases and Patient Management*. Sophia Antipolis; 1999:58.
2. Mukherjee D, Bhatt D, Roe M, Patel V, Ellis S. Direct myocardial revascularization and angiogenesis – how many patients might be eligible? *Am J Cardiol*. 1999;84:598–600.
3. Seiler C. The human coronary collateral circulation. *Heart*. 2003;89:1352–1357.
4. Sawaia N. Embryology of the heart and large vessels. I. Preliminary notes. II – Angiogenesis. *Arq Bras Cardiol*. 1967;20:199–206.
5. Fujita M, Sasayama S, Asanoi H, Nakajima H, Sakai O, Ohno A. Improvement of treadmill capacity and collateral circulation as a result of exercise with heparin pretreatment in patients with effort angina. *Circulation*. 1988;77:1022–1029.
6. Schumacher B, Pecher P, von Specht B, Stegmann T. Induction of neoangiogenesis in ischemic myocardium by human growth factors: first clinical results of a new treatment of coronary heart disease. *Circulation*. 1998;97:645–650.
7. Sellke F, Laham R, Edelman E, Pearlman J, Simons M. Therapeutic angiogenesis with basic fibroblast growth factor: technique and early results. *Ann Thor Surg*. 1998;65:1540–1544.

8. Losordo D, Vale P, Symes J, et al. Gene therapy for myocardial angiogenesis: initial clinical results with direct myocardial injection of phVEGF165 as sole therapy for myocardial ischemia. *Circulation.* 1998;98:2800–2804.
9. Rajagopalan S, Mohler Er, Lederman R, et al. Regional angiogenesis with vascular endothelial growth factor in peripheral arterial disease: a phase II randomized, double-blind, controlled study of adenoviral delivery of vascular endothelial growth factor 121 in patients with disabling intermittent claudication. *Circulation.* 2003;108:1933–1938.
10. Simons M, Annex B, Laham R, et al. Pharmacological treatment of coronary artery disease with recombinant fibroblast growth factor-2: double-blind, randomized, controlled clinical trial. *Circulation.* 2002;105:788–793.
11. Henry T, Rocha-Singh K, Isner J, et al. Intracoronary administration of recombinant human vascular endothelial growth factor to patients with coronary artery disease. *Am Heart J.* 2001;142:872–880.
12. Losordo D, Vale P, Hendel R, et al. Phase 1/2 placebo-controlled, double-blind, dose-escalating trial of myocardial vascular endothelial growth factor 2 gene transfer by catheter delivery in patients with chronic myocardial ischemia. *Circulation.* 2002;105:2012–2018.
13. Laham R, Sellke F, Edelman E, et al. Local perivascular delivery of basic fibroblast growth factor in patients undergoing coronary bypass surgery: results of a phase I randomized, double-blind, placebo-controlled trial. *Circulation.* 1999;100:1865–1871.
14. Unger E, Goncalves L, Epstein S, Chew E, Trapnell C, Cannon Rr, Quyyumi A. Effects of a single intracoronary injection of basic fibroblast growth factor in stable angina pectoris. *Am J Cardiol.* 2000;85:1414–1419.
15. Udelson J, Dilsizian V, Laham R, et al. Therapeutic angiogenesis with recombinant fibroblast growth factor-2 improves stress and rest myocardial perfusion abnormalities in patients with severe symptomatic chronic coronary artery disease. *Circulation.* 2000;102:1605–1610.
16. Rosengart T, Lee L, Patel S, et al. Angiogenesis gene therapy: phase I assessment of direct intramyocardial administration of an adenovirus vector expressing VEGF121 cDNA to individuals with clinically significant severe coronary artery disease. *Circulation.* 1999;100:468–474.
17. Vale P, Losordo D, Milliken C, et al. Randomized, single-blind, placebo-controlled pilot study of catheter-based myocardial gene transfer for therapeutic angiogenesis using left ventricular electromechanical mapping in patients with chronic myocardial ischemia. *Circulation.* 2001;103:2138–2143.
18. Lunde K, Solheim S, Aakhus S, et al. Intracoronary injection of mononuclear bone marrow cells in acute myocardial infarction. *N Engl J Med.* 2006;355:1199–209.
19. Assmus B, Honold J, Schächinger V, et al. Transcoronary transplantation of progenitor cells after myocardial infarction. *N Engl J Med.* 2006;355:1222–1232.
20. Schächinger V, Erbs S, Elsässer A, et al. Intracoronary bone marrow-derived progenitor cells in acute myocardial infarction. *N Engl J Med.* 2006;355:1210–1221.
21. Risau W. Mechanisms of angiogenesis. *Nature.* 1997;386:671–674.
22. Carmeliet P. Angiogenesis in health and disease. *Nature Med.* 2003;9:653–660.
23. Heil M, Schaper W. Insights into pathways of arteriogenesis. *Curr Pharm Biotechnol.* 2007;8:35–42.
24. Heil M, Eitenmüller I, Schmitz-Rixen T, Schaper W. Arteriogenesis versus angiogenesis: similarities and differences. *J Cell Mol Med.* 2006;10:45–55.
25. Carmeliet P. Angiogenesis in life, disease and medicine. *Nature.* 2005;438:932–936.
26. Folkman J. Tumor angiogenesis: therapeutic implications. *N Engl J Med.* 1971;285:1182–1186.
27. Folkman J, Merler E, Abernathy C, Williams G. Isolation of a tumor factor responsible for angiogenesis. *J Exp Med.* 1971;133:275–288.
28. Carmeliet P. Mechanisms of angiogenesis and arteriogenesis. *Nat Med.* 2000;6:389–395.
29. Conway E, Collen D, Carmeliet P. Molecular mechanisms of blood vessel growth. *Cardiovasc Res.* 2001;49:507–521.

30. Bren L. "Frances Oldham Kelsey: FDA medical reviewer leaves her mark on history". In: *FDA Consumer Magazine, US Food and Drug Administration*; 2001.
31. Wang G, Jiang B, Rue E, Semenza G. Hypoxia-inducible factor 1 is a basic-helix-loop-helix-PAS heterodimer regulated by cellular O2 tension. *Proc Natl Acad Sci USA.* 1995;92:5510–5514.
32. Forsythe J, Jiang B, Iyer N, et al. Activation of vascular endothelial growth factor gene transcription by hypoxia-inducible factor 1. *Mol Cell Biol.* 1996;16:4604–4613.
33. Kelly B, Hackett S, Hirota K, et al. Cell type-specific regulation of angiogenic growth factor gene expression and induction of angiogenesis in nonischemic tissue by a constitutively active form of hypoxia-inducible factor 1. *Circ Res.* 2003;93:1074–1081.
34. Annex B, Simons M. Growth factor-induced therapeutic angiogenesis in the heart: protein therapy. *Cardiovasc Res.* 2005;65:649–655.
35. Ribatti D, Vacca A, Presta M. The discovery of angiogeneic factors: a historical review. *General Pharmacol.* 2002;35:227–231.
36. Shing Y, Folkman J, Sullivan R, Butterfield C, Murray J, Klagsbrun M. Heparin affinity: purification of a tumor-derived capillary endothelial cell growth factor. *Science.* 1984;223:1296–1299.
37. Maciag T, Mehlman T, Friesel R, Schreiber A. Heparin binds endothelial cell growth factor, the principal endothelial cell mitogen in bovine brain. *Science.* 1984;225:932–935.
38. Ferrara N, Henzel W. Pituitary follicular cells secrete a novel heparin-binding growth factor specific for vascular endothelial cells. *Biochem Biophys Res Commun.* 1989;161:851–858.
39. Plouët J, Schilling J, Gospodarowicz D. Isolation and characterization of a newly identified endothelial cell mitogen produced by AtT-20 cells. *EMBO J.* 1989;8:3801–3806.
40. Tirziu D, Simons M. Angiogenesis in the human heart: gene and cell therapy. *Angiogenesis.* 2005;8:241–251.
41. Couchman J. Syndecans: proteoglycan regulators of cell-surface microdomains? *Nat Rev Mol Cell Biol.* 2003;4:926–937.
42. Detillieux K, Sheikh F, Kardami E, Cattini P. Biological activities of fibroblast growth factor-2 in the adult myocardium. *Cardiovasc Res.* 2003;57:8–19.
43. Baffour R, Berman J, Garb J, Rhee S, Kaufman J, Friedmann P. Enhanced angiogenesis and growth of collaterals by in vivo administration of recombinant basic fibroblast growth factor in a rabbit model of acute lower limb ischemia: dose-response effect of basic fibroblast growth factor. *J Vasc Surg.* 1992;16:181–191.
44. Asahara T, Bauters C, Zheng L, et al. Synergistic effect of vascular endothelial growth factor and basic fibroblast growth factor on angiogenesis in vivo. *Circulation.* 1995;92(9 Suppl):II365–371.
45. Bernotat-Danielowski S, Sharma H, Schott R, Schaper W. Generation and localisation of monoclonal antibodies against fibroblast growth factors in ischaemic collateralised porcine myocardium. *Cardiovasc Res.* 1993;27:1220–1228.
46. Battler A, Scheinowitz M, Bor A, et al. Intracoronary injection of basic fibroblast growth factor enhances angiogenesis in infarcted swine myocardium. *J Am Coll Cardiol.* 1993;22:2001–2006.
47. Harada K, Grossman W, Friedman M, et al. Basic fibroblast growth factor improves myocardial function in chronically ischemic porcine hearts. *J Clin Invest.* 1994;94:623–630.
48. Yanagisawa-Miwa A, Uchida Y, Nakamura F, et al. Salvage of infarcted myocardium by angiogenic action of basic fibroblast growth factor. *Science.* 1992;257:1401–1403.
49. Unger E, Banai S, Shou M, et al. Basic fibroblast growth factor enhances myocardial collateral flow in a canine model. *Am J Physiol.* 1994;266:H1588–1595.
50. Banai S, Jaklitsch M, Casscells W, et al. Effects of acidic fibroblast growth factor on normal and ischemic myocardium. *Circ Res.* 1991;69:76–85.
51. Lazarous D, Scheinowitz M, Shou M, et al. Effects of chronic systemic administration of basic fibroblast growth factor on collateral development in the canine heart. *Circulation.* 1995;91:145–153.

52. Lazarous D, Shou M, Scheinowitz M, et al. Comparative effects of basic fibroblast growth factor and vascular endothelial growth factor on coronary collateral development and the arterial response to injury. *Circulation*. 1996;94:1074–1082.

53. Seiler C. Human basic fibroblast growth factor induces angiogenesis in hen eggs and rat hearts. *Circulation*. 1999;100:1250–1251.

54. Laham R, Chronos N, Pike M, et al. Intracoronary basic fibroblast growth factor (FGF-2) in patients with severe ischemic heart disease: results of a phase I open-label dose escalation study. *J Am Coll Cardiol*. 2000;36:2132–2139.

55. Ruel M, Laham R, Parker J, et al. Long-term effects of surgical angiogenic therapy with fibroblast growth factor 2 protein. *J Thorac Cardiovasc Surg*. 2002;124:28 34.

56. Grines C, Watkins M, Helmer G, et al. Angiogenic Gene Therapy (AGENT) trial in patients with stable angina pectoris. *Circulation*. 2002;105:1291–1297.

57. Grines C, Watkins M, Mahmarian J, et al. AGTA-S. A randomized, double-blind, placebo-controlled trial of Ad5FGF-4 gene therapy and its effect on myocardial perfusion in patients with stable angina. *J Am Coll Cardiol*. 2003;42:1339–1347.

58. Henry T, Grines C, Watkins M, et al. Effects of Ad5FGF-4 in patients with angina: an analysis of pooled data from the AGENT-3 and AGENT-4 trials. *J Am Coll Cardiol*. 2007;50:1038–1046.

59. Veikkola T, Alitalo K. VEGFs, receptors and angiogenesis. *Semin Cancer Biol*. 1999;9:211–220.

60. Carmeliet P, Ng Y, Nuyens D, et al. Impaired myocardial angiogenesis and ischemic cardiomyopathy in mice lacking the vascular endothelial growth factor isoforms VEGF164 and VEGF188. *Nat Med*. 1999;5:495–502.

61. Shalaby F, Rossant J, Yamaguchi T, et al. Failure of blood-island formation and vasculogenesis in Flk-1-deficient mice. *Nature*. 1995;376:62–66.

62. Fong G, Zhang L, Bryce D, Peng J. Increased hemangioblast commitment, not vascular disorganization, is the primary defect in flt-1 knock-out mice. *Development*. 1999;126:3015–3025.

63. Dumont D, Jussila L, Taipale J, et al. Cardiovascular failure in mouse embryos deficient in VEGF receptor-3. *Science*. 1998;282:946–949.

64. Takeshita S, Zheng L, Brogi E, et al. Therapeutic angiogenesis. A single intraarterial bolus of vascular endothelial growth factor augments revascularization in a rabbit ischemic hind limb model. *J Clin Invest*. 1994;93:662–670.

65. Banai S, Jaklitsch M, Shou M, et al. Angiogenic-induced enhancement of collateral blood flow to ischemic myocardium by vascular endothelial growth factor in dogs. *Circulation*. 1994;89:2183–2189.

66. Tsurumi Y, Takeshita S, Chen D, et al. Direct intramuscular gene transfer of naked DNA encoding vascular endothelial growth factor augments collateral development and tissue perfusion. *Circulation*. 1996;94:3281–3290.

67. Mack C, Patel S, Schwarz E, et al. Biologic bypass with the use of adenovirus-mediated gene transfer of the complementary deoxyribonucleic acid for vascular endothelial growth factor 121 improves myocardial perfusion and function in the ischemic porcine heart. *J Thorac Cardiovasc Surg*. 1998;115:168–176.

68. Hendel R, Henry T, Rocha-Singh K, et al. Effect of intracoronary recombinant human vascular endothelial growth factor on myocardial perfusion: evidence for a dose-dependent effect. *Circulation*. 2000;101:118–121.

69. Henry T, Annex B, McKendall G, et al. The VIVA trial: Vascular endothelial growth factor in Ischemia for Vascular Angiogenesis. *Circulation*. 2003;107:1359–1365.

70. Isner J, Pieczek A, Schainfeld R, et al. Clinical evidence of angiogenesis after arterial gene transfer of phVEGF165 in patient with ischaemic limb. *Lancet*. 1996;348:370–374.

71. Baumgartner I, Pieczek A, Manor O, et al. Constitutive expression of phVEGF165 after intramuscular gene transfer promotes collateral vessel development in patients with critical limb ischemia. *Circulation*. 1998;97:1114–1123.

72. Symes J, Losordo D, Vale P, et al. Gene therapy with vascular endothelial growth factor for inoperable coronary artery disease. *Ann Thor Surg*. 1999;68:830–836.

73. Vale P, Losordo D, Milliken C, et al. Left ventricular electromechanical mapping to assess efficacy of phVEGF(165) gene transfer for therapeutic angiogenesis in chronic myocardial ischemia. *Circulation*. 2000;102:965–974.

74. Fortuin F, Vale P, Losordo D, et al. One-year follow-up of direct myocardial gene transfer of vascular endothelial growth factor-2 using naked plasmid deoxyribonucleic acid by way of thoracotomy in no-option patients. *Am J Cardiol*. 2003;92:436–439.

75. Kastrup J, Jørgensen E, Rück A, et al. Direct intramyocardial plasmid vascular endothelial growth factor-A165 gene therapy in patients with stable severe angina pectoris A randomized double-blind placebo-controlled study: the Euroinject One trial. *J Am Coll Cardiol*. 2005;45:982–988.

76. Gyöngyösi M, Khorsand A, Zamini S, et al. NOGA-guided analysis of regional myocardial perfusion abnormalities treated with intramyocardial injections of plasmid encoding vascular endothelial growth factor A-165 in patients with chronic myocardial ischemia: subanalysis of the EUROINJECT-ONE multicenter double-blind randomized study. *Circulation*. 2005;112(9 Suppl):I157–165.

77. Hedman M, Hartikainen J, Syvänne M, et al. Safety and feasibility of catheter-based local intracoronary vascular endothelial growth factor gene transfer in the prevention of postangioplasty and in-stent restenosis and in the treatment of chronic myocardial ischemia: phase II results of the Kuopio Angiogenesis Trial (KAT). *Circulation*. 2003;107:2677–2683.

78. Stewart D, Hilton J, Arnold J, et al. Angiogenic gene therapy in patients with nonrevascularizable ischemic heart disease: a phase 2 randomized, controlled trial of AdVEGF(121) (AdVEGF121) versus maximum medical treatment. *Gene Ther*. 2006;13:1503–1511.

79. Kalka C, Tehrani H, Laudenberg B, et al. VEGF gene transfer mobilizes endothelial progenitor cells in patients with inoperable coronary disease. *Ann Thor Surg*. 2000;70:829–834.

80. Lu H, Xu X, Zhang M, et al. Combinatorial protein therapy of angiogenic and arteriogenic factors remarkably improves collaterogenesis and cardiac function in pigs. *Proc Natl Acad Sci USA*. 2007;104:12140–12145.

81. Unger E, Sheffield C, Epstein S. Heparin promotes the formation of extracardiac to coronary anastomoses in a canine model. *Am J Physiol*. 1991;260:H1625–1634.

82. Azizkhan R, Azizkhan J, Zetter B, Folkman J. Mast cell heparin stimulates migration of capillary endothelial cells in vitro. *J Exp Med*. 1980;152:931–944.

83. Chiarugi V, Ruggiero M, Porciatti F, Vannucchi S, Ziche M. Cooperation of heparin with other angiogenetic effectors. *Int J Tissue React*. 1986;8:129–133.

84. Damon D, Lobb R, D' Amore P, Wagner J. Heparin potentiates the action of acidic fibroblast growth factor by prolonging its biological half-life. *J Cell Physiol*. 1989;138:221–226.

85. Ehrlich H, Jung W, Costa D, Rajaratnam J. Effects of heparin on vascularization of artificial skin grafts in rats. *Exp Mol Pathol*. 1988;48:244–251.

86. Fujita M, Kihara Y, Hasegawa K, Nohara R, Sasayama S. Heparin potentiates collateral growth but not growth of intramyocardial endarteries in dogs with repeated coronary occlusion. *Int J Cardiol*. 1999;70:165–170.

87. Lobb R, Harper J, Fett J. Purification of heparin-binding growth factors. *Anal Biochem*. 1986;154:1–14.

88. Mueller S, Thomas K, Di Salvo J, Levine E. Stabilization by heparin of acidic fibroblast growth factor mitogenicity for human endothelial cells in vitro. *J Cell Physiol*. 1989;140:439–448.

89. Bashkin P, Doctrow S, Klagsbrun M, Svahn C, Folkman J, Vlodavsky I. Basic fibroblast growth factor binds to subendothelial extracellular matrix and is released by heparitinase and heparin-like molecules. *Biochemistry*. 1989;28:1737–1743.

90. Masuda D, Fujita M, Nohara R, Matsumori A, Sasayama S. Improvement of oxygen metabolism in ischemic myocardium as a result of enhanced external counterpulsation with heparin pretreatment for patients with stable angina. *Heart Vessels*. 2004;19:59–62.

91. Symons J, Firoozmand E, Longhurst J. Repeated dipyridamole administration enhances collateral-dependent flow and regional function during exercise. A role for adenosine. *Circ Res*. 1993;73:503–513.

92. Picano E, Michelassi C. Chronic oral dipyridamole as a ' novel' antianginal drug: the collateral hypothesis. *Cardiovasc Res*. 1997;33:666–670.

93. Belardinelli R, Belardinelli L, Shryock J. Effects of dipyridamole on coronary collateralization and myocardial perfusion in patients with ischaemic cardiomyopathy. *Eur Heart J*. 2001;22:1205–1213.

94. Degenring F, Curnish R, Rubio R, Berne R. Effect of dipyridamole on myocardial adenosine metabolism and coronary flow in hypoxia and reactive hyperemia in the isolated perfused guinea pig heart. *J Mol Cell Cardiol*. 1976;8:877–888.

95. Shryock J, Snowdy S, Baraldi P, et al. A2A-adenosine receptor reserve for coronary vasodilation. *Circulation*. 1998;98:711–718.

96. Ethier M, Chander V, Dobson JJ. Adenosine stimulates proliferation of human endothelial cells in culture. *Am J Physiol*. 1993;265:H131–138.

97. Tornling G, Adolfsson J, Unge G, Ljungqvist A. Capillary neoformation in skeletal muscle of dipyridamole-treated rats. *Arzneimittelforschung*. 1980;30:791–792.

98. Pasyk S, Schaper W, Schaper J, Pasyk K, Miskiewicz G, Steinseifer B. DNA synthesis in coronary collaterals after coronary artery occlusion in conscious dog. *Am J Physiol*. 1982;242:H1031–1037.

99. Teuscher E, Weidlich V. Adenosine nucleotides, adenosine and adenine as angiogenesis factors. *Biomed Biochim Acta*. 1985;44:493–495.

100. Hanna G, Yhip P, Fujise K, et al. Intracoronary adenosine administered during rotational atherectomy of complex lesions in native coronary arteries reduces the incidence of no-reflow phenomenon. *Catheter Cardiovasc Interv*. 1999;48:275–278.

101. Liu G, Thornton J, Van Winkle D, Stanley A, Olsson R, Downey J. Protection against infarction afforded by preconditioning is mediated by A1 adenosine receptors in rabbit heart. *Circulation*. 1991;84:350–356.

102. Leesar M, Stoddard M, Ahmed M, Broadbent J, Bolli R. Preconditioning of human myocardium with adenosine during coronary angioplasty. *Circulation*. 1997;95:2500–2507.

103. Billinger M, Fleisch M, Eberli FR, Garachemani AR, Meier B, Seiler C. Is the development of myocardial tolerance to repeated ischemia in humans due to preconditioning or to collateral recruitment? *J Am Coll Cardiol*. 1999;33:1027–1035.

104. Lambiase P, Edwards R, Cusack M, Bucknall C, Redwood S, Marber M. Exercise-induced ischemia initiates the second window of protection in humans independent of collateral recruitment. *J Am Coll Cardiol*. 2003;41:1174–1182.

105. Bernardo N, Okubo S, Maaieh M, Wood M, Kukreja R. Delayed preconditioning with adenosine is mediated by opening of ATP-sensitive K(+) channels in rabbit heart. *Am J Physiol*. 1999;277:H128–135.

106. Zhao T, Xi L, Chelliah J, Levasseur J, Kukreja R. Inducible nitric oxide synthase mediates delayed myocardial protection induced by activation of adenosine A(1) receptors: evidence from gene-knockout mice. *Circulation*. 2000;102:902–907.

107. Cooke J. NO and angiogenesis. *Atherosclerosis*. 2003;4(suppl):53–60.

108. Hood J, Meininger C, Ziche M, Granger H. VEGF upregulates ecNOS message, protein, and NO production in human endothelial cells. *Am J Physiol*. 1998;274:H1054–1058.

109. Simon B, Cunningham L, Cohen R. Oxidized low density lipoproteins cause contraction and inhibit endothelium-dependent relaxation in the pig coronary artery. *J Clin Invest*. 1990;86:75–79.

110. Inoue N, Venema R, Sayegh H, Ohara Y, Murphy T, Harrison D. Molecular regulation of the bovine endothelial cell nitric oxide synthase by transforming growth factor-beta 1. *Arterioscler Thromb Vasc Biol.* 1995;15:1255–1261.

111. Tiefenbacher C, Chilian W. Basic fibroblast growth factor and heparin influence coronary arteriolar tone by causing endothelium-dependent dilation. *Cardiovasc Res.* 1997;34:411–417.

112. Babaei S, Teichert-Kuliszewska K, Monge J, Mohamed F, Bendeck M, Stewart D. Role of nitric oxide in the angiogenic response in vitro to basic fibroblast growth factor. *Circ Res.* 1998;82:1007–1015.

113. Ziche M, Morbidelli L, Masini E, et al. Nitric oxide mediates angiogenesis in vivo and endothelial cell growth and migration in vitro promoted by substance P. *J Clin Invest.* 1994;94:2036–2044.

114. Dimmeler S, Hermann C, Galle J, Zeiher A. Upregulation of superoxide dismutase and nitric oxide synthase mediates the apoptosis-suppressive effects of shear stress on endothelial cells. *Arterioscler Thromb Vasc Biol.* 1999;19:656–664.

115. Ziche M, Parenti A, Ledda F, et al. Nitric oxide promotes proliferation and plasminogen activator production by coronary venular endothelium through endogenous bFGF. *Circ Res.* 1997;80:845–852.

116. Hudlicka O. Is physiological angiogenesis in skeletal muscle regulated by changes in microcirculation? *Microcirculation.* 1998;5:5–23.

117. Dulak J, Józkowicz A, Dembinska-Kiec A, et al. Nitric oxide induces the synthesis of vascular endothelial growth factor by rat vascular smooth muscle cells. *Arterioscler Thromb Vasc Biol.* 2000;20:659–666.

118. Yu J, deMuinck E, Zhuang Z, et al. Endothelial nitric oxide synthase is critical for ischemic remodeling, mural cell recruitment, and blood flow reserve. *Proc Natl Acad Sci USA.* 2005;102:10999–11004.

119. Mees B, Wagner S, Ninci E, et al. Endothelial nitric oxide synthase activity is essential for vasodilation during blood flow recovery but not for arteriogenesis. *Arterioscler Thromb Vasc Biol.* 2007;27:1926–1933.

120. Fukuda S, Kaga S, Zhan L, et al. Resveratrol ameliorates myocardial damage by inducing vascular endothelial growth factor-angiogenesis and tyrosine kinase receptor Flk-1. *Cell Mol Biol Res.* 2006;44:43–49.

121. Goldstein R, Stinson E, Scherer J, Seningen R, Grehl T, Epstein SE. Intraoperative coronary collateral function in patients with coronary occlusive disease. Nitroglycerin responsiveness and angiographic correlations. *Circulation.* 1974;49:298–308.

122. Piek J, van Liebergen R, Koch K, de Winter R, Peters R, David G. Pharmacological modulation of the human collateral vascular resistance in acute and chronic coronary occlusion assessed by intracoronary blood flow velocity analysis in an angioplasty model. *Circulation.* 1997;96:108–115.

123. Marfella R, Esposito K, Nappo F, et al. Expression of angiogenic factors during acute coronary syndromes in human type 2 diabetes. *Diabetes.* 2004;53:2383–2391.

124. Salloum F, Yin C, Xi L, Kukreja R. Sildenafil induces delayed preconditioning through inducible nitric oxide synthase-dependent pathway in mouse heart. *Circ Res.* 2003;92:595–597.

125. Vidavalur R, Penumathsa S, Zhan L, Thirunavukkarasu M, Maulik N. Sildenafil induces angiogenic response in human coronary arteriolar endothelial cells through the expression of thioredoxin, hemeoxygenase and vascular endothelial growth factor. *Vascul Pharmacol.* 2006;45:91–95.

126. Senthilkumar A, Smith R, Khitha J, et al. Sildenafil promotes ischemia-induced angiogenesis through a PKG-dependent pathway. *Arterioscler Thromb Vasc Biol.* 2007;27:1947–1954.

127. Herrmann L, Bollack C. Bridging defects in large arteries; a problem for arteriogenesis. *AMA Arch Surg.* 1955;71:486–490.

128. Schechter J, Goldsmith P, Wilson C, Weiner R. Morphological evidence for the presence of arteries in human prolactinomas. *J Clin Endocrinol Metab*. 1988;67:713–719.
129. Arras M, Ito W, Scholz D, Winkler B, Schaper J, Schaper W. Monocyte activation in angiogenesis and collateral growth in the rabbit hindlimb. *J Clin Invest*. 1998;101:40–50.
130. Lower R. *Early science in Oxford*. Oxford: Oxford University Press; 1932.
131. Fulton WFM. Arterial anastomoses in the coronary circulation. II. Distribution, enumeration and measurement of coronary arterial anastomoses in health and disease. *Scott Med J*. 1963;8:466–474.
132. Wustmann K, Zbinden S, Windecker S, Meier B, Seiler C. Is there functional collateral flow during vascular occlusion in angiographically normal coronary arteries? *Circulation*. 2003;107:2213–2220.
133. Hoefer I, van Royen N, Buschmann I, Piek J, Schaper W. Time course of arteriogenesis following femoral artery occlusion in the rabbit. *Cardiovasc Res*. 2001;49:609–617.
134. Deindl F, Buschmann I, Hoefer I, et al. Role of ischemia and of hypoxia-inducible genes in arteriogenesis after femoral artery occlusion in the rabbit. *Circ Res*. 2001;89:779–786.
135. Schaper J, König R, Franz D, Schaper W. The endothelial surface of growing coronary collateral arteries. Intimal margination and diapedesis of monocytes. A combined SEM and TEM study. *Virchows Arch A Pathol Anat Histol*. 1976;370:193–205.
136. Eitenmüller I, Volger O, Kluge A, et al. The range of adaptation by collateral vessels after femoral artery occlusion. *Circ Res*. 2006;99:656–662.
137. Tzima E, Irani-Tehrani M, Kiosses W, et al. A mechanosensory complex that mediates the endothelial cell response to fluid shear stress. *Nature*. 2005;437:426–431.
138. Boengler K, Pipp F, Fernandez B, Ziegelhoeffer T, Schaper W, Deindl E. Arteriogenesis is associated with an induction of the cardiac ankyrin repeat protein (carp). *Cardiovasc Res*. 2003;59:573–581.
139. Sarateanu C, Retuerto M, Beckmann J, et al. An Egr-1 master switch for arteriogenesis: studies in Egr-1 homozygous negative and wild-type animals. *J Thorac Cardiovasc Surg*. 2006;131:139–145.
140. Meier P, Antonov J, Zbinden R, et al. Non-invasive gene-expression-based detection of well developed collateral function in individuals with and without coronary artery disease. *Heart*. 2008:Aug 26. [Epub ahead of print].
141. Heil M, Ziegelhoeffer T, Wagner S, et al. Collateral artery growth (arteriogenesis) after experimental arterial occlusion is impaired in mice lacking CC-chemokine receptor-2. *Circ Res*. 2004;94:671–677.
142. Grundmann S, Hoefer I, Ulusans S, et al. Anti-tumor necrosis factor-{alpha} therapies attenuate adaptive arteriogenesis in the rabbit. *Am J Physiol*. 2005;289:H1497–1505.
143. Seiler C, Pohl T, Billinger M, Meier B. Tumour necrosis factor alpha concentration and collateral flow in patients with coronary artery disease and normal systolic left ventricular function. *Heart*. 2003;89:96–97.
144. Seiler C, Pohl T, Wustmann K, et al. Promotion of collateral growth by granulocyte-macrophage colony-stimulating factor in patients with coronary artery disease: a randomized, double-blind, placebo-controlled study. *Circulation*. 2001;104:2012–2017.
145. Heil M, Ziegelhoeffer T, Pipp F, et al. Blood monocyte concentration is critical for enhancement of collateral artery growth. *Am J Physiol*. 2002;283:H2411–2419.
146. Grundmann S, Piek J, Pasterkamp G, Hoefer I. Arteriogenesis: basic mechanisms and therapeutic stimulation. *Eur J Clin Invest*. 2007;37:755–766.
147. Deindl E, Hoefer I, Fernandez B, et al. Involvement of the fibroblast growth factor system in adaptive and chemokine-induced arteriogenesis. *Circ Res*. 2003;92:561–568.
148. Fleisch M, Billinger M, Eberli F, Garachemani A, Meier B, Seiler C. Physiologically assessed coronary collateral flow and intracoronary growth factor concentrations in patients with 1- to 3-vessel coronary artery disease. *Circulation*. 1999;100:1945–1950.
149. Cai W, Koltai S, Kocsis E, et al. Remodeling of the adventitia during coronary arteriogenesis. *Am J Physiol*. 2003;284:H31–40.

150. Cai W, Vosschulte R, Afsah-Hedjri A, et al. Altered balance between extracellular proteolysis and antiproteolysis is associated with adaptive coronary arteriogenesis. *J Mol Cell Cardiol.* 2000;32:997–1011.
151. Stabile E, Burnett M, Watkins C, et al. Impaired arteriogenic response to acute hindlimb ischemia in CD4-knockout mice. *Circulation.* 2003;108:205–210.
152. Hoefer I, Grundmann S, van Royen N, et al. Leukocyte subpopulations and arteriogenesis: specific role of monocytes, lymphocytes and granulocytes. *Atherosclerosis.* 2005;181:285–293.
153. Walter D, Rittig K, Bahlmann F, et al. Statin therapy accelerates reendothelialization: a novel effect involving mobilization and incorporation of bone marrow-derived endothelial progenitor cells. *Circulation.* 2002;105:3017–3024.
154. Ziegelhoeffer T, Fernandez B, Kostin S, et al. Bone marrow-derived cells do not incorporate into the adult growing vasculature. *Circ Res.* 2004;94:230–238.
155. Ito W, Arras M, Winkler B, Scholz D, Schaper J, Schaper W. Monocyte chemotactic protein-1 increases collateral and peripheral conductance after femoral artery occlusion. *Circ Res.* 1997;80:829–837.
156. de Lemos J, Morrow D, Blazing M, et al. Serial measurement of monocyte chemoattractant protein-1 after acute coronary syndromes: results from the A to Z trial. *J Am Coll Cardiol.* 2007;50:2117–2124.
157. van Royen N, Hoefer I, Buschmann I, et al. Effects of local MCP-1 protein therapy on the development of the collateral circulation and atherosclerosis in Watanabe hyperlipidemic rabbits. *Cardiovasc Res.* 2003;57:178–185.
158. van Royen N, Hoefer I, Böttinger M, et al. Local monocyte chemoattractant protein-1 therapy increases collateral artery formation in apolipoprotein E-deficient mice but induces systemic monocytic CD11b expression, neointimal formation, and plaque progression. *Circ Res.* 2003;92:218–225.
159. Shindo J, Ishibashi T, Yokoyama K, et al. Granulocyte-macrophage colony-stimulating factor prevents the progression of atherosclerosis via changes in the cellular and extracellular composition of atherosclerotic lesions in watanabe heritable hyperlipidemic rabbits. *Circulation.* 1999;99:2150–2156.
160. Nimer S, Champlin R, Golde D. Serum cholesterol-lowering activity of granulocyte-macrophage colony-stimulating factor. *JAMA.* 1988;260:3297–3300.
161. Zbinden R, Vogel R, Meier B, Seiler C. Coronary collateral flow and peripheral blood monocyte concentration in patients treated with granulocyte-macrophage colony stimulating factor. *Heart.* 2004;90:945–946.
162. Buschmann I, Hoefer I, van Royen N, et al. GM-CSF: a strong arteriogenic factor acting by amplification of monocyte function. *Atherosclerosis.* 2001;159:343–356.
163. Buschmann I, Busch H, Mies G, Hossmann K. Therapeutic induction of arteriogenesis in hypoperfused rat brain via granulocyte-macrophage colony-stimulating factor. *Circulation.* 2003;108:610–615.
164. Schneeloch E, Mies G, Busch H, Buschmann I, Hossmann K. Granulocyte-macrophage colony-stimulating factor-induced arteriogenesis reduces energy failure in hemodynamic stroke. *Proc Natl Acad Sci USA.* 2004;101:12730–12735.
165. Zbinden S, Zbinden R, Meier P, Windecker S, Seiler C. Safety and efficacy of subcutaneous-only granulocyte-macrophage colony-stimulating factor for collateral growth promotion in patients with coronary artery disease. *J Am Coll Cardiol.* 2005;46:1636–1642.
166. van Royen N, Schirmer S, Atasever B, et al. START Trial: a pilot study on STimulation of ARTeriogenesis using subcutaneous application of granulocyte-macrophage colony-stimulating factor as a new treatment for peripheral vascular disease. *Circulation.* 2005;112:1040–1046.
167. Hill J, Syed M, Arai A, et al. Outcomes and risks of granulocyte colony-stimulating factor in patients with coronary artery disease. *J Am Coll Cardiol.* 2005;46:1643–1648.

168. Jørgensen E, Ripa R, Helqvist S, et al. In-stent neo-intimal hyperplasia after stem cell mobilization by granulocyte-colony stimulating factor Preliminary intracoronary ultrasound results from a double-blind randomized placebo-controlled study of patients treated with percutaneous coronary intervention for ST-elevation myocardial infarction (STEMMI Trial). *Int J Cardiol.* 2006;111:174–177.

169. Zohlnhöfer D, Dibra A, Koppara T, et al. Stem cell mobilization by granulocyte colony-stimulating factor for myocardial recovery after acute myocardial infarction: a meta-analysis. *J Am Coll Cardiol.* 2008;51:1429–1437.

170. Grundmann S, Hoefer I, Ulusans S, et al. Granulocyte-macrophage colony-stimulating factor stimulates arteriogenesis in a pig model of peripheral artery disease using clinically applicable infusion pumps. *J Vasc Surg.* 2006;43:1263–1269.

171. Iwanaga K, Takano H, Ohtsuka M, et al. Effects of G-CSF on cardiac remodeling after acute myocardial infarction in swine. *Biochem Biophys Res Commun.* 2004,325:1353–1359.

172. Yano T, Miura T, Whittaker P, et al. Macrophage colony-stimulating factor treatment after myocardial infarction attenuates left ventricular dysfunction by accelerating infarct repair. *J Am Coll Cardiol.* 2006;47:626–634.

173. Okazaki T, Ebihara S, Takahashi H, Asada M, Kanda A, Sasaki H. Macrophage colony-stimulating factor induces vascular endothelial growth factor production in skeletal muscle and promotes tumor angiogenesis. *J Immunol.* 2005;174:7531–7538.

174. Babamusta F, Rateri D, Moorleghen J, Howatt D, Li X, Daugherty A. Angiotensin II infusion induces site-specific intra-laminar hemorrhage in macrophage colony-stimulating factor-deficient mice. *Atherosclerosis.* 2006;186:282–290.

175. Goumans M, Valdimarsdottir G, Itoh S, Rosendahl A, Sideras P, ten Dijke P. Balancing the activation state of the endothelium via two distinct TGF-beta type I receptors. *EMBO J.* 2002;21:1743–1753.

176. Wahl S, Hunt D, Wakefield L, et al. Transforming growth factor type beta induces monocyte chemotaxis and growth factor production. *Proc Natl Acad Sci USA.* 1987;84:5788–5792.

177. van Royen N, Hoefer I, Buschmann I, et al. Exogenous application of transforming growth factor beta 1 stimulates arteriogenesis in the peripheral circulation. *FASEB J.* 2002;16:432–434.

178. Lutgens E, Gijbels M, Smook M, et al. Transforming growth factor-beta mediates balance between inflammation and fibrosis during plaque progression. *Arterioscler Thromb Vasc Biol.* 2002;22:975–982.

179. Grainger D, Kemp P, Metcalfe J, et al. The serum concentration of active transforming growth factor-beta is severely depressed in advanced atherosclerosis. *Nat Med.* 1995;1:74–79.

180. Grundmann S, van Royen N, Pasterkamp G, et al. A new intra-arterial delivery platform for pro-arteriogenic compounds to stimulate collateral artery growth via transforming growth factor-beta1 release. *J Am Coll Cardiol.* 2007;50:351–358.

181. Judge D, Dietz H. Therapy of Marfan syndrome. *Annu Rev MEd.* 2008;59:43–59.

182. Chung A, Yang H, Radomski M, van Breemen C. Long-term doxycycline is more effective than atenolol to prevent thoracic aortic aneurysm in marfan syndrome through the inhibition of matrix metalloproteinase-2 and -9. *Circ Res.* 2008;102:e73–85.

183. Deindl E, Zaruba M, Brunner S, et al. G-CSF administration after myocardial infarction in mice attenuates late ischemic cardiomyopathy by enhanced arteriogenesis. G-CSF. *FASEB J.* 2006;20:956–958.

184. Werner G, Jandt E, Krack A, et al. Growth factors in the collateral circulation of chronic total coronary occlusions: relation to duration of occlusion and collateral function. Circulation. *Circulation.* 2004;110:1940–1945.

185. Sullivan C, Doetschman T, Hoying J. Targeted disruption of the Fgf2 gene does not affect vascular growth in the mouse ischemic hindlimb. *J Appl Physiol.* 2002;93:2009–2017.

186. Lederman R, Mendelsohn F, Anderson R, et al. Therapeutic angiogenesis with recombinant fibroblast growth factor-2 for intermittent claudication (the TRAFFIC study): a randomised trial. *Lancet.* 2002;359:2053–2058.

187. Czepluch F, Bergler A, Waltenberger J. Hypercholesterolaemia impairs monocyte function in CAD patients. *J Intern Med.* 2007;261:201–204.
188. Landmesser U, Engberding N, Bahlmann F, et al. Statin-induced improvement of endothelial progenitor cell mobilization, myocardial neovascularization, left ventricular function, and survival after experimental myocardial infarction requires endothelial nitric oxide synthase. *Circulation.* 2004;110:1933–1939.
189. Pourati I, Kimmelstiel C, Rand W, Karas R. Statin use is associated with enhanced collateralization of severely diseased coronary arteries. *Am Heart J.* 2004;146:876–881.
190. Dincer I, Ongun A, Turhan S, Ozdol C, Ertas F, Erol C. Effect of statin treatment on coronary collateral development in patients with diabetes mellitus. *Am J Cardiol.* 2006;97:772–774.
191. Zbinden S, Brunner N, Wustmann K, Billinger M, Meier B, Seiler C. Effect of statin treatment on coronary collateral flow in patients with coronary artery disease. *Heart.* 2004;90:448–449.
192. Laflamme M, Zbinden S, Epstein S, Murry C. Cell-based therapy for myocardial ischemia and infarction: pathophysiological mechanisms. *Annu Rev Pathol.* 2007;2:307–339.
193. Asahara T, Murohara T, Sullivan A, et al. Isolation of putative progenitor endothelial cells for angiogenesis. *Science.* 1997;275:964–967.
194. Asahara T, Masuda H, Takahashi T, et al. Bone marrow origin of endothelial progenitor cells responsible for postnatal vasculogenesis in physiological and pathological neovascularization. *Circ Res.* 1999;85:221–228.
195. Luttun A, Carmeliet P. De novo vasculogenesis in the heart. *Cardiovasc Res.* 2003;58:378–389.
196. Peichev M, Naiyer A, Pereira D, et al. Expression of VEGFR-2 and AC133 by circulating human CD34(+) cells identifies a population of functional endothelial precursors. *Blood.* 2000;95:952–958.
197. Jackson K, Majka S, Wang H, et al. Regeneration of ischemic cardiac muscle and vascular endothelium by adult stem cells. *J Clin Invest.* 2001;107:1395–1402.
198. Reyes M, Dudek A, Jahagirdar B, Koodie L, Marker P, Verfaillie C. Origin of endothelial progenitors in human postnatal bone marrow. *J Clin Invest.* 2002;109:313–315.
199. Gill M, Dias S, Hattori K, et al. Vascular trauma induces rapid but transient mobilization of VEGFR2(+)AC133(+) endothelial precursor cells. *Circ Res.* 2001;88:167–174.
200. Shintani S, Murohara T, Ikeda H, et al. Mobilization of endothelial progenitor cells in patients with acute myocardial infarction. *Circulation.* 2001;103:2776–2779.
201. Takahashi T, Kalka C, Masuda H, et al. Ischemia- and cytokine-induced mobilization of bone marrow-derived endothelial progenitor cells for neovascularization. *Nat Med.* 1999;5:434–438.
202. Gehling U, Ergün S, Schumacher U, et al. In vitro differentiation of endothelial cells from AC133-positive progenitor cells. *Blood.* 2000;95:3106–3112.
203. Hattori K, Dias S, Heissig B, et al. Vascular endothelial growth factor and angiopoietin-1 stimulate postnatal hematopoiesis by recruitment of vasculogenic and hematopoietic stem cells. *J Exp Med.* 2001;193:1005–1014.
204. Kalka C, Masuda H, Takahashi T, et al. Transplantation of ex vivo expanded endothelial progenitor cells for therapeutic neovascularization. *Proc Natl Acad Sci U S A.* 2000;97:3422–3427.
205. Kawamoto A, Gwon H, Iwaguro H, et al. Therapeutic potential of ex vivo expanded endothelial progenitor cells for myocardial ischemia. *Circulation.* 2001;103:634–637.
206. Fuchs S, Baffour R, Zhou Y, et al. Transendocardial delivery of autologous bone marrow enhances collateral perfusion and regional function in pigs with chronic experimental myocardial ischemia. *J Am Coll Cardiol.* 2001;37:1726–1732.
207. Orlic D, Kajstura J, Chiment S, et al. Bone marrow cells regenerate infarcted myocardium. *Nature.* 2001;410:701–705.
208. Urbich C, Dimmeler S. Endothelial progenitor cells: characterization and role in vascular biology. *Circ Res.* 2004;95:343–353.

209. Kinnaird T, Stabile E, Burnett M, Epstein S. Bone-marrow-derived cells for enhancing collateral development: mechanisms, animal data, and initial clinical experiences. *Circ Res.* 2004;95:354–363.
210. van Vliet P, Sluijter J, Doevendans P, Goumans M. Isolation and expansion of resident cardiac progenitor cells. *Expert Rev Cardiovasc Ther.* 2007;5:33–43.
211. Chen S, Fang W, Ye F, et al. Effect on left ventricular function of intracoronary transplantation of autologous bone marrow mesenchymal stem cell in patients with acute myocardial infarction. *Am J Cardiol.* 2004;94:92–95.
212. Wollert K, Meyer G, Lotz J, et al. Intracoronary autologous bone-marrow cell transfer after myocardial infarction: the BOOST randomised controlled clinical trial. *Lancet.* 2004;364:141–148.
213. Meyer G, Wollert K, Lotz J, et al. Intracoronary bone marrow cell transfer after myocardial infarction: eighteen months' follow-up data from the randomized, controlled BOOST (BOne marrOw transfer to enhance ST-elevation infarct regeneration) trial. *Circulation.* 2006;113:1287–1294.
214. Janssens S, Dubois C, Bogaert J, et al. Autologous bone marrow-derived stem-cell transfer in patients with ST-segment elevation myocardial infarction: double-blind, randomised controlled trial. *Lancet.* 2006;367:113–121.
215. Meluzín J, Mayer J, Groch L, et al. Autologous transplantation of mononuclear bone marrow cells in patients with acute myocardial infarction: the effect of the dose of transplanted cells on myocardial function. *Am Heart J.* 2006;152:975.e9–15.
216. Kang H, Lee II, Na S, et al. Differential effect of intracoronary infusion of mobilized peripheral blood stem cells by granulocyte colony-stimulating factor on left ventricular function and remodeling in patients with acute myocardial infarction versus old myocardial infarction: the MAGIC Cell-3-DES randomized, controlled trial. *Circulation.* 2006;114 (1 Suppl):I145–151.
217. Ruan W, Pan C, Huang G, Li Y, Ge J, Shu X. Assessment of left ventricular segmental function after autologous bone marrow stem cells transplantation in patients with acute myocardial infarction by tissue tracking and strain imaging. *Chin Med J (Engl).* 2005;118:1175–1181.
218. Ge J, Li Y, Qian J, et al. Efficacy of emergent transcatheter transplantation of stem cells for treatment of acute myocardial infarction (TCT-STAMI). *Heart.* 2006;92:1764–1767.
219. Meier P, Gloekler S, Zbinden R, et al Beneficial effect of recruitable collaterals: a 10-year follow-up study in patients with stable coronary artery disease undergoing quantitative collateral measurements. *Circulation.* 2007;116:975–983.
220. Ripa R, Jø rgensen E, Wang Y, et al. Stem cell mobilization induced by subcutaneous granulocyte-colony stimulating factor to improve cardiac regeneration after acute ST-elevation myocardial infarction: result of the double-blind, randomized, placebo-controlled stem cells in myocardial infarction (STEMMI) trial. *Circulation.* 2006;113:1983–1992.
221. Zohlnhöfer D, Ott I, Mehilli J, et al. Stem cell mobilization by granulocyte colony-stimulating factor in patients with acute myocardial infarction: a randomized controlled trial. *JAMA.* 2006;295:1003–1010.
222. Engelmann M, Theiss H, Hennig-Theiss C, et al. Autologous bone marrow stem cell mobilization induced by granulocyte colony-stimulating factor after subacute ST-segment elevation myocardial infarction undergoing late revascularization: final results from the G-CSF-STEMI (Granulocyte Colony-Stimulating Factor ST-Segment Elevation Myocardial Infarction) trial. *J Am Coll Cardiol.* 2006;48:1712–1721.
223. Harada M, Qin Y, Takano H, et al. G-CSF prevents cardiac remodeling after myocardial infarction by activating the Jak-Stat pathway in cardiomyocytes. *Nat Med.* 2005;11:305–311.
224. Hirsch A, Nijveldt R, van der Vleuten P, et al. Intracoronary infusion of autologous mononuclear bone marrow cells in patients with acute myocardial infarction treated with primary PCI: Pilot study of the multicenter HEBE trial. *Catheter Cardiovasc Interv.* 2008;71:273–281.

225. Murray C. The physiological principle of minimum work: I. The vascular system and the cost of blood volume. *Proc Natl Acad Sci USA*. 1926;12:207–214.
226. Murray C. The physiological principle of minimum work: II. Oxygen exchange in capillaries. *Proc Natl Acad Sci USA*. 1926;12:299–304.
227. Seiler C, Kirkeeide RL, Gould KL. Basic structure-function relations of the epicardial coronary vascular tree. Basis of quantitative coronary arteriography for diffuse coronary artery disease. *Circulation*. 1992;85:1987–2003.
228. Kassab G. Scaling laws of vascular trees: of form and function. *Am J Physiol*. 2006;290:H894–903.
229. Kamiya A, Togawa T. Adaptive regulation of wall shear stress to flow change in canine carotid artery. *Am J Physiol*. 1980;239:H14–H21.
230. Seiler C, Kirkeeide R, Gould K. Measurement from arteriograms of regional myocardial bed size distal to any point in the coronary vascular tree for assessing anatomic area at risk. *J Am Coll Cardiol*. 1993;21:783–797.
231. Windecker S, Allemann Y, Billinger M, et al. Effect of endurance training on coronary artery size and function in healthy men: an invasive followup study. *Am J Physiol*. 2002;282:H2216–2223.
232. Mittleman M, Maclure M, Tofler G, Sherwood J, Goldberg R, Muller J. Triggering of acute myocardial infarction by heavy physical exertion. Protection against triggering by regular exertion. Determinants of Myocardial Infarction Onset Study Investigators. *N Engl J Med*. 1993;329:1677–1683.
233. Currens J, White P. Half a century of running. Clinical, physiologic and autopsy findings in the case of Clarence DeMar ("Mr. Marathon"). *N Engl J Med*. 1961;265:988–993.
234. Mann G, Spoerry A, Gray M, Jarashow D. Atherosclerosis in the Masai. *Am J Epidemiol*. 1972;95:26–37.
235. Rose G, Prineas R, Mitchell J. Myocardial infarction and the intrinsic calibre of coronary arteries. *Br Heart J*. 1967;29:548–552.
236. Haskell W, Sims C, Myll J, Bortz W, St Goar F, Alderman E. Coronary artery size and dilating capacity in ultradistance runners. *Circulation*. 1993;87:1076–1082.
237. Spaan J, Piek J, Hoffman J, Siebes M. Physiological basis of clinically used coronary hemodynamic indices. *Circulation*. 2006;113:446–55.
238. Gould K, Lipscomb K, Hamilton G. Physiologic basis for assessing critical coronary stenosis. Instantaneous flow response and regional distribution during coronary hyperemia as measures of coronary flow reserve. *Am J Cardiol*. 1974;33:87–94.
239. Zbinden R, Zbinden S, Windecker S, Meier B, Seiler C. Direct demonstration of coronary collateral growth by physical endurance exercise in a healthy marathon runner. *Heart*. 2004;90:1350–1351.
240. Eckstein R. Effect of exercise and coronary artery narrowing on coronary collateral circulation. *Circ Res*. 1957;5:230–235.
241. Heaton W, Marr K, Capurro N, Goldstein R, Epstein S. Beneficial effect of physical training on blood flow to myocardium perfused by chronic collaterals in the exercising dog. *Circulation*. 1978;57:575–581.
242. Neill W, Oxendine J. Exercise can promote coronary collateral development without improving perfusion of ischemic myocardium. *Circulation*. 1979;60:1513–1519.
243. Scheel K, Ingram L, Wilson J. Effects of exercise on the coronary and collateral vasculature of beagles with and without coronary occlusion. *Circ Res*. 1981;48:523–530.
244. Schaper W. Influence of physical exercise on coronary collateral blood flow in chronic experimental two-vessel occlusion. *Circulation*. 1982;65:905–912.
245. Cohen M, Yipintsoi T, Scheuer J. Coronary collateral stimulation by exercise in dogs with stenotic coronary arteries. *J Appl Physiol*. 1982;52:664–671.
246. Roth D, White F, Nichols M, Dobbs S, Longhurst J, Bloor C. Effect of long-term exercise on regional myocardial function and coronary collateral development after gradual coronary artery occlusion in pigs. *Circulation*. 1990;82:1778–1789.

247. White F, Bloor C, McKirnan M, Carroll S. Exercise training in swine promotes growth of arteriolar bed and capillary angiogenesis in heart. *J Appl Physiol.* 1998;85:1160–1168.
248. Indermühle A, Vogel R, Meier P, et al. The relative myocardial blood volume differentiates between hypertensive heart disease and athlete's heart in humans. *Eur Heart J.* 2006;27:1571–1578.
249. Stewart K, Hiatt W, Regensteiner J, Hirsch A. Exercise training for claudication. *N Engl J Med.* 2002:1941–1951.
250. Heberden W. Commentaries on the history and cure of diseases. In: Wilius F, Kays T, eds. *Classics of Cardiology.* New York: Dover; 1961:220–224.
251. Ferguson R, Petitclerc R, Choquette G, et al. Effect of physical training on treadmill exercise capacity, collateral circulation and progression of coronary disease. *Am J Cardiol.* 1974;34:764–769.
252. Kennedy C, Spiekerman R, Lindsay MJ, Mankin H, Frye R, McCallister B. One-year graduated exercise program for men with angina pectoris. Evaluation by physiologic studies and coronary arteriography. *Mayo Clin Proc.* 1976;51:231–236.
253. Conner J, LaCamera FJ, Swanick E, Oldham M, Holzaepfel W, Lyczkowskyj O. Effects of exercise on coronary collateralization – angiographic studies of six patients in a supervised exercise program. *Med Sci Sports.* 1976;8:145–151.
254. Nolewajka A, Kostuk W, Rechnitzer P, Cunningham D. Exercise and human collateralization: an angiographic and scintigraphic assessment. *Circulation.* 1979;60:114–121.
255. Niebauer J, Hambrecht R, Marburger C, et al. Impact of intensive physical exercise and low fat diet on collateral vessel formation in stable angina pectoris and angiographically confirmed coronary artery disease. *Am J Cardiol.* 1995;76:771–775.
256. Belardinelli R, Georgiou D, Ginzton L, Cianci G, Purcaro A. Effects of moderate exercise training on thallium uptake and contractile response to low-dose dobutamine of dysfunctional myocardium in patients with ischemic cardiomyopathy. *Circulation.* 1998;97:553–561.
257. Senti S, Fleisch M, Billinger M, Meier B, Seiler C. Long-term physical exercise and quantitatively assessed human coronary collateral circulation. *J Am Coll Cardiol.* 1998;32:49–56.
258. Zbinden R, Zbinden S, Meier P, et al. Coronary collateral flow in response to endurance exercise training. *Eur J Cardiovasc Prev Rehabil.* 2007;14:250–257.
259. Sdringola S, Nakagawa K, Nakagawa Y, et al. Combined intense lifestyle and pharmacologic lipid treatment further reduce coronary events and myocardial perfusion abnormalities compared with usual-care cholesterol-lowering drugs in coronary artery disease. *J Am Coll Cardiol.* 2003;41:263–272.
260. Patel S, Breall J, Diver D, Gersh B, Levy A. Bradycardia is associated with development of coronary collateral vessels in humans. *Coron Artery Dis.* 2000;11:467–472.
261. Wright A, Hudlicka O. Capillary growth and changes in heart performance induced by chronic bradycardial pacing in the rabbit. *Circ Res.* 1981;49:469–478.
262. Brown M, Davies M, Hudlicka O. The effect of long-term bradycardia on heart microvascular supply and performance. *Cell Mol Biol Res.* 1994;40:137–142.
263. Zheng W, Brown M, Brock T, Bjercke R, Tomanek R. Bradycardia-induced coronary angiogenesis is dependent on vascular endothelial growth factor. *Circ Res.* 1999;85:192–198.
264. Lei L, Zhou R, Zheng W, Christensen L, Weiss R, Tomanek R. Bradycardia induces angiogenesis, increases coronary reserve, and preserves function of the postinfarcted heart. *Circulation.* 2004;110:796–802.
265. Downey J, Kirk E. Inhibition of coronary blood flow by a vascular waterfall mechansim. *Circ Res.* 1975;36:753–760.
266. Brown B, Gundel W, Gott V, Covell J. Coronary collateral flow following acute coronary occlusion: a diastolic phenomenon. *Cardiovasc Res.* 1974;8:621–631.

267. Müller K, Lübbecke F, Schaper W, Walter P. Effect of intraaortic balloon counter-pulsation (IABP) on myocardial infarct size and collateral flow in an experimental dog model. *Intensive Care Med.* 1982;8:131–137.
268. Sato M, Saito T, Mitsugi M, et al. Effects of cardiac contraction and coronary sinus pressure elevation on collateral circulation. *Am J Physiol.* 1996;271:H1433–1440.
269. Ido A, Hasebe N, Matsuhashi H, Kikuchi K. Coronary sinus occlusion enhances coronary collateral flow and reduces subendocardial ischemia. *Am J Physiol.* 2001;280:H1361–1367.
270. Banai S, Ben Muvhar S, Parikh K, et al. Coronary sinus reducer stent for the treatment of chronic refractory angina pectoris: a prospective, open-label, multicenter, safety feasibility first-in-man study. *J Am Coll Cardiol.* 2007;49:1783–1789.
271. Kinnaird T, Stabile E, Zbinden S, Burnett M, Epstein S. Cardiovascular risk factors impair native collateral development and may impair efficacy of therapeutic interventions. *Cardiovasc Res.* 2008;78:257–264.
272. van Weel V, de Vries M, Voshol P, et al. Hypercholesterolemia reduces collateral artery growth more dominantly than hyperglycemia or insulin resistance in mice. *Arterioscler Thromb Vasc Biol.* 2006;26:1383–1390.
273. Epstein S, Stabile E, Kinnaird T, Lee C, Clavijo L, Burnett M. Janus phenomenon: the interrelated tradeoffs inherent in therapies designed to enhance collateral formation and those designed to inhibit atherogenesis. *Circulation.* 2004;109:2826–2831.
274. Schirmer S, Fledderus J, Bot P, et al. Interferon-beta signaling is enhanced in patients with insufficient coronary collateral artery development and inhibits arteriogenesis in mice. *Circ Res.* 2008;102:1286–1294.
275. Luo Y, Zhou H, Krueger J, et al. Targeting tumor-associated macrophages as a novel strategy against breast cancer. *J Clin Invest.* 2006;116:2132–2141.
276. Lewis C, Pollard J. Distinct role of macrophages in different tumor microenvironments. *Cancer Res.* 2006;66:605–612.
277. Peters B, Diaz L, Polyak K, et al. Contribution of bone marrow-derived endothelial cells to human tumor vasculature. *Nat Med.* 2005;11:261–262.
278. Baklanov D, Moodie K, McCarthy F, et al. Comparison of transendocardial and retrograde coronary venous intramyocardial catheter delivery systems in healthy and infarcted pigs. *Catheter Cardiovasc Interv.* 2006;68:416–423.
279. Imada T, Tatsumi T, Mori Y, et al. Targeted delivery of bone marrow mononuclear cells by ultrasound destruction of microbubbles induces both angiogenesis and arteriogenesis response. *Arterioscler Thromb Vasc Biol.* 2005;25:2128–2134.
280. Vogel R, Indermuhle A, Reinhardt J, et al. The quantification of absolute myocardial perfusion in humans by contrast echocardiography: algorithm and validation. *J Am Coll Cardiol.* 2005;45:754–762.
281. Leong-Poi H, Christiansen J, Heppner P, et al. Assessment of endogenous and therapeutic arteriogenesis by contrast ultrasound molecular imaging of integrin expression. *Circulation.* 2005;111:3248–3254.
282. Mazur A, Deylig A, Schaper W, Meinertz T, Ito W. Biopanning of single-chain antibodies expressing phages reveals distinct expression patterns of angiogenic and arteriogenic vessels. *Endothelium.* 2003;10:277–284.

Index

Printed in the United States of America